D1237124

PREPARING NURSES FOR DISASTER MANAGEMENT

Joanne C. Langan, PhD, RN
Saint Louis University School of Nursing

Dotti C. James, PhD, RN
Saint Louis University School of Nursing

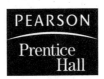

Upper Saddle River, New Jersey 07458

Library of Congress Cataloging-in-Publication Data
Langan, Joanne C.
    Preparing nurses for disaster management / Joanne C. Langan & Dotti C. James.
        p. ; cm.
    Includes bibliographical references and index.
    ISBN 0-13-178069-7
    1. Disaster nursing.
    [DNLM: 1. Disaster Planning. 2. Nursing Process. WY 154 L271p 2005] I. James, Dotti
C. II. Title.
RT108.L365 2005
616.02'5—dc22   2004001636

Publisher: Julie Levin Alexander
Publisher's Assistant: Regina Bruno
Editor-in-Chief: Maura Connor
Acquisitions Editor: Pamela Fuller
Editorial Assistants: Malgorzata Jaros-White and Eileen Monaghan
Director of Manufacturing and Production: Bruce Johnson
Managing Production Editor: Patrick Walsh
Production Liaison: Cathy O'Connell
Production Editor: Robin Reed, Carlisle Communications
Manufacturing Manager: Ilene Sanford
Manufacturing Buyer: Pat Brown
Design Director: Cheryl Asherman
Cover Designer: Blair Brown
Senior Design Coordinator: Maria Guglielmo Walsh
Director of Marketing: Karen Allman
Executive Marketing Manager: Nicole Benson
Channel Marketing Manager: Rachele Strober
Media Editor: John Jordan
Media Production Manager: Amy Peltier
Media Project Manager: Stephen Hartner
Composition: Carlisle Communications
Printer/Binder: Courier/Westford
Cover Printer: Phoenix Color

This book was set in 10/12 Goudy by Carlisle Communications, LTD. and was printed and bound by Courier Westford. The cover was printed by Phoenix Color.

Notice: Care has been taken to confirm the accuracy of information presented in this book. The authors, editors, and the publisher, however, cannot accept any responsibility for errors or omissions or for consequences from application of the information in this book and make no warranty, express or implied, with respect to its contents.

    The authors and publisher have exerted every effort to ensure that drug selections and dosages set forth in this text are in accord with current recommendations and practice at time of publication. However, in view of ongoing research, changes in government regulations, and the constant flow of information relating to drug therapy and drug reactions, the reader is urged to check the package inserts of all drugs for any change in indications of dosage and for added warnings and precautions. This is particularly important when the recommended agent is a new and/or infrequently employed drug.

Pearson Education Ltd.
Pearson Education Singapore, Pte. Ltd.
Pearson Education Canada, Ltd.
Pearson Education—Japan

Pearson Education Australia PTY, Limited
Pearson Education North Asia Ltd.
Pearson Educacíon de Mexico, S.A. de C.V.
Pearson Education Malaysia, Pte. Ltd.
Pearson Education, Upper Saddle River, New Jersey

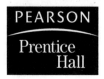

10 9 8 7 6 5 4 3 2 1
ISBN: 0-13-178069-7

DEDICATION

We dedicate this book to all disaster nurses, rescue personnel, planning teams, volunteers, and those behind the scenes who work diligently to prevent and mitigate the impact of disasters.

To our friends whose love and support have sustained us throughout this endeavor.

To my daughters, Becky and Stephanie
>   *DCJ*

To my loving and supportive husband, John, and children John II (wife, Marissa), Christina (husband, Chad), Becky, and Justin
>   *JCL*

CONTENTS

CHAPTER 4 Promoting Mental Health: Predisaster and Postdisaster 55

Dorcas E. McLaughlin, Ruth B. Murray, and Julie Benbenishty

CHAPTER 5 Preparing Nursing Administrators, Faculty, and Students for Disasters 79

Joanne C. Langan, Vered Kater, and Ayala Aharoni

CHAPTER 6 Preparing Staff and Inactive Registered Nurses to Manage Casualties 95

Dotti C. James, Joanne C. Langan, Helen Sandkuhl, and Julie Benbenishty

CHAPTER 7   Management and Preparation for Battlefield Casualties   125

Michelle R. Mandy

CHAPTER 8   Preparing Community Health Nurses and Nurses in Ambulatory Health Centers   143

Dotti C. James

CHAPTER 9   Considerations for Vulnerable Populations   159

Joanne C. Langan and Dotti C. James

CHAPTER 10   Preparing Nurses to Plan and Care for Children During Disaster Situations   177

Nina K. Westhus, Diana Fendya, and Vered Kater

CHAPTER 11   The Role of the Infection Control Nurse in Disaster Preparedness   199

Terri Rebmann

CHAPTER 12   Disaster as the Personal Experience   219

Joanne C. Langan and Vered Kater

APPENDIX A   Agencies and Acronyms   235

APPENDIX B   Test Your Knowledge Answers   237

APPENDIX C   Decontamination Forms and Volunteer Log   241

FOREWORD

On September 11, 2001, we, the Executive Advisory Board of the Saint Louis University School of Nursing (SLUSON), had just concluded our meeting when an assistant dean of the school came in to inform us of the horrendous event that had just taken place in New York City. As people all over the country were doing, each member of the board struggled, trying to comprehend this unspeakable crime on the United States.

Life went on. We went on aware that something horrible had happened, trying desperately to return to normal. We went about our varied activities of teaching, research, and service. At the next advisory board meeting, however, one of the members asked what the School of Nursing was doing to prepare our faculty and students for bioterrorism or natural disasters or the aftermath. It struck me that there was something we *could* do. The school's involvement began at a faculty meeting in April 2002, when I asked for a task force to study bioterrorism and disaster preparedness. Several faculty indicated an interest in pursuing the idea of what we could do to be of assistance should any heinous crime or natural disaster occur. At that meeting many faculty, including Drs. Joanne Langan and Dotti James, began a discussion of actions to be taken in the event of a mass casualty incident here in our community.

Sheila Manion, of the Saint Louis University Development Office, and I began to organize meetings throughout the summer of 2002. In these meetings we developed a plan to inform people of our intent to pursue ways we could be of assistance should a disaster occur. Sheila and I had an appointment to visit an alumna and mentioned the school's interest in disaster preparedness. We met with Elsie Roth, a SLUSON baccalaureate graduate and retired nurse. She became intensely involved with us from the first moment we mentioned this and insisted we visit Israel to study terrorism and disasters. Israel is one of the places where the experts are, unfortunately, due to experience with attacks on its citizens. Elsie knew exactly where to go and how to get there—the Hadassah medical system in Jerusalem. The medical complex there is the largest treatment center, teaching hospital, research, and rehabilitation facility in the Middle East. Here, nurses handle the aftershocks of terrorism and live with the threat every day. Mrs. Roth volunteered to contact the director of the Hadassah nursing councils in the United States to assist in planning the trip to Jerusalem. The Hadassah Medical Organization operates relief programs all over the world, and the nursing councils are part of this organization. Barbara Sabin, the director, agreed with Mrs. Roth that Jerusalem was the place to go. Ms. Sabin contacted Orli Rotem Pickerd, Director of Hadassah Nursing Services, and Dr. Miri Rom, Dean of the Henrietta Szold Hadassah-Hebrew University School of Nursing, to see if they would develop a curriculum to educate American nurses. They agreed. Mrs. Roth volunteered to lead the group to Israel.

Dr. Greg Evans, Director of the Institute for Bio-Security at Saint Louis University School of Public Health, was contacted. Drs. James and Langan wanted to know what was available for nurses interested in learning more about bioterrorism and disaster education. Dr. Evans informed them that the center develops educational materials for doctors and public health professionals but had nothing specifically for nurses. Therein lies the gap in educational opportunities. A proactive approach to prepare practicing nurses, faculty members, and students for disaster events was needed. Terri Rebmann, an infectious disease specialist from the Institute, also joined the group. A five-person team was formed.

During the one-week stay in Israel, an intensive learning program included hands-on experience working in protective suits, education at a gas mask distribution center, and tutorials in coordinating first aid and transportation for large numbers of victims. The team also received lessons in psychosocial issues such as breaking bad news to families and pointers on dealing with post-traumatic stress disorder in victims, families, and health care workers.

It became obvious that large numbers of nurses were interested in education about disaster preparedness and mass casualty events. SLUSON decided to offer an online disaster preparedness certificate program. In addition, Drs. Langan and James recognized the need for a book to address issues in disaster preparedness specific to nurses in a variety of practice sites, with diverse groups of clients with special needs. This is important, as nurses will be called upon to be leaders in caring for disaster victims. Nurses will play key roles in disaster relief in emergency departments, obstetrics, pediatrics, or general medical-

surgical units in the hospital, in residential facilities, ambulatory care, or at home in their communities.

We are indebted to these authors for anticipating the need and going beyond their teaching roles to write this book.

Joan Hrubetz, PhD, RN
Professor and Dean
Saint Louis University
School of Nursing

PREFACE

This textbook addresses issues in disaster preparedness specific to nurses in a variety of practice sites. This is important for nurses who will be leaders in caring for disaster victims. Nurses will play key roles in disaster relief whether they work full time, part time, or at home in their communities.

Nurses will be expected to help victims, rescuers, family members, and friends who are directly or indirectly involved in mass casualty events. The public expects professional nurses to provide skilled, competent care after natural and man-made disasters. Therefore, nurses have the responsibility to learn basic disaster preparedness.

This textbook will introduce nurses and students to basic disaster nursing. It is a compilation of research and nurses' personal experiences in disaster and trauma care, from the authors' experiences and from other experts in bioterrorism and disaster preparedness. We were part of a team who traveled to Israel to study with nurses and health care professionals who deal with terrorism and disasters on a daily basis. Many effective disaster planning and response systems are in place in other countries. We welcome comments from nurses in these countries and will compile this information in later editions of *Preparing Nurses for Disaster Management*. Our education is ongoing. We must prepare our families, neighbors and communities to respond appropriately to terrorism and disasters of all types.

Chapter 1 presents a general overview of types of disasters; conventional and nonconventional terrorism, and chemical, biological, and nuclear terrorist agents. Chapters 2 and 3 contain practical advice for planning and organizing health care agencies for disasters, including assessing community and organizational vulnerability, identifying agencies involved in disaster response, and agencies and personnel who are integral in coordinating rescue efforts. Chapter 4 explores mental health theory and explains how nurses promote mental health before and after disasters. Chapters 5 through 11 deal with preparing nurses in a variety of practice settings to assist patients and victims with diverse needs to prepare for the trauma of disasters. The final chapter shares stories from persons who live in the aftermath of disasters. Selected chapters include Nursing Vignettes, commentaries from nurses who have experienced disasters, or respond to terrorism on a daily basis.

This textbook will assist educators to integrate disaster preparedness within existing curricula. The tests, case studies, and discussion questions will identify areas needing reinforcement or additional education. In addition, agencies will use this book as a foundation for staff and employee development.

Joanne Langan
Dotti James

ACKNOWLEDGMENTS

We gratefully acknowledge all who have contributed to the creation and completion of this book. We would like to specifically acknowledge:

Dean Joan Hrubetz for her support in making our trip to Israel possible;

Elsie Roth for her vision in linking the Saint Louis University School of Nursing and the Henrietta Szold Hadassah School of Nursing, and for her belief in the power of nursing;

Dean Miri Rom and the faculty of the Henrietta Szold Hadassah-Hebrew University School of Nursing, Dean Ruth Kaplan and the faculty of the Assaf Harofeh Medical Center School of Nursing, and the Hadassah Medical Organization for their dedication to excellence and saving lives;

Freda DeKeyser for her coordination of Israeli faculty and contributors;

The staff of St. Joseph Hospital of Kirkwood and the Emergency Preparedness Team for their commitment to public health, safety and contributions;

Jeff Hamilton of St. John's Mercy Medical Center, St. Louis, for his contributions;

St. Louis Metropolitan Medical Response System (SLMMRS), Dr. Karen Webb, Dr. Greg Evans, Bruce Clements, and the Institute for Bio-Security at Saint Louis University School of Public Health for their input and expertise;

Teresa Dunleavy of the Saint Louis University Cancer Center for sharing her knowledge;

All of the nurses and the Roth family for sharing their stories about the disaster experience;

Mary Shapiro for listening to our ideas and encouraging the development of the book, and Gosia Jaros-White for her constant vigilance and assistance; and

All of those with the foresight to plan and prepare a response to terrorism and disasters.

CONTRIBUTING AUTHORS AND REVIEWERS

CONTRIBUTING AUTHORS

Ayala Aharoni, RN, MPH
Chapter 5
Coordinator of Trauma and Emergency Nursing
Henrietta Szold Hadassah-Hebrew University
School of Nursing
Jerusalem, Israel

Julie Benbenishty, BA, RN
Chapters 2, 4, and 6
Research Coordinator
Intensive Care Department
Hadassah Medical Organization
Jerusalem, Israel

Diana G. Fendya, MSN(R), RN
Chapter 10
Trauma/Acute Care Specialist
Emergency Services for Children National
Resource Center
Washington, DC

Vered Kater, RN, BA, MSN
Chapters 5, 10, and 12
Nurse Educator
Henrietta Szold Hadassah-Hebrew University
School of Nursing
Jerusalem, Israel
Clinical Instructor in Nursing
Saint Louis University School of Nursing
St. Louis, Missouri

Dorcas E. McLaughlin, PhD, APRN, BC, CP
Chapter 4
Assistant Professor
Saint Louis University
School of Nursing
St. Louis, Missouri

Michelle R. Mandy, RN, MPA, BSN, TNS, CMC
Chapter 7
Clinical Instructor
Saint Louis University
School of Nursing
St. Louis, Missouri

Ruth Murray, EdD, APRN, BC, FAAN
Chapter 4
Professor; Coordinator, Psychiatric/Mental Health
Nursing Graduate Specialty
Saint Louis University
School of Nursing
St. Louis, Missouri

Terri Rebmann, MSN, RN, CIC
Chapter 11
Infectious Disease Specialist
Saint Louis University
Institute for Bio-Security at Saint Louis University
School of Public Health
St. Louis, Missouri

Helen Sandkuhl, RN, MSN, CEN, TNS
Chapter 6
Director of Nursing, Emergency Services
Saint Louis University Hospital
St. Louis, Missouri

Nina Westhus, PhD, RN
Chapter 10
Assistant Professor
Saint Louis University
School of Nursing
St. Louis, Missouri

REVIEWERS

Janet G. Alexander, EdD, MSN, BSN
Associate Professor
Samford University
Ida V. Moffett School of Nursing
Birmingham, Alabama

Joan Bickes, MSN, CHN, APRN, BC
Assistant Professor
Wayne State University
College of Nursing
Detroit, Michigan

Gail M. Burns, RN, MSN
Instructor
College of Mount St. Joseph
Cincinnati, Ohio

Brenda Cobb, PhD, MSN
Associate Professor
Medical College of Georgia
School of Nursing
Augusta, Georgia

Elizabeth Scannell-Desch, PhD, RN, MSN, BSN
Assistant Professor
Rutgers University
College of Nursing
Newark, New Jersey

Barbara Dunn, RN, MSN
Assistant Professor
Armstrong Atlantic State University
Department of Nursing
Savannah, Georgia

Barbara Gaffke, PhD, MSN, BSN, APN, CS
Director of Administration and Leadership—
Graduate Nursing Program
DePaul University
Department of Nursing
Chicago, Illinois

Kim Gregg, RN, MSN, CRNP
Nursing Instructor
Jacksonville State University
Jacksonville, Alabama

Sheila Q. Hartung, PhD, RN, BC
Assistant Professor
Bloomsburg University
Bloomsburg, Pennsylvania

Patricia Leary, MS
Allied Health Instructor
Ferris State University
Big Rapids, Michigan

Thomas Terndrup, MD
Professor and Chair
University of Alabama at Birmingham
School of Medicine
Department of Emergency Medicine
Birmingham, Alabama

R. Steven Tharrat, MD, MPUM
Professor of Internal Medicine
University of California at Davis
Division of Pulmonary and Critical Care
Sacramento, California

ABOUT THE AUTHORS

Dotti C. James, PhD, RN is an Associate Professor at Saint Louis University School of Nursing. She traveled as part of a team to the Henrietta Szold Hadassah Hebrew University School of Nursing and the Hadassah Medical Centers in Israel to learn about preparing health care providers to manage mass casualty events. She has spoken at area colleges, hospitals, skilled-care facilities, and professional and first responder organizations about various aspects of preparing for and responding to terrorism. She is currently a faculty member in the Disaster Preparedness Online Certificate Program for Nurses, covering topics such as organization of the disaster response, management of casualties, and considerations for vulnerable populations. Dr. James coordinates the online and onsite Perinatal Nursing Graduate Specialty. Her research interests include developing an evidence base for intrapartal nursing interventions, the effectiveness of educational strategies and techniques, and nursing attitudes and awareness about victims of violence. She has received awards for Excellence in Classroom Teaching from Saint Louis University and the Emerson Electric Company. Dr. James has served in leadership roles in local, regional, and national professional organizations, and is a contributing author to three texts.

Joanne C. Langan, PhD, RN is an Assistant Professor at Saint Louis University School of Nursing. She received a BS in Education from Quincy University and a BSN from the University of Southern Mississippi. Dr. Langan earned MSN and PhD degrees in Nursing Administration and a Nursing Education Certificate from George Mason University. While a faculty member at GMU, she was the Co-Project Director for the Washington Regional Academic and Community Consortium and the Project Director of the Partnerships for Quality Education. At Saint Louis University, Dr. Langan is the coordinator of the traditional students' Public Health Nursing course. Research and areas of interest include Faculty Practice and nursing student learning, the Nursing Shortage, Community Partnerships in Graduate Medical and Nursing Education, and Disaster Preparedness. She is a contributing author for two Community-Based Nursing Practice books. She was a member of a team who received intensive education at the Henrietta Szold Hadassah Hebrew University School of Nursing and the Hadassah Medical Centers in Israel and is developing modules and curriculum as a faculty member of a Bioterrorism/Disaster Preparedness Certificate Program. Dr. Langan is a consultant/member of the Emergency Preparedness Team at St. Joseph Hospital of Kirkwood.

INTRODUCTION

In writing about disaster preparedness these days, one almost always begins with a reference to the events of September 11, 2001. The day of the attacks in New York, Washington, DC, and Pennsylvania proved to be a watershed in the awareness of Americans and people the world over to the growing danger presented by terrorism of all sorts. The subsequent anthrax letters and political tensions in the Middle East only aggravated fears, and made it clear to all how ill-prepared we were to deal with such attacks and disasters, both man-made and natural. As director of the Institute for Bio-Security at Saint Louis University School of Public Health, it has been my goal to create and disseminate as efficiently as possible the educational information that would fill some of those gaps, and help us to be ready for future health emergencies. In the process of this work, I have met many dedicated and highly trained individuals whose mission has been, like mine, to facilitate the education, training, and treatment of those whose lives have been touched by such disasters, and to prepare us for any future attacks. The nurses of Saint Louis University are just such a dedicated group, and it is an honor to write this introduction to their textbook. The articles, case studies, exercises, and other resources it provides will go a long way toward expanding the understanding of the role of nurses in all levels of disaster preparedness.

Over the past few years, we have all become familiar with the ramifications of cutbacks in nursing staff at hospitals and other health care institutions. However, few are aware how these cutbacks can affect disaster preparedness. Until recently, as Dr. Langan notes in her opening chapter, planning for bioterrorist events in the United States has largely excluded all members of the health profession. Now, it has been recognized that in the event of bioterrorist attack, health professionals will be the first responders because victims will require prophylaxis and medical treatment. And since nurses are the largest group of health professionals, they will, in fact, be at the forefront of a bioterrorist event, and will bear much of the brunt of coordinating the response.

In the fall of 2002, I saw this reality played out before my eyes when I traveled with four of the authors/contributors of this text to Hadassah Hospital in Jerusalem, Israel, in order to learn more about how a society copes with the problems of terrorist attacks, and how to best prepare our health professionals to do so. During five days of intensive seminars, discussions, simulations, and drills, we were repeatedly reminded of what is often forgotten in American hospitals—namely, the importance of the nurses' roles in preparing for and coping with all sorts of disasters. Their training must prepare them for multiple roles including everything from triage to directing patient care to victims of disaster, coordinating incident command, and handling mental health problems of victims and their families. Truly, as Michelle Mandy notes in her historical survey of battlefield nursing, these professionals are consummate multitaskers: "When faced with unusual situations the nurse must improvise, adapt, and overcome to meet the needs of the patient." Indeed, nurses are educated for this purpose, and are thus ideally positioned to play leadership roles during all phases of a disaster, from planning and preparing a disaster plan, to responding to the disaster and its aftermath. Dr. Dotti James in her chapter, "Organization of the Disaster Response," discusses these various roles, particularly as they relate to consequence management.

As Terri Rebmann notes in her chapter, "Role of the Infection Control Nurse in Disaster Preparedness," bioterrorist events will not be suddenly evident as in the case of a bomb or outright attack, rather, victims will appear at clinics and hospital emergency rooms with various symptoms that must be quickly diagnosed and treated. Nurses, especially those working in infectious disease, are already trained to be suspicious of unusual symptoms, and to maintain a constantly high level of surveillance—they are thus best situated to pick up the first indications of a bioterrorist event and set in action the necessary response. Their community-based networks will provide the ideal basis for communicating important information to those impacted by attacks, and for relaying information back to those working out of treatment centers.

While my trip to Israel taught me a great deal about the professional role that nurses can and should have in preparing for and responding to various disasters, it also showed me what personal dedication and passion to a cause can do. These nurses lead regular exercises to prepare for the eventuality of biological or chemical terrorist attacks while dealing with the day-to-day terror of suicide bombings. I am proud to count disaster nurses among my colleagues and my friends.

R. Gregory Evans, PhD
Professor
Saint Louis University School of Public Health
Director, Institute for Bio-Security at Saint Louis
University School of Public Health

CHAPTER 1

Disasters: A Basic Overview

Joanne C. Langan

LEARNING OBJECTIVES

1. Define *disaster* and *terrorism*.
2. Differentiate intentional versus accidental disasters.
3. Express the value of all nurses having a working knowledge of disaster planning and response.
4. Differentiate conventional versus nonconventional terrorism.

5. Discuss methods of dissemination of chemical, biological, and nuclear terrorist agents.
6. Analyze terrorist events of the past five years and the factors that affected the degree of each event's damage.

MEDIALINK www.prenhall.com/langan

Resources for this chapter can be found on the Companion Website at http://www.prenhall.com/langan. Click on Chapter 1 to select the activities for this chapter.

CHAPTER OUTLINE

Know Your Terms
Audio Glossary
Web Links
    Government Resources
    Nursing Resources
MediaLink Applications
    Essay Questions: Terrorism

GLOSSARY

Biological terrorism/bioterrorism. The use and dissemination of various kinds of microbes or toxins with the intent to intimidate or coerce a government or civilian population to further political or social objectives; humans, animals, and plants are often targets

Chemical terrorism. Attacks meant to cause mass devastation in which terrorist organizations release toxins; chemical attacks meant primarily to terrorize, blackmail, or cause economic damage; a specific attack in a particular product, particularly a food product

Chemical warfare agents. Highly toxic chemicals that can be disseminated as vapors, gases, liquids, or aerosols or adsorbed to dust particles

Conventional weapons. More frequently used weapons of terrorism such as bombs and guns

Dirty bomb. See *radiological dispersion bomb*

Disaster. An occurrence, either natural or man made, that causes human suffering and creates human needs that victims cannot alleviate without assistance

Domestic terrorism. Terrorist acts by individuals or groups within a given country, without foreign direction or involvement

Emergency stage. Involves the immediate response to the effects of the disaster, immediate community provides assistance or aid because outside sources of aid have not yet arrived

Hazardous materials. Substances that, because of their chemical, biological, or physical nature, pose a potential risk to life, health, or property if released

Impact stage. A time when the disaster event has occurred and the community experiences the immediate effects; the community is rapidly assessed for damage, types and extent of injuries suffered, and immediate needs of the community

International terrorism. Terrorist acts directed by foreign groups who transcend national boundaries, affecting people in several countries

Ionizing radiation. Causes the long-term destructive force of the dirty bomb, an ion's electrical charge may lead to unnatural chemical reactions inside the cells, break DNA chains, either causing DNA strand death or DNA mutations; unlikely ill effects in very small doses

Mass casualty incident. A situation with 100 or more casualties, significantly overwhelms available emergency medical services, facilities, and resources

Mitigation. Action taken to prevent or reduce the harmful effects of a disaster on human health or property, involves future-oriented activities to prevent subsequent disasters or to minimize their effects

Multiple casualty incident. Disaster in which there are more than 2 but fewer than 100 persons injured

Nonconventional weapons. Less frequently used weapons of terrorism such as chemical, nuclear, and biological categories

Nondisaster stage. Also known as the interdisaster stage, the time for prevention, planning, preparedness, and mitigation activities; the threat of a disaster is still in the future

Nuclear terrorist attack. An incident in which a terrorist organization uses a nuclear device to cause mass murder and devastation, includes the use or threat of the use of fissionable radioactive materials in an attack, or an assault on a nuclear power plant for the purpose of causing extensive and/or irreversible environmental damage

Post-Traumatic Stress Disorder (PTSD). An anxiety disorder that can develop after exposure to a terrifying event or ordeal in which grave physical harm occurs or is threatened

Predisaster stage. Occurs when there is knowledge about an impending disaster; activities include warning, preimpact mobilization, and evacuation if appropriate

Radiation sickness. One of the results of DNA mutation inside cells exposed to ionizing radiation; can be deadly, but survivable with bone marrow transplantation

Radiological dispersion bomb. The most accessible nuclear device to be used by a terrorist, consists of a conventional explosive such as trinitrotoluene (TNT) packed with radioactive waste by-products from nuclear reactors, discharges deadly radioactive particles into the environment; also called a *dirty bomb*

Reconstruction stage. Restoration, reconstitution, and mitigation take place, rebuilding, replacing lost or damaged property, returning to school and work; when life returns to some semblance of "normal," another name for *recovery stage*

Recovery stage. See *reconstruction stage*

Terrorism. The systematic use of terror, the deliberate creation and exploitation of fear for bringing about political change

Trauma. Physical injury caused by violent or disruptive action, or by the introduction into the body of a toxic substance, or a psychic injury resulting from a severe emotional shock

INTRODUCTION

Prior to September 11, 2001, little was done to prepare public and private health care workers for bioterrorism threats and the aftermath of actual incidents. "The very group that would handle the consequences of an attack has yet to receive widespread education on the topic" (Agency for Healthcare Research and Quality, 2001). Since the 9-11 events, the value of bioterrorism education, and disaster preparedness education in general, is no longer in question.

Disaster preparedness education is imperative for people of varying disciplines, especially in service and health care organizations. This textbook will discuss a variety of disciplines and their roles in disaster preparedness and response, but the main focus is the preparation of nurses. Nurses play key roles in disaster relief whether they are in the emergency department, obstetrics, pediatrics, or general medical surgical units in the hospital, in residential facilities, ambulatory care, or simply at home in their communities.

WHY NURSES NEED TO BE PREPARED

Recent newspaper headlines from Washington, DC, include topics such as smallpox vaccinations, nerve gas, and nuclear weapons. People throughout the world are sharing an increased awareness of the vulnerability to terrorism.

The United States has made bioterrorism preparedness a priority for government and military agencies. Until recently, the public and private health care sectors had been largely excluded from the nation's bioterrorism preparatory efforts. However, health care professionals are among the essential personnel in addressing preparations for terrorism and disasters and in dealing with the consequences of an attack.

Nurses comprise the largest group of health care professionals. Many nurses wanted to respond to the tragic events of September 11, 2001. Some did not know how to respond; and others simply left their homes and converged on the site of the World Trade Center disaster. In both cases, we have learned that nurses may have been better utilized had they been taught the best means to communicate with the disaster management teams, and specific skills to implement with the victims and their families. Nurses want to know what is expected of them and how they can learn what they need to know in the event of an emergency, disaster, or mass casualty event. Nurses in all states can link into the National Nurse Response Team (NNRT), International Nursing Coalition for Mass Casualty Education (INCMCE), American Red Cross (ARC), Medical Reserve Corps (MRC), and Disaster Medical Assistance Teams (DMATs) to learn about organizational efforts to prepare nurses to respond to mass casualty events. See subsequent chapters for more information regarding specific actions to prepare nurses.

A set of core emergency preparedness competencies exists for public health workers, created by Dr. Gebbie of Columbia University School of Nursing, Center for Health Policy (2001). These core competencies were used as the model for the core emergency and disaster preparedness competencies outlined for nurses in general. See Box 1–1.

While these core competencies for nurses might seem overwhelming, they are extremely important. Nurses have the knowledge and skills to perform complex tasks. However, because many of the tasks of disaster preparedness and response are specific to the situation, nurses need additional education to learn the best methods to prepare and respond. In August, 2003, the INCMCE published the "Educational Competencies for Registered Nurses Related to Mass Casualty Incidents". According to the American Nurses Association (ANA), "The aim of nursing actions is to assist patients, families, and communities to improve, correct, or adjust to physical, emotional, psychosocial, spiritual, cultural, and environmental conditions for which they seek help" (*Nursing's Social Policy Statement, 1995*). Nurses have the flexibility and the ability to assimilate the new skills and demands necessary to prepare for and respond to disastrous situations effectively.

People have suffered through unexpected events that cause massive destruction, injury, and death throughout the ages. Disasters are of even greater concern today than in the past, due to several factors. The frequency of disaster events has increased; human populations are more densely populated, increasing the potential for exposure to disaster events as they occur; and people are more likely to build, live, and work in areas with high disaster potential (Comerio, 1998). Recent events have demonstrated the willingness of some groups to undertake meticulous planning to engineer massive disasters to achieve their political goals. Long-term effects of these events can be minimized when extensive preparations for disasters are made and effective responses to disasters are conducted.

BOX 1–1   Core Emergency and Disaster Preparedness Competencies for Nurses

1. Describe the agency's role in responding to a range of emergencies that might arise.
2. Describe the chain of command in emergency response.
3. Identify and locate the agency's emergency response plan (or the pertinent portion of it).
4. Describe emergency response functions or roles and demonstrate them in regularly performed drills.
5. Demonstrate the use of equipment (including personal protective equipment) and the skills required in emergency response during regular drills.
6. Demonstrate the correct operation of all equipment used for emergency communication.
7. Describe communication roles in emergency response.
8. Identify the limits of your own knowledge, skills, and authority, and identify key system resources for referring matters that exceed these limits.
9. Apply creative problem-solving skills and flexible thinking to the situation, within the confines of your role, and evaluate the effectiveness of all actions taken.
10. Recognize deviations from the norm that might indicate an emergency and describe appropriate action.
11. Participate in continuing education to maintain up-to-date knowledge in relevant areas.
12. Participate in evaluating every drill or response and identify necessary changes to the plan.

(Gebbie and Qureshi, 2002)

BOX 1–2   Determination of Compliance with the Standard of Conduct at 244 CMR 9.03(15)

Prohibiting Patient Abandonment

When the Board evaluates a complaint of patient abandonment, it will determine whether a patient abandonment has occurred based on information demonstrating that the licensed nurse:

A. accepted responsibility for the nursing care of a patient or group of patients;

B. voluntarily withdrew from caring for the patient or patients with any ongoing nursing care need;

C. failed to give reasonable notice to an appropriate person that she or he was withdrawing from caring for the patient or patients so that arrangements could be made for continuation of safe care; and

D. failed to report essential information to an appropriate person.

The following situation is an example of patient abandonment:

A nurse accepts an assignment of patient care and then leaves the facility. The appropriate licensed nursing staff does not know that the nurse is not in the facility, nor has the nurse given a status report on her patient or patients to another nurse who assumes responsibility for patient care (Massachusetts Board of Registration in Nursing, 2000).

The health of the public is our first concern. *Nursing: Scope and Standards of Practice* (ANA, 2004), *Nursing's Social Policy Statement* (1995), and the *Code of Ethics for Nurses* (2001) contribute to a description and understanding of nursing's accountability to the public. This accountability includes the nurse's obligation to acquire and maintain current knowledge and competency in nursing practice. We cannot deny that the threat of bioterrorism, terrorist acts, and disasters is real. The learning curve is steep in this field of study. Nurses must learn their role in disaster preparedness and response and how to integrate this role with the myriad of personnel called upon in mass casualty events.

When disasters occur, it may be a natural reaction for some persons to wish to leave the health care facility to be with loved ones and friends. This concern is very real. However, nurses must be cognizant of the determination of compliance with the standard of conduct prohibiting patient abandonment by a licensed nurse. See your facility policy for specifics, and Box 1–2 for an example.

When nurses are educated in disaster preparedness and are familiar with their agency's disaster preparedness plan, they have the information necessary to react appropriately in a disastrous situation. This preparation will help nurses to realize the community's resources and the comprehensive systems in place to plan for and respond to disaster events. These systems should include a means for nurses to contact family and friends to determine their safety as well as a call-in system to provide relief for nurses who are exhausted from the disaster relief effort. With the knowledge that realistic, supportive assistance plans are in place, nurses will realize and fulfill the vital role they play in maintaining or restoring the health of the community in which they work or dwell.

Whether you are a health care professional in an acute care setting, make home visits, or work in ambulatory care or residential centers, we are all in this together. We need your individual expertise in the concerted effort in disaster planning and response. The process of learning about disaster planning and mitigation is ongoing. The dynamic state of preparation will continually be revised and updated in anticipation of known and unknown threats to the public's health and well-being. Some of these disaster threats will now be discussed.

NATURAL AND MAN-MADE DISASTERS

The American Red Cross (ARC) defines **disaster** as an "occurrence, either natural or man-made, that causes human suffering and creates human needs that victims cannot alleviate without assistance" (ARC, 1975). Noji defines disasters similarly, but more simply, as "events that require extraordinary efforts beyond those needed to respond to everyday emergencies" (1997).

Natural disasters are events caused by nature or emerging diseases, and they can have serious consequences (Box 1–3). For example, after natural disaster Hurricane Isabel in 2003, President George W. Bush declared federal disasters in North Carolina, Maryland, and Virginia. This event resulted in 18 deaths and an initial estimate of $1 billion in damage (Tharpe & Dart, 2003).

Man-made disasters are complex emergencies, technological disasters, material shortages, and other disasters not caused by natural hazards (Noji, 1997). Man-made or human-generated disasters include war; chemical, biological, radiological, and nuclear terrorism; transportation accidents; group violence such as riots; food or water contamination; deforestation; and building collapses.

Man-made disasters may be either accidental or deliberate. A wrecked tanker truck or railroad car carrying dangerous chemicals that overturns due to a collision are both man-made disasters, yet are considered accidental. Terrorist bombings, the release of sarin gas into a Tokyo subway, and the deliberate crashing of three planes into the World

---

BOX 1–3   Examples of Natural Disasters

- Epidemics
- Famine
- Hurricane
- Tornado
- Storm
- Flood
- Earthquake
- Wind-driven water

- Tidal wave
- Volcanic eruption
- Landslide
- Mudslide
- Snowstorm
- Avalanche
- Drought

Trade Center and the Pentagon are man-made and planned; they were not accidental.

Hazardous materials are substances that, because of their chemical, biological, or physical nature, pose a potential risk to life, health, or property, if they are released. Potential hazards can occur during any stage of use from production and storage to transportation, use, or disposal. Production and storage of hazardous materials occur in chemical plants, gas stations, hospitals, and other sites. Hazardous materials accidents can range from a chemical spill on a highway, to groundwater contamination by naturally occurring methane gas, to a household hazardous materials accident. Radiological accidents involving a specific hazardous material are also a concern to the public's health.

In 1979, a cooling malfunction caused part of the core to melt in the number two reactors at Three Mile Island power station near Harrisburg, Pennsylvania. Some radioactive gas was released two days after the accident. Deficient control room instrumentation and inadequate emergency response training proved to be root causes of the accident (World Nuclear Association, 2001).

Until 1953, chemicals of unknown kind and quantity were buried at the Love Canal landfill. After 1953, the site was covered with earth. Over a period of time, about 100 homes were built and an elementary school opened. Chemical odors filled the basements of homes bordering the landfill. This indiscriminate disposal of toxic materials caused the planned exodus of 235 families and the expense of public monies and efforts to contain the disaster and restore a degree of normalcy to the lives of those affected (University of Idaho Cooperative Extension System, 2002).

Disaster events may be a combination of man-made and natural causes. For example, if a person leaves a campsite without properly dousing the campfire, the ensuing forest fire would be considered man-made, yet may be exacerbated by a dry summer season and strong blowing winds, which are natural elements.

Another distinction among disasters is one in which there are more than two but fewer than 100 persons injured. This is considered a **multiple casualty incident.** A **mass casualty incident** is a situation with 100 or more casualties. Mass casualty incidents significantly overwhelm

available emergency medical services, facilities, and resources (Beachley, 2000). Affected communities will require the assistance of neighboring communities, states, and possibly the federal government. Both multiple and mass casualty incidents may be caused by natural or man-made disasters such as terrorism. See Box 1–4.

TERRORISM

Terrorism is the systematic use of terror. To terrorize is to fill with terror, scare, to coerce by threat or violence. According to Hoffman (1998), terrorism is the "deliberate creation and exploitation of fear for bringing about political change." All terrorist acts have one key element in common—violence or the threat of violence. Terrorism is designed to have psychological effects that reach a much wider audience than the immediate victims or object of an attack. Through their use of dramatic, bloody, and destructive acts of violence, terrorist groups choose to frighten and intimidate large populations such as rival ethnic or religious groups, a country and its political leadership, or the international community. These high-profile acts draw attention to the terrorists and their cause. As Hoffman (2003) states, "Through the publicity generated by their violence, terrorists seek to obtain the leverage, influence, and power they otherwise lack."

Terrorist acts include murder, kidnapping, bombing, and arson. These acts have been defined in both national and international law as crimes. Most countries around the world regard terrorism as a crime and they state this explicitly in legal statutes.

The legal system and code of law of the United Kingdom has influenced those of the United States, Canada, and Israel. The United Kingdom's legislation, "Terrorist Act 2000" states that terrorism is "the use of threat of action . . . designed to influence the government or to intimidate the public or a section of the public . . . for the purpose of advancing a political, religious or ideological cause" (Hoffman, 1998).

The United States Code, Title 18, Section 2331 is a federal statute that defines terrorism as "violent acts or acts

BOX 1–4   Lessons Learned From Multiple Casualty and Mass Casualty Incidents

A fire in the Cocoanut Grove nightclub in Boston on November 28, 1942, claimed the lives of 492 people and injured 166. It is considered the worst nightclub fire disaster in history. With approximately 1,000 people in attendance, the club exceeded its 600-person capacity. It is believed the fire started when a young man lit a match to replace a light bulb that had been removed by a patron. Artificial palm trees and drapery quickly caught fire. The entire building was engulfed in 15 minutes. People were unable to exit the club as frantic patrons quickly blocked the two revolving doors (Maihos, 2003).

What have we learned from this tragedy and what has been done?

1. Revolving doors were later required to have flanking exits.
2. Emergency lighting became a rule.
3. Exit lights became required.
4. Occupant capacity placards were also established as a new rule.
5. Fire sprinklers, first introduced in 1874 to protect warehouses, came into widespread use as a way to provide life safety for buildings. The Life Safety Code originated from the Cocoanut Grove fire.
6. Autopsies revealed lung damage in victims that might have been related to the refrigerator coolant, methyl chloride. It is believed that methyl chloride poisoning from the cooling system in a corner of the nightclub was a cause of some of the deaths in the fire (Maihos, 2003).

In more recent tragedies in February 2003, 21 persons in a Chicago club and 96 persons in a West Warwick, Rhode Island, club were killed due to crowd crushing and inability to find exits in a fire respectively. Many lessons were learned from these tragedies. Firefighters and crowd control experts advise the following in an effort to save lives of those who may need to escape crowded places.

1. Be aware of your surroundings. Find all of the exits, not just those most obvious such as the one through which you entered.
2. If exits are blocked, notify at least one of the building's employees. It is against fire code. If you choose to stay, stay near accessible exits.
3. If you are disabled, do not allow yourself to be placed in areas which may prove to be difficult for you to evacuate.
4. The front row may not be the best place in times of disaster, especially if the crowd pushes toward the entertainers. Choose the periphery.
5. Do not panic, run, or shout during an emergency evacuation. Conserve your energy for survival.
6. If you are attempting to leave a burning building, crouch down or crawl low to the ground. More deaths are caused by smoke inhalation than the fire itself.
7. If you are on fire, stop, drop, and roll. This will squelch the fire and eliminate the oxygen the fire needs to burn.
8. If you cannot see due to dark and heavy smoke, back up to the wall and follow it to an exit.
9. Do not attempt to save persons who have fallen if it causes you to be caught in a stampede.
10. Wear some kind of identifiable clothing that is easily seen by your friends so that they can locate you in a crowd.
11. Before entering a building or club, choose a meeting place outside of the building where you can meet your friends in case you lose sight of each other on the inside.

Follow your instincts—if a situation does not feel safe, leave.

(Chicago Tribune, 2003; CNN, 2003; Roth, 2003)

---

dangerous to human life that . . . appear to be intended (i) to intimidate or coerce a civilian population; (ii) to influence the policy of a government by intimidation or coercion; or (iii) to affect the conduct of a government by assassination or kidnapping" (U.S.C., 2002).

Canada's Anti-terrorism Act (Bill C-36) designates "terrorist activity" as

an act or omission . . . that is committed in whole or in part for a political, religious, or ideological purpose, objective or cause and in whole or in part with the intention of intimidating the public, or a segment of the public, with regard to its security, including its economic security, or compelling a person, a government or a domestic or an international organization to do or to refrain from doing any act, whether the person, government or organization is inside or outside Canada . . . (House of Commons of Canada, 2001, p. 3)

Israeli law does not address terrorism specifically (Hoffman, 1998). However, the Prevention of Terrorism Ordinance Number 33 defines a terrorist organization as "a body of persons resorting in its activities to acts of violence calculated to cause death or injury to a person or to threats of such acts of violence" (Ben-Gurion & Rosenblueth, 1948).

Terrorist activity is categorized as domestic or international. Individuals or groups within a given country, without foreign direction or involvement, perpetrate **domestic terrorism.** White supremacist activities against African

---

BOX 1–5   Conventional Terrorist Weapons: Car Bomb

Excerpts from a FEMA Report dated April 20, 1995 at Noon, EDT follow:

Situation: On April 19, 1995, at 9:05 am, in Oklahoma City, OK, one car bomb destroyed the Alfred P. Murrah Federal Building. The building normally housed approximately 500 people, and it is estimated that there were 250 visitors on the day of the bombing.

Casualties: As of 5:00 am EDT, April 20, the Public Health Service reports 29 confirmed dead, between 150 and 200 injured, and 140 missing.

Mass Care: A ten-block area around the explosion area was evacuated. The American Red Cross (ARC) is setting up a shelter for those from a large apartment complex of approximately 600 apartments. ARC is sending in two additional canteens to support local chapter operations. The ARC has activated their Disaster Health and Mental Health people to possibly deploy to Oklahoma City.

Resource Support: This part of the Federal Response Plan was activated at 1:00 am EDT, on April 20, 1995, at FEMA Headquarters to support the efforts in identifying, locating, and acquiring the necessary assets required to provide logistical/resource support.

Health and Medical: The Department of Veterans Affairs has dispatched medical professionals to augment local hospital personnel and psychiatric crisis teams to work with both the injured and onlookers.

Urban Search and Rescue: Two Urban Search and Rescue teams with specially trained personnel consisting of rescue, medical and search components have arrived in Oklahoma City. These teams are from AZ and CA. Teams from VA and New York City will arrive today at 2:30 pm. Two additional teams from MD and Los Angeles County, CA have also been activated and are awaiting transportation.

Donations: The American Red Cross has a national toll-free number to call to offer donations: 1-800-HELP-NOW.

Media Inquiries: All media inquiries are to be referred to FEMA Headquarters, Office of Emergency Information and Public Affairs. (pp. 1–3)

Americans, Jews, and other ethnic and religious groups are examples of domestic terrorism. **International terrorism,** in contrast, is directed by foreign groups and may transcend national boundaries, affecting people in several countries (Federal Emergency Management Agency [FEMA], 1997).

CONVENTIONAL TERRORIST WEAPONS

Currently, terrorists use **conventional weapons** such as bombs and guns more frequently than the chemical, nuclear, and biological nonconventional terrorist weapons. Car and truck bombs have become powerful weapons, especially in suicide attacks. The Oklahoma City bombing of April 19, 1995, is a prime example of a car bomb causing a major disaster. See Box 1–5.

Terrorists use both explosive bombings and incendiary bombings such as Molotov cocktails. A suicide bomber/terrorist using an explosive bomb is an all-too frequent occurrence in Israel. Terrorists have also made use of letter and parcel bombs. Other "weapons of choice" such as handguns, rifles, and semiautomatic weapons have been used in assassinations, snipings, armed attacks, and massacres. A variety of grenades may be used, ranging from hand grenades to the rocket-propelled device. A few terrorist groups are known to possess surface-to-air, shoulder-fired missiles that can bring down helicopters, fighter aircraft, and civilian airliners (United Nations Office for Drug Control and Crime Prevention, 2002).

NON-CONVENTIONAL TERRORIST WEAPONS

Non-conventional terrorist weapons include those in chemical, biological, and nuclear categories. Each of these types of weapons is explained below, as well as preparations for each kind of attack.

Chemical Terrorism

Chemical terrorism is grouped into two main types.

1. Attacks meant to cause mass devastation, in which the terrorist organization releases a toxin in congested population centers, bodies of water, and unventilated areas, to create as many victims as possible.
2. Chemical attacks meant primarily to terrorize, blackmail, or cause economic damage; a specific attack in a particular product—particularly a food product—mainly by introducing a toxic chemical substance into the product itself (Ganor, 1998).

Three ways to spread a chemical or biological agent are through the air, municipal water supply, and food supply.

Air Dissemination

The most feared dissemination of terrorist agents is through the air. The following techniques are used to spread agents through the air.

1. Bomb or missile explosion, spreading the chemical or biological agent over a wide area.
2. Crop-duster or other aircraft spraying the agent over a city.
3. Car or truck drives through the city spraying a fine mist along city streets in crowded areas.
4. Small bombs or aerosol canisters are released in crowded areas like subways, sports arenas or convention centers. (Brain, 2003, p. 1)

The effects of this type of nonconventional terrorism were seen when the toxic gas, sarin, began wafting through the tunnels of Japan's subway system in Tokyo and Yokohama in 1995, killing several people and injuring dozens of others. Acts of chemical terrorism are likely to be overt due to the fact that their effects tend to be immediate and obvious. Biological terrorism tends to be covert in that its effects are more insidious and may occur over lengthy incubation periods. (See section on biological terrorism below.) The anthrax letters sent in the United States in 2001 may be considered an overt attack because they were announced. A covert attack, most likely in the form of an aerosolized release, is more likely to cause more illness and death due to the delayed recognition of the attack. Some chemical agents are capable of covert dissemination in food and water.

Food and Water Dissemination

Various organizations in different parts of the world have laced food products with chemicals in order to sabotage marketing of them and terrorize consumers. A chemical substance was found injected into citrus fruit exported from Israel to European markets. This was done to cause economic damage to Israel (Ganor, 1998).

The Rajneeshee religious cult in The Dalles, Oregon planned to infect residents with *Salmonella* on election day to influence the results of county elections. They contaminated salad bars at 10 restaurants with *S. ty-phimurium* on several occasions before the election. This was done to practice for the attack before the election day. At least 751 cases of salmonellosis were documented in a county that typically reports less than five cases per year. Bioterrorism was considered unlikely. It was only when the Federal Bureau of Investigation (FBI) investigated the cult for other criminal violations that the source of the outbreak became known. A vial of *S. ty-phimurium* identical to the outbreak strain was found in a laboratory on the cult's property. Eventually, members of the cult admitted to contaminating the salad bars and putting the bacteria into a city water supply tank (Mc-Dade & Franz, 1998).

The FBI later released a bulletin to state and local law enforcement agencies cautioning that terrorists might use two naturally occurring toxins—solanine and nicotine—to poison U.S. food or water supplies. Solanine is found in potatoes that are old or have been over-exposed to sunlight and nicotine is found in tobacco plants. Although the FBI said there were no known uses of either toxin by extremist groups, in May 2003, a man from Michigan pleaded guilty to lacing 250 pounds of ground beef with an insecticide containing nicotine. This act of terrorism, an attempt to get a supermarket co-worker in trouble, sickened 92 people (Anderson, 2003).

The World Health Organization (WHO) has published a 45-page booklet, *Terrorist Threats to Food: Guidance for Establishing and Strengthening Prevention and Response Systems.* It warns of the potential addition of pesticides, viruses, and parasites into food as a means of deliberately harming populations. The example of the intentional food attack in Oregon with *Salmonella* is cited (Schlundt, 2003).

Another potential mode of dissemination is through the water supply. One of the main threats to the nation's water supply is contamination by chemical, biological or radiological agents. "Supply interruptions include the destruction of, or interference with reservoir dams, water towers, pumping stations, intakes, treatment plants, infrastructure, and fire hydrants. Water pressure in the lines could be reduced to zero, thereby denying the population drinking water" (Lancaster-Brooks, 2002). A number of measures are being taken to monitor the water systems and to prevent the kind of panic and disruption that could be caused by the denial of water to the population for any period of time.

The Environmental Protection Agency (EPA) is working with state and local governments to protect the drinking water supply from terrorist attacks. In the Public Health Security and Bioterrorism Preparedness and Response Act of 2002, the Safe Drinking Water Act was amended. Specific actions that community water systems and the U.S. EPA must take to improve the security of the nation's drinking water infrastructure are outlined. *EPA's Strategic Plan for Homeland Security* addresses utilities' vulnerabilities to possible attack, encourages the use of scientific information and technologies for water security, and outlines actions to improve security and to respond effectively in the event that an incident occurs (U.S. EPA, 2002).

Chemical Warfare Agents

Chemical warfare agents are highly toxic chemicals that can be disseminated as vapors, gases, liquids, or aerosols or adsorbed to dust particles (Tucker, 2000). Chemical weapons are categorized by the major organ system affected. These categories include blister or vesicant agents, such as mustard, that affect the skin and lungs; chemicals that affect the blood such as arsine, hydrogen chloride, and hydrogen cyanide; and agents such as chlorine gas, nitrogen oxide, sulfur trioxide—chlorosulfonic acid, and zinc

---

BOX 1–6   Likely Chemical Agents: FBI Critical Agent List

The chemicals listed have been used as weapons by terrorists. These agents were used based on ease of acquisition, dissemination and damage that could be inflicted.	Ammonia Hydrogen Sulfide Sulfur Dioxide	Arsine Methyl Isocyanate Fluorine	Chlorine Phosgene	Cyanides Phosphine

---

Source: NIJ/FBI Chemical/Biological Agent Threat Assessment, 2002 unpublished data presented April 2002, at the National Disaster Medical System Conference in Atlanta, Georgia.

---

oxide that affect the respiratory system. Other categories of chemical agents include those that cause mental incapacitation such as LSD and phenothiazines; those that affect the central and peripheral nervous systems such as sarin and V-gas; those that are used for riot control such as tear gas; and those that induce vomiting such as adamsite and ciphenylcyanoarsine (Centers for Disease Control and Prevention [CDC], 2001). See Box 1–6.

Preparation for Chemical Attacks

The CDC continually updates information regarding preparation for chemical attacks. Public health responsibilities in this area include developing capabilities for detecting and responding to chemical attacks, educating first responders and health care personnel regarding chemical terrorism, and obtaining and storing supplies of chemical antidotes. The U.S. military has developed some diagnostic processes for chemical injuries. Public health authorities continue to review existing diagnostic information and to develop new diagnostic tools. The education of the public about potential effects and actions to be taken in the case of chemical attacks is also essential.

Biological Terrorism

Biological terrorism is "the use and dissemination of biological weapons (various kinds of microbes) in population centers, by various means, in order to cause morbidity and numerous casualties" (Ganor, 1998, p. 4). Unlike chemical terrorism, biological weapons are not designed and ordinarily cannot be used for specific, circumscribed attacks; their principle purpose is mass devastation, and is often political in nature. The results of a biological attack are not immediate; they become apparent several hours or days later. Biological weapons are not as common, accessible, or available as chemical weapons.

See Box 1–7 for general information on chemical-biological agents.

Preparation for Biologic Attacks

Two of the main responsibilities of state and local public health preparedness personnel and disaster response planners are the assessment of existing surveillance systems capable of identifying unusual disease patterns and the availability of expertise and resources needed to respond to chemical or biological terrorist attacks.

Specific preparation for biological attacks as recommended by the Centers for Disease Control and Prevention (2000) include these categories:

- Surveillance and response capabilities
- Diagnostic services and tests, vaccines and appropriate treatments
- Communication systems
- Education of health care providers and public health professionals
- Education of the general public
- Obtaining and storing drugs and vaccines

The National Center for Infectious Diseases expanded these guidelines in 2001 to include specific roles of health care providers in the recognition, reporting, and treatment of high-priority biological agents. Laboratory personnel are advised to test findings on cultures that would normally be discarded as contaminants when they occur in suspicious circumstances. Unusual clusters of laboratory results are to be reported. Unusual specimens are to be sent to specialty laboratories as directed.

Radiological and Nuclear Terrorism

A **nuclear terrorist attack** is an incident in which a terrorist organization uses a nuclear device to cause mass murder and devastation. This type of terrorism also includes the use or threat of the use of fissionable radioactive materials in an attack, or an assault on a nuclear power plant for the purpose of causing extensive and/or irreversible environmental damage. In the last case, the terrorist organization does not need to develop, acquire or gain control of a nuclear bomb to cause extensive damage. The terrorist organization can cause great damage and havoc by using conventional weapons against one of the many nuclear reactors in the world. This type of action would seriously damage the reactor. Once this occurs, radioactive matter is released into the atmosphere and has the potential to endanger large population centers (U.S. Department of State, 2002). Terrorist organizations consider the use of nuclear weapons a major advantage because they can inflict wide-scale damage and command worldwide media attention (Ganor, 1998).

BOX 1–7 Chemical-Biological Agents

Biological agents can be dispersed by an aerosol spray, which must be inhaled. However, these agents can also be used to contaminate food, water and other products. Attention to basic food hygiene when traveling abroad is very important.

A. Some chemical agents may be volatile—evaporating rapidly to form clouds of agent. Others may be persistent. These agents may act directly on the skin, lungs, eyes, and respiratory tract or be absorbed through your skin and lungs causing injury. Choking and nerve agents damage the soft tissue in these organs.

B. When properly used, appropriate masks are effective protection to prevent the inhalation of either biological or chemical agents; however this assumes an adequate warning. Gas masks alone do not protect against agents that act through skin absorption. Those who wish to acquire protective equipment for personal use should contact commercial vendors.

C. There is an incubation period after exposure to biological agents. It is essential that you seek appropriate care for illnesses acquired while traveling abroad to assure prompt diagnosis and treatment.

D. One of the biological agents is the spore-forming bacterium that causes Anthrax, an acute infectious disease. It should be noted, however, that effective dispersal of the Anthrax bacteria is difficult.

- Anthrax is treatable if that treatment is initiated promptly after exposure. The post-exposure treatment consists of certain antibiotics administered in combination with the vaccine.
- An anthrax vaccine that confers protective immunity does exist, but is not readily available to private parties. Efficacy and safety of use of this vaccine for persons under 18 or over 65 and pregnant women have not been determined.
- The anthrax vaccine is produced exclusively by Bioport under contract to the Department of Defense. Virtually all vaccine produced in the United States is under Defense Department contract primarily for military use and a small number of other official government uses.
- For additional information, please consult your health care provider or local health authority.

Note: From *Fact Sheet: Chemical-Biological Agents* by U.S. Department of State, October 2001, Washington, DC. Retrieved September 11, 2002, from *http://travel.state.gocbw.htm*

It is believed that the **radiological dispersion bomb** is the most accessible nuclear device to be used by a terrorist. Another name for this simple device is **dirty bomb.** It consists of a conventional explosive such as trinitrotoluene (TNT) packed with radioactive waste by-products from nuclear reactors. Upon detonation, the dirty bomb would discharge deadly radioactive particles into the environment. This type of device is cheaper than a nuclear bomb and radioactive waste material is relatively easy to obtain. Radioactive waste is found throughout the world and is typically not as well guarded as nuclear weapons (Blair, 2001; Harris, 2003).

The dirty bomb uses the gas expansion as a means of propelling radioactive material over a wide area. It is not very destructive in its own right, compared to the amount of damage inflicted by the rapidly expanding, hot gas of high explosives. When the dirty bomb explodes, the radioactive material spreads in the wind like a dust cloud reaching a far wider area than the initial explosion (Harris, 2003).

As Harris (2003) explains, the long-term destructive force of the dirty bomb would be caused by the **ionizing radiation** from the radioactive material. In a person's body, an ion's electrical charge may lead to unnatural chemical reactions inside the cells. The charge can break DNA chains. Cells with broken DNA strands either die or the DNA develops a mutation. Diseases develop as the result of widespread cell death. Radiation sickness may be the re-

sult of a number of steps that progress as a result of DNA mutation within cells.

1. If the DNA mutates, a cell may become cancerous.
2. The cancer may spread.
3. Cells may malfunction.
4. This may result in a wide variety of symptoms collectively referred to as **radiation sickness.**
5. Radiation sickness can be deadly but people can survive it, especially if they receive a bone marrow transplant.

(Harris, 2003)

People are exposed to ionizing radiation frequently, but in small doses. Some of the sources of this everyday exposure are outer space, natural radioactive isotopes, and X ray machines. Although these encounters with radiation have the potential to cause cancer, it is unlikely as the exposure is in such small doses. A person's risk of cancer and radiation sickness would be increased by exposure to a dirty bomb and the subsequent rise in radiation levels above normal. The fatal effects of the dirty bomb may not be apparent in the short term after exposure, but could kill people years later (Harris, 2003).

Preparation for Radiological and Nuclear Attacks
Within the United States, several strategies are in place to mitigate the possibility of nuclear terrorism. These strategies include: (1) the buildup of intelligence capabilities that

warn of potential attacks; (2) shoring up possible sources of nuclear material; (3) increased monitoring of ports; (4) inspection of containers coming into the country; (5) increased airline and airport security; (6) increased security around nuclear power plants; (7) expanded perimeters of restricted airspace; and (8) the deployment of Nuclear Emergency Search Teams (NEST), a group of highly trained and knowledgeable individuals who assist in locating and disarming weapons if a credible threat of a dirty bomb or a full-fledged nuclear weapon occurs. The preferred action is prevention and intervention to secure any sources of nuclear terrorism before they enter the country (Blair, 2001).

Although prevention and intervention are important aspects of disaster planning and response, one must understand all stages of the disaster response.

STAGES OF DISASTER RESPONSE

Disasters evolve in five stages: the nondisaster or interdisaster stage, the predisaster stage, the impact stage, the emergency stage, and the reconstruction or rehabilitation stage (Noji, 1997). See Figure 1–1. The **nondisaster stage** is the time for planning and preparation, as the threat of a disaster is still in the future. Communities should use this time for vulnerability analyses and capability inventories. This is also a time for prevention, preparedness, and mitigation activities. According to Malilay (1997), **mitigation** is the action taken to prevent or reduce the harmful effects of a disaster on human health or property. Mitigation may take the form of reinforcing highway overpasses, developing communication strategies as backup systems to what is currently in place, and educating professionals and the public regarding preparation and response to disasters.

The **predisaster stage** occurs when there is knowledge about an impending disaster, but it has not yet occurred. Activities during this stage include warning, preimpact mobilization, and evacuation if appropriate. The **impact stage** is a time when the disaster event has occurred and the community experiences the immediate effects. The community is rapidly assessed for damage, and the types and extent of injuries suffered as well as the immediate needs of the community are determined. The **emergency stage** involves the immediate response to the effects of the disaster. Early in the response to the community, the immediate community provides assistance or aid, because outside sources of aid have not yet arrived. Later, assistance from outside of the affected area arrives and search and rescue operations commence as well as first aid, emergency medical assistance, establishment or restoration of communication and transportation, assessment of infectious diseases and mental health problems and evacuation of residents, if necessary. In the **reconstruction** or **recovery stage,** restoration, reconstitution and mitigation take place. Restoration includes rebuilding, replacing lost or damaged property, returning to school and work, and continuing life without

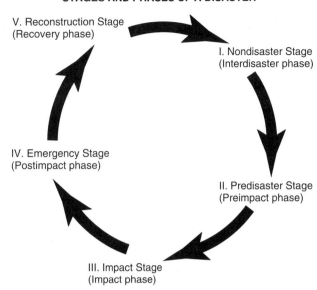

STAGES AND PHASES OF A DISASTER

V. Reconstruction Stage (Recovery phase)

I. Nondisaster Stage (Interdisaster phase)

IV. Emergency Stage (Postimpact phase)

II. Predisaster Stage (Preimpact phase)

III. Impact Stage (Impact phase)

Figure 1–1. The stages of a disaster are cyclical. Postdisaster, the planning cycle begins again, with evaluation of the current disaster plan and community response, debriefing with all disaster response agencies and personnel, and modifying disaster plans based on lessons learned. *Illustration by Christina Langan Dalton*

those who were killed in the disaster. Reconstitution occurs when the life of the community returns to some semblance of "normal." The final stage of recovery after a disaster is mitigation. This involves future-oriented activities to prevent subsequent disasters or to minimize their effects. For example, increased security and surveillance measures are efforts aimed at preventing subsequent terrorist activities and their effects (Clark, 2003). See Table 1–1.

DISASTER MANAGEMENT AGENCIES AND ORGANIZATIONS

Many agencies are involved in disaster relief efforts. Local governments and communities are the obvious first responders. Nurses should follow the disaster plan of their communities and the local Emergency Management Agency (Beachley, 2000). This includes having a disaster plan of your own. You must be able to take care of yourself and your family before you may feel ready to help others outside of your family. The Civil Defense Preparedness Agency takes the lead in organizing plans for public safety, utilities, and the local American Red Cross. Mock drills are essential to practice before the threat of a real disaster. Mock drills allow flaws in a disaster plan to be more readily seen. Modifications may be made to the plan before it is actually implemented in a real disaster event. Practice also helps improve staff skill. State resources include the state police, and the National Guard, which may be called out by the governor. If federal resources are needed, FEMA will coordinate

TABLE 1–1. STAGES AND PHASES OF A DISASTER

Nondisaster Stage (Interdisaster phase) period of time before the threat of a disaster materializes
Characterized by:
Planning and preparation
- Planning—coordinated by Emergency Management Agency, involves government agencies, public safety, private organizations, and health care entities
Vulnerability analysis
Capability inventory
Prevention, preparedness, and mitigation activities
- Mitigation—legislating specific building codes, land use restrictions
- Assessment and inventory of resources for special equipment, supplies, personnel necessary to support an emergency response
Education of professionals and the public related to disaster prevention and preparation

Predisaster Stage (Preimpact phase) when a disaster event is imminent but not yet occurred
Characterized by:
Warning
- Warning Opportunity—emergency preparedness plan is put into effect
- Emergency operations centers are opened by state or local Emergency Management Agency (EMA) also referred to as the Office of Emergency Preparedness (OEP)
Preimpact Mobilization—action aimed at averting the disaster or minimizing its effects
- Seeking shelter from effects of disaster
- Evacuating people from areas threatened by the disaster
- Implementing plans to deal with the effects of a disaster
- Sandbagging, boarding up windows, tying down equipment
- Off-duty health care personnel might be called to health facilities in preparation for treating anticipated casualties

Impact Stage (Impact phase) disaster event has occurred and its immediate effects are experienced by the community, lasts until the threat of further destruction has passed and the emergency plan is in effect
Characterized by:
Assessment
- The impact of the disaster with an inventory of the immediate needs of the community
- The nature, extent and geographic area of disaster
- Number of persons requiring shelter
Estimate needed emergency resources
Enduring hardship or injury and trying to survive
Triage injured persons
Established and coordinated morgue facilities
Organized search and rescue activities

Emergency Stage (Postimpact phase) immediate response to the effects of the disaster, begins at end of impact phase and ends when there is no longer any immediate threat of injury or destruction
Isolation phase—immediate response to community needs arises from community members themselves
Relief phase—assistance provided from sources outside of the area affected by the disaster
Characterized by:
Incident command is established if it was not established in the warning phase
Search and rescue
First aid, emergency medical assistance
Establishment or restoration of modes of communication and transportation
Surveillance for public health effects of the disaster
Evacuation of community members from affected areas and those residents vulnerable to further disaster
Emergency Response

- Debris removal
- Provision of temporary housing

Reconstruction Stage (Recovery phase) returning the community to equilibrium
Recovery begins during the emergency phase and ends with the return of normal community order and functioning, timeframe for reconstruction may span years
Characterized by:
Residents repair or rebuild housing
Physical reordering of communications
Restoration of public services, utilities, roads, and general physical environment
Agricultural activities resume
Replacement and Reconstruction of capital stock
Initiation of improvements and developmental reconstruction that stimulate economic growth and local development
Restoration—occurs within first six months of a disaster, reestablishment of a basic way of life
- Schools reopen
- Residents return to work
Reconstitution—several months to several years depending on the degree of damage sustained in the disaster, when life of the community has returned, as far as possible, to normal, in extreme cases, reconstitution may never occur
Mitigation—future-oriented activities to prevent subsequent disasters or to minimize their effects
- Engineering action to prevent the likelihood of subsequent floods
- Disaster response plan created
- Increased security measures
- Irradiating mail
- Cycle the community back into the nondisaster stage

(Adapted from Beachley, 2000; Clark, 2003; Landesman, 2001)

---

federal assistance. The American Red Cross has the legal power to establish immediate intervention programs, especially if the president declares an area a major disaster. The American Red Cross offers damage assessment, mass care, health services, family services, and disaster welfare inquiry services. These services are offered to victims of disasters free of charge and are financed by donations.

TRAUMA

Nurses working with disaster victims can expect to see trauma, and need to have an understanding of both physical and psychological trauma. **Trauma** is the "physical in-

jury caused by violent or disruptive action, or by the introduction into the body of a toxic substance, or a psychic injury resulting from a severe emotional shock" (Anderson, Anderson, & Glanze, 1994, p. 1581). An example of physical injury may occur as a result of blunt trauma or penetration injuries of the abdomen. Blunt trauma to the abdomen occurs with falls, assaults with blunt objects, crush injuries, and explosions. Penetrating trauma to the abdomen is sustained with knife attacks, gunshot wounds or other missiles. In Israel, the use of radiology is stressed as a diagnostic tool, as many terrorist bombing victims suffer trauma injuries that are not immediately known on gross examination. For example, a young man seemed to suffer no major injury as he appeared at the emergency department following a

BOX 1–8   Implications for Nurses When Working with Victims of Disasters

The nurse should concentrate on the victim whose perception of the disaster is the most overwhelming. If clients complain of several symptoms that suggest PTSD syndrome, further assessment must be done to confirm the diagnosis. Continue the assessment of the client and ask if other PTSD syndrome symptoms have been experienced. Several factors increase one's risk of long-term impairment as a result of experiencing a traumatic event. According to the CDC (2003), the nurse should also assess for the following factors:

1. Proximity to the event. Closer exposure to actual event leads to greater risk (dose-response phenomenon).
2. Multiple stressors. More stress or an accumulation of stressors may create more difficulty.
3. History of trauma.
4. Meaning of the event in relation to past stressors. A traumatic event may activate unresolved fears or frightening memories.
5. Persons with chronic mental illness or psychological disorders.

---

bomb attack. On examination of his X rays, however, it was discovered that three-inch nails were embedded in his neck and thigh, lying parallel to his femur.

Psychic trauma is no less important to assess than physical trauma. Factors that have an impact on a person's reactions to disasters include the existence and length of a warning period and the person's physical proximity to the actual site of the disaster. The closer an individual is to the actual site and the longer he or she is exposed to the immediate site, the greater the psychological distress the individual will experience. The victim's perception of the disaster is the strongest influence on the type of psychological response to a disaster that an individual will experience (Richtsmeir and Miller, 1985). The experience for the individual is directly related to the degree to which he or she is directly affected. A victim who perceives the disaster to be less severe than it is will be expected to have a less severe psychological reaction than a person who perceives the disaster and its effects as catastrophic. See Box 1–8.

Post-traumatic stress disorder (PTSD) is defined by the National Institute of Mental Health (NIMH) (2004) as an anxiety disorder that can develop after exposure to a terrifying event or ordeal. The disorder may be triggered following violent personal assaults, natural or human-caused disasters, accidents, or military combat in which grave physical harm occurs or is threatened. Other incidents that may trigger PTSD symptoms are terrorist attacks, being tortured, being a prisoner of war, severe automobile accidents or being diagnosed with a life-threatening illness (American Psychiatric Association, 2000).

There are many signs and symptoms indicative of PTSD. Many people with PTSD re-experience the traumatic event through flashbacks, memories, nightmares or frightening thoughts when they are exposed to events or objects which remind them of the trauma. Other symptoms include emotional numbness, sleep disturbances, depression, anxiety, irritability or outbursts of anger and feelings of intense guilt. Most people with PTSD persistently avoid any stimuli associated with the trauma. PTSD is typically diag-

nosed when symptoms last more than one month and is best diagnosed by a mental health professional (NIMH, 2004).

PTSD syndrome is a very real phenomenon for the injured and noninjured victims, their families, significant others, friends, and health care workers. Remember to check on coworkers at frequent intervals. The health care worker is not immune to the devastating effects of the disaster and its aftermath. Although many rescuers, health care workers, and volunteers may wish to work long hours for many days, limits must be placed on the amount of sustained exposure. It has been suggested that no relief worker or volunteer remain in the rescue mode greater than two weeks. Offer debriefings, therapy, and support to all classifications of victims—the injured, noninjured, family members, significant others, friends, rescue and health care workers, as well as volunteers. See Chapter 4 for detailed information on promoting mental health.

SUMMARY

The United States and all nations of the world have become acutely aware of the varying degrees of vulnerability to terrorist attacks. Disasters of many kinds affect everyone, and everyone can do something to be prepared for both anticipated and unexpected disasters. Nurses have a unique opportunity to learn about disasters and their vital roles in emergency preparedness and response. These roles will be played out in places of employment and in the community, including neighborhoods and private residences.

Many issues must be well thought out when considering the major topic of disasters. The concepts of trauma and mental health issues surrounding disastrous events, planning, and responding to disasters are covered in greater depth in subsequent chapters. Later chapters will also address special concerns that nurses will encounter when assisting multiple types of patients in various settings.

CASE STUDY

Train Explosion

A commuter train with multiple cars is rushing its way between the city and the suburbs at approximately 6:15 p.m. on a Wednesday evening. The cars are particularly crowded with a class of high school seniors who just completed a day in the city on a field trip and the usual rush hour workers returning home. Suddenly, when the train is about 0.25 mile from the suburban station, a large blast is heard, and the train car lights blink and go out. The cars are completely dark, the smell of fire and smoke is overwhelming and the passengers begin to cough and choke on the fumes. They scream and pound on the exit doors to try to escape.

Answer the following questions and give the rationale for your responses.

1. What type of disaster do you suspect is happening here?
2. What types of injuries would you expect the victims to suffer?
3. Would you estimate a multiple casualty incident or a mass casualty incident?
4. With the estimated number of victims involved, would you anticipate that this community would require assistance outside of its own personnel and resources?

TEST YOUR KNOWLEDGE

1. A situation with a large number of casualties, usually greater than 100 persons, that overwhelms available emergency medical services, facilities, and resources is a
   A. Multiple casualty incident
   B. Mass casualty incident

2. An example of a natural disaster is
   A. Three Mile Island
   B. War
   C. Love Canal
   D. Volcanic eruption

3. The production and storage of hazardous materials occur in
   A. Chemical plants
   B. Gas stations
   C. Hospitals
   D. All of the above

4. Hazardous materials are substances that pose a potential risk to life, health, or property if they are released.
   A. True
   B. False

5. The planned exodus of 235 families from Love Canal was the result of
   A. A nuclear power plant accident
   B. The indiscriminate disposal of toxic materials
   C. A biological experiment gone awry
   D. The governor's plan to build a shopping center at that site

6. Car and truck bombs are typically considered as
   A. Conventional terrorist weapons
   B. Nonconventional terrorist weapons

7. An example of an accidental disaster is
   A. A car loaded with bombs that steers into a bus loaded with passengers
   B. A fuel tanker that runs aground due to poor visibility in a storm
   C. Anthrax spores that are disseminated to a large population through the mail
   D. A toxic agent that is discovered in a jar of baby food

8. Chemical weapons are categorized by the major organ system affected.
   A. True
   B. False

9. The final stage of recovery after a disaster, which involves future-oriented activities to prevent subsequent disasters or to minimize their effects, is called
   A. Reconstruction
   B. Recovery
   C. Mitigation
   D. Reconstitution

10. Symptoms associated with PTSD include all of the following *except*
   A. Emotional numbness
   B. Sleep disturbances and nightmares
   C. Feelings of intense joy, now that the traumatic event is past
   D. Irritability and outbursts of anger

See Test Your Knowledge answers in Appendix B.

EXPLORE 🌐 MEDIALINK

Interactive resources and an audio glossary for this chapter can be found on the Companion Website at http://www.prenhall.com/langan. Click on Chapter 1 to select the activities for this chapter.

REFERENCES

Agency for Healthcare Research and Quality. (2001). *Training of clinicians for public health events relevant to bioterrorism preparedness*. Rockville, MD: Author.

American Nurses Association. (1995). *Nursing's social policy statement*. Washington, DC: Author.

American Nurses Association. (2004). *Nursing: Scope and standards of practice*. Washington, DC: Author.

American Nurses Association. (2001). *Code of ethics for nurses*. Washington, DC: Author.

American Psychiatric Association (APA). (2000). *Diagnostic and statistical manual of mental disorders* (4th ed.). Washington, DC: Author.

American Red Cross (ARC). (1975). *Disaster relief program*, 2235. Washington, DC: Author.

Anderson, C. (2003, September 5). Terrorists could target U.S. food and water supplies, FBI cautions. *St. Louis Post-Dispatch*, p. A13.

Anderson, K. N., Anderson, L. E., & Glanze, W. D. (1994). *Mosby's medical, nursing, and allied health dictionary* (4th ed.). St. Louis: Mosby.

At least 96 killed in nightclub inferno. (2003, February 21). CNN. Retrieved October 7, 2003 from http://www.cnn.com/2003/US/Northeast/02/21/deadly.nightclub.fire/

Beachley, M. (2000). Nursing in a disaster. In C. M. Smith & F. A. Maurer, (Eds.). *Community health nursing* (pp. 424–445). Philadelphia: W. B. Saunders.

Ben-Gurion, D. & Rosenblueth, F. (1948). *Prevention of terrorism ordinance No. 33 of 5708–1948*. Retrieved February 22, 2003 from http://www.ict.org.il/counter_ter/law/lawdet.cfm?lawid=11

Blair, B. G. (2001). *Center for defense information terrorism project: What if the terrorists go nuclear?* Retrieved August 29, 2003 from http://www.cdi.org/terrorism/nuclear.cfm

Brain, M. (2003). *How biological and chemical warfare work*. Retrieved September 6, 2003 from http://people.howstuffworks.com/biochem-war5.htm

Centers for Disease Control and Prevention (CDC). (2000). Strategic planning workgroup. Biological and chemical terrorism: Strategic plan for preparedness and response. *Morbidity and Mortality Weekly Report*, 49 (RR-4), 1–14.

Centers for Disease Control and Prevention (CDC). (2001). *Agents/diseases*. Retrieved October 25, 2001 from http://wwwbt.cdc.gov/agentagentlist.asp

Centers for Disease Control and Prevention (CDC). (2003). *Coping with a traumatic event. Information for health professionals*. Retrieved June 12, 2003 from http://www.cdc.gov/masstrauma/factsheets/professionals/coping_with_trauma.htm

Clark, M. J. (2003). Care of clients in disaster settings. In M. J. Clark (Ed.), *Community health nursing*, (4th ed.) (pp. 623–653). Upper Saddle River, NJ: Pearson Education.

Columbia University School of Nursing. Center for Health Policy. (2001). *Core public health worker competencies for emergency preparedness and response*. [Brochure]. Retrieved August 5, 2002 from http:/cpmcnet.columbia.edu/dept/nursing/academics-programs/sub-specialties/epr.html

Comerio, M. (1998). *Disaster hits home: New policy for urban housing recovery*. Berkley, CA: University of California Press.

Federal Emergency Management Situation Report. (1995, April 20). *Oklahoma City bombing*. Retrieved June 12, 2003 from http://www.disaster.net/historical/ok/fema.html

Federal Emergency Management Agency (FEMA). (1997). *Backgrounder: Terrorism*. Retrieved October 25, 2001 from http://www.fema.gov

Ganor, B. (1998, April 25). *Non-conventional terrorism: chemical, nuclear, biological*. Retrieved November 24, 2002 from http://www.ict.org.il/articles/articledet.cfm?articleid=1

Gebbie, K. M., & Qureshi, K. (2002). Emergency and disaster preparedness: Core competences for nurses. *American Journal of Nursing*, 102(1), 46–51.

Harris, T. (2003). *How dirty bombs work*. Retrieved August 27, 2003 from http://people.howstuffworks.com/dirty-bomb1.htm

Hoffman, B. (1998). *Inside terrorism*. New York: Columbia University Press.

Hoffman, B. (2003). Terrorism. *Microsoft Encarta Online Encyclopedia 2003*. Retrieved February 22, 2003 from http://encarta.msn.com/encnet/frefpages/RefArtTextOnly.asp?refid=761564344&print=3

House of Commons of Canada. (2001, November 28). BillC-36, Part II.1, 83.01. Retrieved July 8, 2004 from http://www.parl.gc.ca/37/1/parlbus/chambus/house/bills/government/C-36/C-36_3/90168b

International Nursing Coalition for Mass Casualty Education. (2003, August). *Educational competencies for registered nurses related to mass casualty incidents*. Retrieved May 11, 2004 from http://www.aacn.nche.edu/Education/INCMCECompetencies.pdf

International Terrorism, Definitions. (2002, May 10). U. S. C. Title 18, Part I, Chapter 113B, Sec. 2331. Retrieved February 23, 2003 from http://www4.law.cornell.edu/cgi-bin/htm_hl?DB=uscode18&STEMMER=EN&words=1

Lancaster-Brooks, R. (2002). *Water terrorism among ambitious range of topics Presented at BCWWWA Conference*. Retrieved September 1, 2003 from http://www.esemag.com/0602/bcwwa.html

Landesman, L. Y. (2001). Essentials of disaster planning. In L. Y. Landesman (Ed.), *Public health management of disasters* (pp. 109–119). Washington, DC: American Public Health Association.

Malilay, J. (1997). Floods. In E. K. Noji (Ed.), *The public health consequences of disasters* (pp. 287–301). New York: Oxford University Press.

Maihos, J. (2003). *Cocoanut Grove fire*. Retrieved September 6, 2003 from http://boston.about.com/library/weekly/aa022203a.htm

Massachusetts Board of Registration in Nursing. (2000). *Standard of Conduct Policy 01-01, Determination of Compliance with the Standard of Conduct at 244 CMR 9.03(15) Prohibiting Patient Abandonment*. Retrieved August 26, 2003 from http://www.state.ma.us/reg/boards/rn/misc/nwrgaban.htm

McDade, J. E., & Franz, D. (1998). *Bioterrorism as a public health threat*. Retrieved September 1, 2003 from http://www.cdc.gov/ncidod/eid/vol14no3/mcdade.htm

National Institute of Mental Health. (2004, April 9). *Posttraumatic stress disorder (PTSD)*. Retrieved May 2, 2004 from http://www.nimh.nih.gov/publicat/ptsdfacts.cfm

Noji, E. K. (1997). The nature of disaster: General characteristics and public health effects. In E. K. Noji (Ed.), *The public health consequences of disasters* (pp. 3–20). New York: Oxford University Press.

Richtsmeir, J. L., & Miller, J. R. (1985). Psychological aspects of disaster situation. In L. M. Garcia (Ed.), *Disaster nursing*. Rockville, MD: Aspen.

Roth, K. (2003, February 25). *How to keep yourself safe if there is a crowd crush or fire at a club.* Retrieved October 7, 2003 from http://www.vh1.com/news/articles/1470144/02252003/id_0.jhtml

Schlundt, J. (2003). *WHO publishes guidance to minimize terrorist threats to food.* Retrieved September 1, 2003 from http://www.who.int/mediacentre/statements/nfpl/en/print.html

Terrorism Act 2000. (2000). Retrieved February 22, 2003 from http://www.hmso.gov.uk/acts/acts2000/00011—b.htm

Tharpe, J., & Dart, B. (2003, September 20). Isabel cuts swath of suffering, with 18 dead. *St. Louis Post-Dispatch,* p. 28.

Tribune coverage of the E2 tragedy. (2003, May 25). *Chicago Tribune.* Retrieved October 7, 2003 from http://www.chicagotribune.com/news/chi-nightclubtragedy-gallery,0,4597060.storygallery

Tucker, J. B. (2000). Introduction. In J.B. Tucker (Ed.), *Toxic terror: Assessing terrorist use of chemical and biological weapons* (pp. 1–14). Cambridge, MA: MIT Press.

United Nations Office for Drug Control and Crime Prevention. (2002). *Conventional terrorist weapons.* Retrieved January 5, 2003 from http://www.undcp.org/odccp/terrorism_weapons_conventional.html

U.S. Department of State, Washington, D. C. (October, 2001). *Fact sheet: Chemical-biological agents.* Retrieved September 11, 2002 from http://travel.state.gov/cbw.html

U.S. Department of State. (2002). *Fact sheet: Guidance for responding to radiological and nuclear incidents.* Washington, DC. Retrieved September 11, 2002 from http://travel.state.gov/nuclear_incidents.html

U.S. Environmental Protection Agency (U.S. EPA). (2002). *Water infrastructure security.* Retrieved September 1, 2003 from http://www.epa.gov/safewater/security/index.html

University of Idaho Cooperative Extension System. (2002). *Hazardous materials accidents.* Retrieved January 5, 2003 from http://www.uidaho.edu/bae/disaster/haz/hazmat.html

Washington State Department of Health. (2003). *Protecting the nation's water supplies from terrorist attack.* Retrieved September 1, 2003 from http://www.doh.wa.gov/ehp/dw/Publications/epa_terrorism_factsheet.htm

World Nuclear Association. (2001). *Three Mile Island: 1979.* Retrieved January 5, 2003 from http://www.world-nuclear.org/info/inf36.htm

CHAPTER 2

Planning for Disasters

Joanne C. Langan and Julie Benbenishty

LEARNING OBJECTIVES

1. Identify various agencies that may be involved in pre-disaster planning.
2. List at least five principles of disaster preparedness.
3. Describe your own emergency preparedness plan.
4. Determine your role in disaster planning in your agency or in your community.

MEDIALINK www.prenhall.com/langan

Resources for this chapter can be found on the Companion Website at http://www.prenhall.com/langan. Click on Chapter 2 to select the activities for this chapter.

CHAPTER OUTLINE

Know Your Terms
Audio Glossary
Web Links
    Plan Development Tools and Resources
    Partners in Planning: Federal and Local Resources
MediaLink Applications
    Case Study: Disaster Role Play

GLOSSARY

Agent-specific planning. A strategy for disaster planning, the approach communities take when they plan for threats most likely to occur in their region

All-hazards approach. A strategy for disaster planning, the approach communities take to plan for the common problems and tasks that arise in the majority of disasters; the level of preparedness is maximized for the effort and expenditures involved

Burn specialty team. Highly specialized DMAT staffed by physicians and nurses with specific training and experience in treating severely burned patients

Capability inventory. Assesses a community's resources and its ability to cope with the consequences of disasters

Damage assessment. Gathering of information about the physical damage resulting from a disaster; an American Red Cross program

Disaster Medical Assistance Team (DMAT). Group of professional and paraprofessional medical personnel designed to provide emergency medical relief during a disaster or other event

Disaster Mortuary Operation Team (DMORT). Specialty DMAT, provides mortuary services

Disaster welfare inquiry service. Gathering information about the disaster area, what and who were affected and individuals killed or injured, information available to concerned relatives through their local ARC chapter

Family services. An emergency assistance program to help families return to some form of normalcy by providing food, clothing, shelter, and medical needs including eyeglasses, dentures, procurement of prescriptions, household furnishings, and occupational supplies and equipment; an American Red Cross program

Hazard vulnerability chart. Tool used in planning for disasters; addresses types of emergencies, probability of each emergency's occurrence, human impact, property impact, business impact, and internal and external resources; high scores indicate that the agency should develop additional contingency plans

Health services. Tending to the emotional and medical needs of victims and disaster workers; an American Red Cross program

Mass care. Providing shelter, food, and supplies for victims of disasters; an American Red Cross Program

National Disaster Medical System (NDMS). A cooperative asset-sharing partnership between HHS, the Department of Defense, the Department of Veterans Affairs, FEMA, state and local governments, private businesses, and civilian volunteers to ensure that resources are available to provide medical services following a disaster that overwhelms the local health care resources

National Medical Response Team (NMRT). Specialized DMAT, equipped and trained to provide medical care for victims of weapons of mass destruction, particularly chemical and biological agents

Off-gassing. Vaporization of toxic substances from contaminated materials

Office of Emergency Preparedness (OEP). Within the U.S. Department of Health and Human Services, has departmental responsibility for managing and coordinating federal health, medical, and health-related social services and recovery to major emergencies and federally declared disasters such as natural and technological disasters, major transportation accidents, and terrorism

Strategic National Stockpile (SNS). Works with governmental and nongovernmental partners to upgrade the nation's public health capacity to a national emergency; ensures that federal, state, and local entities are able to receive, stage, and dispense antibiotics, chemical antidotes, antitoxins, life-support medication, intravenous administration and airway maintenance supplies, and medical/surgical items

Triage. "To sort," a method of assigning priorities for treatment and transport for injured citizens

Twelve-hour push packages. Preassembled sets of supplies, pharmaceuticals, and medical equipment ready for quick delivery

Vendor-managed inventory. Pharmaceuticals and/or medical supplies that can be tailored to a specific event and shipped within 24 to 36 hours

Veterinary Medical Assistance Team (VMAT). Specialized DMAT, provides veterinary services

Vulnerability analysis. Assesses the potential consequences of disasters that are likely to occur within the community

INTRODUCTION

Disaster planning is a continuous, dynamic effort. Planning is made prior to the disaster, for events during and after the disaster as well as for evaluating and modifying the plans for future efforts. A concerted effort by each community to participate in disaster planning will ensure that lives are saved. Coordination of efforts is key. Specific agencies are assigned specific responsibilities, roles, and communication patterns. Planning needs to happen daily and those who will be involved in implementing the plan must know the plan well to reach a state of "readiness." Although reality may play out in a totally different manner than the best disaster plans anticipate, priority emphasis to planning for disasters is essential.

DISASTER PLANNING—SO WHAT?

Every region of the United States is vulnerable to disasters. As Landesman (2001) explains, "Immigration, imported goods, rapid international transportation, emerging and resident pathogens, and terrorism (chemical, nuclear, and biological) increase the potential for technological disasters and epidemic spread of disease" (p. 110). Furthermore, incidents that affect the economic health of the United States affect the country's ability to recover from disasters and exacerbate the plight of the needy. The costs of all types of disasters take their toll in human death and suffering as well as in economic terms.

Coordinated efforts among agencies provide for a smoother response in an actual disaster situation (Paris, 2000). Clark (2003) emphasizes the benefit of contingency plans. Performance of critical functions will be less disrupted if different scenarios are anticipated. For example, if a community plans for victims to be brought to a specific hospital and that hospital becomes contaminated or is unable to accept casualties, then an alternative must be sought. If there is no alternative plan, the community has difficulty adapting, the victims will suffer and more lives may be lost.

During our travels to Israel, experts there shared a great deal about their disaster plans and how they are executed. References to this learning experience will be made throughout the chapter. Additionally, this chapter will discuss disaster preparedness plans for individuals, families, aggregates, and communities and a number of agencies involved in planning will be introduced.

FIVE STAGES OF DISASTERS

As discussed in Chapter 1, the five stages of disasters are the nondisaster or interdisaster stage, the predisaster stage, the impact stage, the emergency stage, and the reconstruction or rehabilitation stage (Noji, 1997). The first, or nondisaster, stage occurs before the threat of a disaster becomes real. It is a time of planning, preparation, and assessing community vulnerability to likely disasters and determining community ability to withstand the consequences of various disasters. In addition to prevention and preparedness activities, mitigation activities are undertaken to prevent or reduce the harmful effects of a disaster on human health or property (Malilay, 1997). Examples of mitigation include construction of buildings to withstand the force of natural hazards, and retrofitting or reinforcing major highway overpasses. In the event of disasters that cannot be prevented, such as major brush fires, communication strategies can be developed to enhance the response capabilities, thus mitigating the extent of the damage. Education of both professionals and the public regarding disaster prevention and planning is another important activity to be achieved during the nondisaster planning stage.

The predisaster stage is the time during which a disaster event is certain to occur but has not yet happened. It is the warning or threat stage. The activities during this stage include warning, preimpact mobilization, and evacuation (Noji, 1997).

The impact stage is described as a time when the disaster has occurred and the community is experiencing its effects. The fourth emergency stage is when the community comes to the aid of its members and, later, assistance is provided from agencies outside of the affected area. Finally, the reconstruction or recovery stage includes the ac-

tivities of restoration, reconstitution, and mitigation. The affected community begins the cleanup and rebuilding and attempts to return to normalcy (Clark, 2003).

This chapter will concentrate on the first two stages of disasters and the activities that these stages encompass. The remaining stages of disaster response will be addressed in Chapter 3.

PREDISASTER PLANNING

The key to effective disaster management is predisaster planning and preparation. Beachley (2000) states "the purpose of disaster planning is to put into place the policies, procedures and guidelines necessary to protect lives and limit the extent of injuries. A comprehensive emergency management plan addresses four major areas: mitigation, preparedness, response, and recovery" (p. 430). Chapter 11 explains these four major areas in depth.

A comprehensive disaster plan requires the coordinated, cooperative effort among many people, agencies, and levels of government. Planning will call on familiarity with possible disaster agents based on previous experiences, as well as experiences of others from various regions and countries. Sharing past experiences and information will help improve building techniques, public awareness campaigns, and early warning systems to reduce the impact of disasters.

Buy-In and Communication of Plan

Initially, local authorities organize the disaster response in the first 48 hours. State and federal support will be forthcoming when it is determined that the local response effort will become overwhelmed. All persons expected to respond to a disaster should be represented in the planning of the disaster response. Disaster plans must be acceptable to the elected officials, to the departments that will implement them, and to those for whom the plans are written.

It is imperative that all persons and agencies who may be involved in the disaster response be involved in the planning. If all become involved in the planning, there is greater buy-in to the plan and the information is shared. Representatives from local health departments and regional offices need to be involved in both the development and the communication of the plan. An agency's plan must coordinate with the community's plan. For example, the incident command structure that is chosen by the hospital should be the same as the community's choice. In this way, the disaster plan is optimally effective, because the communication and coordination of the plan is not hampered.

Planning requires appropriate "technology to forecast events, engineering to reduce risks, public education about potential hazards, a coordinated emergency response, and a systematic assessment of the effects of a disaster to better prepare for the future" (Merchant, 1986). All major areas of disaster planning are shared by local, state, federal, and voluntary agencies. Because many health care professionals will be called upon to respond and work collaboratively with a number of organizations in a disaster situation or mass casualty event, it is necessary to review key agencies involved in the planning phase.

Agencies as Resources in Plan

Numerous disaster agencies can be tapped as community resources when creating a plan. These include the Federal Emergency Management Agency (FEMA), U.S. Army Corps of Engineers, Department of Health and Human Services (HHS), American Red Cross (ARC) (an International Disaster Relief agency), United Nations Headquarters of the Disaster Relief Organization, Pan American Health Organization (PAHO), International Reserve Committee, and local volunteer organizations such as the Boy Scouts of America, Goodwill Industries, Volunteers of America, and Church of the Brethren. (See Appendix A for organizational acronyms.) National agencies have state and local offices that respond to disasters; the most immediate response is logically from the local groups and offices. The state may request aid from other states or the federal government if the disaster exceeds local and state resources and private and volunteer organizations.

Local Governments and Communities

Communities must have an emergency operations plan. Local disaster response organizations include local area government agencies such as fire departments, police departments, public health departments, public works departments, emergency services, and the local branch of the American Red Cross. Local disaster response plans include action plans for various types of disaster situations, designation of an overall incident commander,

and identification of community resources. The local emergency management agency is also represented in the state emergency management planning efforts (Beachley, 2000).

Area hospitals develop their own action plans for handling small community disasters. A committee should be convened to create, implement, practice, evaluate, and modify hospital-based disaster plans. This committee plays a vital role in the overall effectiveness of a facility's plan. It is virtually impossible for an individual to take on the task of planning in the facility without the support and input from a variety of members. Departments that should be represented are hospital epidemiology, infection control, emergency department, nursing, security, administration, facilities engineering, occupational health, environmental health, housekeeping, food and nutrition, the local FBI, Emergency Medical Service (EMS) personnel, and the police and public health. It is essential that a committee leader be selected to guide the discussions, plans and actions even though the planning committee chair may vary from hospital to hospital. See Figure 2–1.

Voluntary Agencies

Volunteers and volunteer agencies are considered assets as the disaster plan takes shape. Volunteer agencies are additional resources to be used as the need arises. Local health care professionals may be called on to volunteer their services during an emergency. As stated, nurses will be in great demand to deliver disaster relief. One need not be an emergency department nurse to be invited to help. Nurses in all kinds of service areas will be tapped as well as those in the community who may not be currently employed. Neighbors, friends, and communities traditionally seek nurses out for health care information and advice. As Willshire and Hassmiller (2002) explain, nurses are uniquely

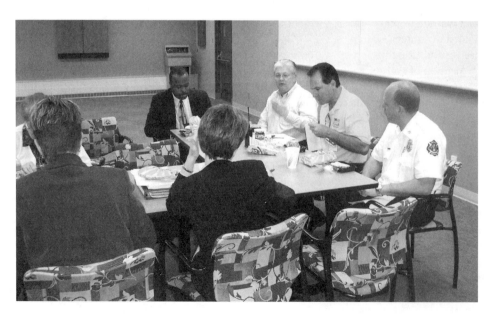

Figure 2–1. Meeting among local emergency medical service personnel, police, and hospital personnel. *(Courtesy of Joanne Langan.)*

positioned to provide information regarding disaster preparedness to the community. Their special knowledge, skills, and abilities make them key providers of disaster relief services. Nurses are especially well prepared to meet the health needs of victims and their families as well as disaster responders.

The American Red Cross is a voluntary agency that was granted a charter in 1905 by the U.S. Congress. The charter gives the ARC the authority to act as the primary voluntary national disaster relief agency for the American people. The ARC acts to coordinate the disaster relief efforts of a variety of voluntary agencies. The ARC has created five major programs to meet the human needs of a disaster. These postdisaster activities are described in Chapter 3.

State Governments

The state emergency operations plan is developed and coordinated by the state governments. They also establish a State Emergency Management Agency (SEMA), to coordinate the state response to a disaster event. Coordination of response services will be necessary if the disaster affects multiple areas (Beachley, 2000).

Federal Government

FEMA was established in 1979 as the coordinating agency for all available federal disaster assistance. This agency works closely with state and local governments by funding emergency programs and providing technical guidance and training.

Planning Tools/Resources

Numerous planning resources and documents are available to assist communities in developing or revising disaster plans. The Association for Professionals in Infection Control and Epidemiology/Centers for Disease Control and Prevention (APIC/CDC) *Bioterrorism Readiness Plan: A Template for Healthcare Facilities* is just one of the planning tools readily available to agencies that wish to have a guide in creating their own disaster preparedness plans. The introduction to this document provides key advice. Institution-specific response plans should be prepared in partnership with local and state health departments. Many of the bioterrorism planning components may be incorporated into existing disaster preparedness and other emergency management plans. Should a bioterrorism event be suspected, a network of communication must be activated to involve infection control (IC) personnel, health care administration, local and state health departments, the FBI field office, and the CDC. Existing local emergency plans should be reviewed and a multidisciplinary approach outlined that includes local EMS, police and fire departments, and media relations in addition to health care providers and IC professionals. A bioterrorism scenario can be incorporated into

the annual disaster preparedness drills held at many facilities to test and refine bioterrorism readiness plans at each facility. Other planning resources include:

- A local public health agency primer developed by the National Association of County and City Health Officials (NACCHO) in 2001;
- *Model Emergency Response Communication Plan for Infectious Disease Outbreaks and Bioterrorist Events*, published by the Association of State and Territorial Directors of Health Promotion and Public Health Education in 2000; and
- *Health and Medical Services Support Plan for the Federal Response to Acts of Chemical and Biological Terrorism*, published by the Department of Health and Human Services. See MediaLink for further resources.

Assessing Community Vulnerability and Capabilities

As discussed earlier, the nondisaster or interdisaster stage is the period of time before the threat of a disaster materializes. This period of time is also when communities should plan and prepare for potential disasters. Just as in the nursing process, the first process in planning is assessment. The community identifies potential disaster risks and maps their locations in the community. For example, a map may show the locations of nuclear power or chemical plants, rivers, dams, bridges, hospitals, schools, nursing homes, and emergency facilities.

The community will also assess the potential consequences of disasters that are likely to occur within the community and its ability to cope with these consequences. These functions are called **vulnerability analysis** and **capability inventory.** How well a community is able to adapt or respond to a disaster is largely dependent on the inventory of its resources that will be needed in the event of a variety of disasters (Clark, 2003). A **hazard vulnerability chart** is a useful tool to organizations in planning for disasters. See Box 2-1.

Community agencies must also work with the emergency management sector to assess (1) the status of the health and health risks of the community, (2) the status of health care facilities, (3) the protection of vital records, (4) the potential requirements for public shelters, (5) the available resources for alternative emergency and primary care, and (6) the availability of and procedures for obtaining state and federal assistance (Landesman, 2001).

In assessing the overall health of a community, the following issues must be examined.

1. Prevalent disease and persons with special needs who will need assistance related to evacuation and continuity of care
2. Ability of the affected population to obtain prescription medication

Box 2–1   Hazard Vulnerability Chart

A hazard vulnerability chart typically addresses the following elements:

Type of emergency—identifies types of emergencies that have an historical, a geographic, technological, or other likelihood of occurrence in a specific area

Probability—rates the likelihood of each emergency's occurrence

Human impact—analyzes the potential human impact of each emergency, the potential for death or injury

Property impact—considers the potential property losses and damages, considering cost to replace, cost to set up temporary replacements, and cost to repair

Business impact—considers the potential impact on the agency's ability to provide services to patients; assesses

the impact of employees' inability to report to work, patients' inability to reach the facility, interruption of critical supplies, ability to reach patients or transport them, and the impact on utility services supplying the agency

Internal and external resources—examines each type of emergency from beginning to end by asking, "Do we have the needed resources and capabilities to respond?" and "Will external resources be able to respond to us for this emergency as quickly as we may need them, or will they have other priority areas to serve?"

High scores indicate the likelihood that the agency should develop additional contingency plans.

(American Society for Healthcare Engineering, n.d., p.1)

---

3. Building safety and ability to protect victims from injury, the elements, and hazardous material release
4. Ability to maintain air quality, food safety, sanitation, waste disposal, vector control, and water systems (Landesman, 2001, p. 116)

Facility Assessment

Health care facilities need to assess their ability to meet patient needs and maintain communication, water, power, and other basic functions in the event of a disaster. Hospital, long-term care, and residential care facilities' disaster plans must include the rapid discharge or evacuation of patients. These facilities may be asked to admit disaster victims or may be unable to operate due to damage sustained. Plans need to include communications with poison control centers and the maintenance of health care services such as dialysis, intravenous medications, in-home services and medical supplies at all of the relocation sites.

A tool that may be very effective in assessing facilities is the "Mass Casualty Disaster Plan Checklist: A Template for Healthcare Facilities," originally written by the security team for the 2000 Olympics in Sydney, Australia, to assess its readiness for disasters. This document was modified by the APIC Bioterrorism Task Force and became a Center for the Study of Bioterrorism and Emerging Infections (Institute for Bio-Security at Saint Louis University School of Public Health) and APIC document (see MediaLink resources).

The "Mass Casualty Disaster Plan Checklist" is a template used to assess facilities as they prepare for incidents that result in mass casualties. This 18-page document has 25 sections, some of which include:

- Hospital disaster control command center
- Identification of authorized personnel
- Alerting system

- Security
- Media
- Education and training
- Incident Command System

Keep in mind that assessments and background data need to be obtained for both victims and rescue personnel. Public health departments will collect this data including medical needs, lodging, water, sanitation, and feeding arrangements.

Resource Assessment

Resources to be assessed include personnel, supplies, equipment, and information. The success of a disaster plan could depend on how the plan outlined the process to rapidly deliver resources to the locations most in need.

Strategic National Stockpile Program

On March 1, 2003, the National Pharmaceutical Stockpile (NPS) became the Strategic National Stockpile (SNS). The SNS works with governmental and nongovernmental partners to upgrade the nation's public health capacity to respond to a national emergency. Its critical mission is to ensure that federal, state, and local entities are able to receive, stage, and dispense antibiotics, chemical antidotes, antitoxins, life-support medications, intravenous administration and airway maintenance supplies, and medical/surgical items (CDC, 2003).

DISASTER PLANNING: PREPARATION

Resource Management

Personnel and Supplies

A comprehensive disaster plan should also discuss the procedures for locating specialty resources: physicians, nurses, search and rescue teams and dogs, devices to locate trapped victims, heavy equipment and tools, dialysis centers, equipment to treat crush victims, laboratories to analyze hazardous chemicals or biological agents, radiation detection instruments, and hazardous materials response teams with appropriate protective clothing and gear.

Health and medical services resources required in the response to a chemical or biological terrorist incident are urgently needed within the first few hours of the incident. Resource requirements are highly specialized and include medical response personnel with specialized training; chemical-biological-specific medical supplies and equipment; transportation, logistical, and administrative systems support; and communication system support. What is the plan to get these resources into place?

The Department of Health and Human Services's "Health and Medical Services Support Plan for the Federal Response to Acts of Chemical and Biological Health Terrorism" (1996) states that

If activated as a support agency to the Department of Health and Human Services (HHS)(Emergency Support Function [ESF] #8) in accordance with the Federal Response Plan (FRP), General Services Administration (GSA), and representatives of HHS, Department of Veterans Affairs (VA), Department of Defense (DOD) and the Department of Transportation (DOT) will coordinate arrangements for the procurement and transportation of medical equipment and supplies. (p.25)

Smith and Maurer (2000) discuss in the following excerpt the disaster response plan and the responsibilities of nurses to be knowledgeable about agency resources, equipment, and supplies.

a response plan should be concerned with delivering emergency health care as efficiently and as quickly as possible. To that end, nurses should know in advance all community medical and social agency resources that will be available during a disaster. They should know where equipment and supplies have been stored and their prearranged role and rendezvous site. (p. 435)

Checking Supplies

Beachley (2000) advises that emergency personnel and all disaster responders be very familiar with the equipment and supplies they will use in the event of an actual disaster. In addition to mock disaster drills that allow personnel to practice procedures and set up equipment, a periodic check of equipment and supplies should be part of the response plan. Some of the supplies are perishable and need to be restocked at regular intervals. If supplies are not actually unpacked at regular intervals, health care personnel may be disconcerted during a disaster to find damaged, destroyed, or outdated supplies.

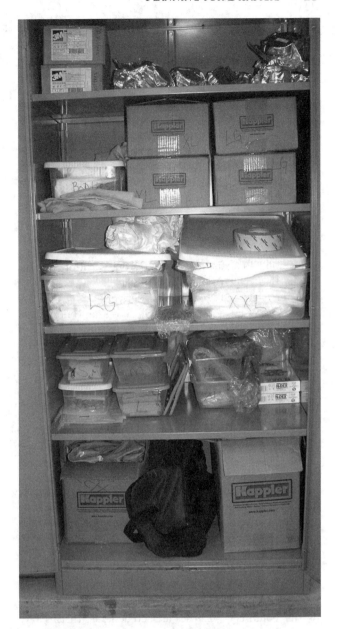

Figure 2–2. Examples of disaster management supplies gathered and stored in lockers inside the ambulance bay at a large Midwestern hospital. Stocks of supplies must be periodically checked and rotated to ensure supplies are still available and expiration dates have not passed.

In Israel, extra carts of supplies are ready to go for any disaster event. Nurses routinely check the carts for outdated medicines and restock them. This effort not only keeps the medicines current, but also keeps the nurses familiar with the inventory of supplies on the carts. See Figure 2–2.

The cost and acquisition of supplies, and related expenses such as education and training should be shared. Landesman (2001) encourages disaster planners to ensure that the disaster preparedness plan identifies state and federal assistance programs for reimbursement and that it establishes procedures to verify full reimbursement for disaster-related health care.

Bioethical Concerns and Use of Resources

Disaster preparedness plans should include some education or seminar sessions dealing with bioethical issues. For instance, in the event of a mass casualty incident, difficult decisions may have to be made regarding the use of limited resources. Which patients would receive treatment and which would not? For example, how would a hospital with a limited number of ventilators decide who would be given ventilator treatment and who would be denied or removed from ventilator equipment? These difficult issues need to be addressed. Planning should include not only education and seminars but also written guidelines. These guidelines should be directly related to the categorizing or triaging of victims. This planning must take place quickly as these decisions should be well thought out. The time required for these types of decisions is a luxury not afforded during a real-time event.

Disaster Alert and Notification Network

Most agencies have a disaster notification network to alert personnel. Staff must follow a protocol of notification so that all available personnel are alerted or called to duty when the need arises. Some personnel may not be reachable. A contingency plan allows the communication network to continue to function. For example, if a nurse is called but cannot be reached, what should the caller do? The notification process would continue until a person answers and can continue the notification process. If a caller stops making calls after leaving a message on an answering machine, it is likely that the subsequent nurses on the list will not be notified.

If possible, when disasters are predictable or probable, health care personnel should be prewarned or placed on alert. Having personnel on alert status reduces the response time during the actual disaster.

Reporting Site

Plans must be made to direct volunteers and professional responders. Check-in or staging areas will be used to verify the volunteers' licenses and credentials. In this way proper deployment of human resources can be achieved most efficiently. Agencies and individuals will plan in advance to assign specific tasks and responsibilities especially in areas where there is no clear-cut statutory or contractual responsibility.

Another important element of a response plan during preparations is the designation of an alternative reporting site for health care workers. In the event of a major disaster, some designated sites may be destroyed or damaged. A good plan will include alternative response sites to which workers can report.

Directing the Flow of Traffic and Patients

Disaster plans must include the organization of the flow of both vehicular traffic and patients. To avoid mass chaos, the perimeter of health care facilities must be secured when receiving victims of a mass casualty event. If decontamination is necessary, the decontamination area must be clearly delineated from the clean areas and be located where the **off-gassing** (the release of gases or hazardous liquids into the environment) will not contaminate the entrance to the hospital or emergency area.

Decontamination

Decontamination education must be specific, and your agency's disaster plan should include details about who will be prepared to act as the decontamination team, where and how personal protective equipment can be obtained, where it is stored, when training will be given and how often it will be reinforced. Additionally, it should include a list of agents (chemical, radiation, nuclear) that will most likely require the decontamination process.

Every victim suspected of exposure to an agent with a risk of secondary contamination to others must be decontaminated. Disaster plans should include the procedures for gross decontamination as well as the technical decontamination. The purchase of and practice in the use of radiation and nuclear contamination detection equipment must be included in the disaster plan.

Another interesting aspect of Israel's plan is that they teach nonprofessional staff how to decontaminate victims so that the physicians and nurses may be available to perform more highly skilled interventions. Nursing students would be excellent health team members to learn the decontamination process and assist in the disaster relief effort at the decontamination shelter area. Specific details of the decontamination process are addressed in Chapter 6.

Personnel Identification

It is often confusing to know who is responsible for specific duties during a disaster response. The disaster plans should include a means to identify response personnel. It is important that nurses, physicians, chaplains, social workers, police, security personnel, housekeeping staff, and others be identified. This is especially significant when decontamination is taking place. With all of the required personal protective equipment including the impermeable suit and gas mask, it is virtually impossible to identify the person inside the suit. In Israel, persons receiving patients wear brightly colored vests with their position such as "doctor" or "nurse" clearly attached in large letters so that everyone may easily identify them. Additionally, some hospitals in the United States have adopted color-coded vests and caps to coordinate with the triage level or team to which they are assigned (Figure 2–3). All personnel who will be actively involved in disaster response and patient treatment must be made aware of this system and how it is to be implemented before a disaster event occurs.

Patient Tracking

Patient tracking becomes complicated due to the fact that most persons who evacuate their homes do not seek lodging in public shelters where the American Red Cross will register their presence. Many victims get to hospitals by

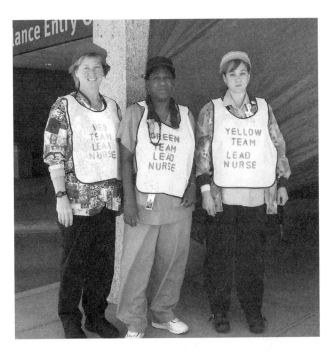

Figure 2–3. Triage nurses in color-coded vests and hats. *(Courtesy of Joanne Langan.)*

private means, and emergency medical services have an incomplete record of injuries. No single agency serves as a central repository of information about the location of victims from area hospitals, morgues, shelters, jails, or other locations. Therefore, a plan must be created to track patients as they enter health care facilities seeking care for their disaster-related injuries.

Mitigation

Mitigation activities are undertaken to lessen the severity of disasters or to minimize their effect on human lives and property. Reinforcing existing structures or building new structures to withstand the forces of a disaster are examples of mitigation. Another example of mitigation is recruiting and preparing volunteers to step in to assist community members in the preparation and prevention of disasters and to assist in disaster relief efforts.

Bomb Shelters

When structures in Israel were built, bomb shelters were included in the design. For example, one apartment house basement in Israel is actually a bomb shelter for about eight families. A long-term care facility in Israel has a bomb shelter room on each floor. One bomb shelter room that is particularly interesting doubles as the physical therapy room. The hospital emergency departments have reinforced walls and air filter systems built into specially designed bomb shelter windows. Disaster plans in the United States should include the construction or the identification of such safe rooms.

Volunteers

Volunteers are valuable assets during the disaster preparation phase and during disaster relief and recovery efforts. Aspects to consider about the volunteer effort during mitigation are as follows.

1. **Recruiting.** Volunteer nurses are always in demand by the American Red Cross and other community agencies. Agencies in need of nurses actively recruit in community newspapers, on radio and television stations, and through word of mouth.
2. **Education.** The American Red Cross will provide orientation and educational materials to prepare nurses for disasters. A number of nursing organizations are actively involved in offering education in the format of continuing education, case studies on the World Wide Web (Sigma Theta Tau), seminars, conferences, books, and online and printed journal articles.
3. **Retention.** Retaining volunteers is a difficult task in any organization. Hopefully, the same motivation that caused the volunteers to join an effort will sustain them throughout the time they are needed.
4. **Maintaining skills.** The only way to maintain the skills necessary for disaster response is to practice repeatedly. Participating in mock disasters, continuous reading of updated protocols, and the practice of skills are just a few ways to maintain these skills.

It must be emphasized that volunteers are integral assets in disaster response. However, all volunteers must be certified as having the credentials they purport to have and the disaster training necessary to be most effective. If background checks are not accomplished prior to the disaster, the volunteers may be asked to help in a nonsecure area, for obvious security reasons.

The American Red Cross is very active in disaster relief, especially in shelters and minor first aid injury responses. Some nurses may choose to volunteer on EMS-type response teams.

Education

Another key area of activity in the planning period is the education of professionals and the public regarding disaster prevention and preparation. It is unfortunate that many deny the need for disaster planning when they are not faced with the immediate threat of a disaster.

Nurses in the community should plan to prepare other nurses, individuals, and families in the community. Nurses in acute care facilities should also be educated for disasters. Nurses who work in specialized areas such as the OR and OB may be asked to float to other, less familiar areas to help with patient management. Operating rooms will cease to perform elective surgeries during a disaster and nurses will be deployed to areas with the most need.

Beachley (2000) states that public education efforts should be geared toward safety, self-help, and first aid measures in the event of a disaster event. The education programs should "include information about proper storage of food and water, rotation of canned goods so that they are used before expiring and boiling water if equipment is available, or using bottled water when tap water is not safe to drink and plumbing is not working" (p. 436). Using the mass media to educate the public can be an effective public health tool. Public education such as injury prevention, a common occurrence especially during cleanup efforts, and monitoring carbon monoxide exposure from charcoal and unvented heaters can prove to be valuable (Landesman, 2001).

It is essential that the public know what types of supplies are needed in a first aid kit. The public will need help in becoming prepared to address trauma injuries such as fractures, bleeding, and burns. Knowledge of first aid basics will help families cope with the most common injuries in a disaster. See Box 2–2 for recommended items to include in a disaster supplies kit.

Family Personal Preparedness Plan

Each family in the community should be encouraged to have a personal preparedness plan. This plan is especially pertinent for nurses and health care professionals who may be expected to respond in the event of a mass casualty incident. Just as passengers are given the instructions on the correct sequence of events in using oxygen on the airlines (adults place the oxygen masks on themselves before placing on their children), responders must have their own families organized before they can expect to take care of others. In this way, they may better concentrate on caring for others, knowing their own families are safe and properly prepared.

A family disaster plan is available from the American Red Cross (2001). See Box 2–3 for what every individual should know following in an emergency.

Evacuation

Another vital element in disaster planning is teaching the public about evacuation. When advance warnings are possible, evacuation can be the most effective lifesaving strategy in a disaster. The U.S. Weather Bureau usually is responsible for the detection and assessment of threatening weather. The sheriff's office is often the organization that makes the decision to order an evacuation and commercial radio and television stations typically warn the public. The warnings must be clear and consistent, come from a credible warning source, be repeated frequently, and include specific information that allows the listener to determine his or her imminent danger. Additionally, the warning must include specific information on self-protective actions (World Health Organization, 1989). The goal in these warnings is that the population at risk should take the threat seriously and take appropriate action based on the warning. Unfortunately, this goal is not always achieved. See Nursing Vignette 2–1.

At the Shelter

Nurses may wish to teach residents in the community about the types of supplies to bring with them to designated shelters. By taking the following items with them to the shelter, emergency shelter supplies will not be depleted as quickly and shelter living may be a bit more comfortable. The suggested items to take to the shelter include food, blankets, pillows, prescription medication, personal

---

BOX 2–2   Items to Include in Disaster First Aid Kit

- Aspirin or nonaspirin pain reliever, adult and child formulas
- Alcohol preps or antiseptic spray
- Antacid (low sodium) tablets
- Eyewash
- Hydrogen peroxide
- Isopropyl alcohol
- Antidiarrheal agent (such as Kaopectate)
- Laxative
- Emetic agent (such as Ipecac, for use if advised by Poison Control Center)
- Activated charcoal (for use if advised by Poison Control Center)
- Cleansing agent or bar of soap
- Moistened towelettes
- Gauze pads, assorted sizes
- Gauze rolls
- Adhesive tape
- Adhesive bandages
- Latex gloves
- Lubricant (such as petroleum jelly)
- Triangular bandages
- Scissors
- Tweezers
- Sewing needle and thread
- Safety razor blades
- Safety pins assorted sizes
- Sunscreen
- Thermometer
- Tongue blades

Adapted from American Red Cross. (March 1992). Your family disaster supplies kit. Washington, DC: Author.

Box 2-3   Essential in the Event of a Disaster

What to Know and Do
- How and where to turn off utilities
- How to escape and where to go
- Where to meet with family members in case of separation (e.g., a neighbor's house)
- Plans for care of pets (pets are not allowed in shelters)
- Safety precautions for various kinds of disasters (e.g., fire, hurricane, etc.)

A List of Necessary Items, Including
- Medications
- Dentures
- Eyeglasses
- Special food or infant formula
- Sturdy shoes
- Identification
- Checkbook
- Credit cards

- Driver's license
- Blankets
- Important papers
- Favorite toys
- Extra clothing for children
- Clothing for cold or inclement weather

Additional Items That May be Necessary to Have in the Event of a Disaster Include
- Emergency phone numbers
- Working flashlight
- First aid kit
- Battery-operated radio
- Extra batteries
- Prescription medications
- Physician names, addresses, phone numbers
- Persons to be notified in an emergency
- Medical information such as allergies, blood types

Adapted from American Red Cross (2001). Terrorism: Preparing for the unexpected. Washington, DC: Author.

Nursing Vignette 2-1   Personal Evacuation Story–Gulf Coast of Mississippi

Joanne C. Langan

While we were living on the Gulf Coast of Mississippi in 1985, we received a warning of a hurricane and the recommendation to evacuate. The skies were gray and threatening. We quickly boarded the windows, removed all lightweight lawn furniture, decorations, and equipment to avoid the possibility of such items being hurled as projectiles in heavy winds. Next, we loaded the car with food, bottled water, clothes, diapers, and emergency contact numbers. We did not have any pets at the time. My husband was a naval officer and was ordered to return to his duty station to await further military assignment. Many of the military wives and I joined the caravan of cars for the trip to hotels or motels in Northern Mississippi. After 24 hours of being away and the threat of a hurricane avoided, we received the "all clear," returned home and began to enjoy the beautiful sunny skies of our Labor Day weekend. During our Sunday picnic, an unexpected second warning for a hurricane was issued. This time, it was less believable because of the gorgeous warm weather and sunny skies. Because my husband was ordered to return for duty

again, I was not about to stay in the house by myself with three small children with the threat of a hurricane and the ensuing tornadoes. I loaded up again and headed to Alabama to visit relatives. Some of the neighbors chose not to evacuate a second time in the same weekend, as they did not believe the warnings. Hurricane Elena struck our town with its full fury less than five hours after our evacuation. A number of tornadoes followed, causing a great deal of damage to the homes in our neighborhood. One little neighbor boy whose family chose to stay in their home during this disaster event chewed ulcers into the sides of his mouth. Another young child hid in his closet when heavy winds howled outside and had recurrent nightmares. Luckily, no one was killed in our neighborhood, but we were without electricity for five days and safe drinking water for seven. We heard the constant whir of the power saws for months as people tried to remove the numerous trees that had crushed our homes and reconstruction took place. The moral to my story: When evacuation warnings are issued, take them seriously and get out!

grooming items, portable chairs, and a radio (ARC, 1991). With enough warning before evacuation, families might also consider taking diversionary recreational equipment such as crossword puzzles, card games, drawing materials and toys (Hayes, Goodwin, and Miars, 1990).

Nurse and Other Health Care Personnel Evacuation

While a disaster is happening, the impact stage, nurses and other health care personnel are advised to stay in place and not to attempt to provide heroic disaster relief until the situation has calmed down. Nurses and emergency personnel may be asked to evacuate the site of the pending disaster in weather-related or predictable disasters such as hurricanes or tornadoes. In this way, they can remain safe and be available to offer assistance after the disaster has struck.

Health care agencies need to carefully plan for the personal needs of their personnel when they develop disaster response plans. Health care workers often find it difficult to evacuate from the danger area. Many may be torn between their duty to go to their places of employment and treat patients and the need to be with their own family members. Health care agency administrators need to communicate clear expectations of health care personnel. All health care personnel, including nurses, need to determine in advance which course of action they intend to take and communicate this clearly with the agency administrators.

Family Care Center

Child care and a family care shelter should be part of the health care agency's plan. While in Israel, the travel team learned of a research study conducted with hospital nurses as subjects. The majority of nurses stated that they would not respond to terrorist/emergency or disaster relief calls if they had no child care in place (Kater, Braverman, & Chowers, 1992). The hospital devised a plan to convert an employee lounge into a child care center for nurses responding to the call for disaster volunteers. With the knowledge that their children would be cared for while the nurses worked, most nurses stated that they would be willing to assist disaster victims. Nurses and health care workers, in general, will require the services of persons willing to assist in watching and protecting their children, elderly parents, and special needs family members. We suggest calling this special, safe area a family care center. Having this type of center written into an agency's disaster plan will greatly enhance the number of employees willing to respond in an emergency. Interestingly, a separate study conducted in the United States found that the second most frequent reason given for health care employees refusing to respond to emergency calls is pet care (J. Hamilton, personal communication, May 14, 2003). Perhaps the best way to prepare employees in this regard would be to ask them to have pet kennels ready or to have prearranged pet sitters available in emergency situations.

Transportation and Communication Strategies

The disaster plan must also consider alternative transportation and modes of communication. Health care personnel may not be able to report to their assigned agencies on their own in cases of floods, earthquakes, and snowstorms. For example, nurses in Northern Virginia needed to take advantage of volunteer drivers in four-wheel drive vehicles to get them to work at the hospital after heavy snows, and an excellent system was devised. Nurses who could not rely on their own transportation to get them to the hospital called into a control center to request transportation to the hospital. Volunteer drivers reported to the control center and were dispatched to the nurses' homes. This effort required planning so that drivers were able to pick up nurses located in the same geographic area.

Alternate means of communication must be addressed in the disaster plan. If telephone service is interrupted, phones and beepers will not function. Local radio stations, ham radio operators, and telephone company representatives can assist in developing realistic communication plans for the organization. This specific planning will allow for communication among the organization, its personnel, other community organizations, and the county or city emergency operations center (EOC) during a disaster event. If the disaster warrants it, communications may also reach to the state EOC. In a large-scale disaster, such as with a weapons of mass destruction or terrorist attack, FEMA will respond and the Federal Response Plan (FRP) may be activated.

Sharing information among organizations is often difficult due to the large amount of equipment needed and the number of people involved. Two-way radios are often the only reliable form of communication across distances. If ground and cellular telephone systems are working, they may be congested or overloaded. Due to Health Insurance Portability and Accountability Act (HIPAA) regulations, hospitals may not share a list of victims with other hospitals or families, but the list may be shared with the health department (Landesman, 2001).

ESSENTIALS AND PRINCIPLES OF DISASTER PLANNING

Flexibility

In her book, *Public Health Management of Disasters* (2001), Landesman explains that disaster plans should be based on what people are likely to do rather than on the expectation that the public will behave "according to the plan." Because there are many laws, organizations, populations, technologies, hazards, resources, and people involved in disaster response, it is vital that disaster plans are flexible and easy to change.

Plans should be general enough to cover all potential disaster events. When separate plans exist for different types of disasters, there is potential for confusion regarding roles and responsibilities. However, all possible types of disasters must be considered, such as specific actions to be taken for chemical and biological disasters, bombings, and other more traditional disasters (Clark, 2003).

Extended Authority

Landesman (2001) recommends that disaster plans provide for some authority at the lowest levels of the organization because workers at these levels must make many decisions during the disaster impact and postimpact phases. Disasters of all types often require decision making that exceeds the routine bureaucratic capacities and information processing of the normal day-to-day management structure. Disaster plans are able to optimize the resources of each agency if they do not rely on the top-down approach to decision-making. Nurses in Israel are given extended power in decision making in cases of terrorist events, because they are in the front lines of disaster relief and there are not enough physicians to safely lead each response group. The Israeli nurses assume leadership responsibilities and need the power to make decisions rapidly and offer care that might typically be rendered by physicians under normal circumstances. The decision to grant extended authority must be made prior to the impact phase of a disaster. In this way, expectations, duties, and responsibilities will be clear.

Agent-Specific Versus All-Hazards Approach to Planning

There are two strategies for disaster planning according to Landesman (2001). The first, called **agent-specific planning,** is the approach communities take when they plan for threats most likely to occur in their region. For example, planning for hurricanes on the Gulf Coast is more useful than planning for earthquakes. Persons are typically more motivated by what they perceive locally as the most viable threats in their specific location.

The second approach is called the **all-hazards approach** to disaster planning. Because many disasters pose similar problems and require similar tasks, an all-hazards approach involves planning for the common problems and tasks that arise in the majority of disasters. The level of preparedness is maximized for the effort and expenditures involved.

Sharing Information with the Public

The need for each facility to designate one or two spokespersons is not to be overlooked in the disaster plan. The media will demand information at all hours, day and night. Standard responses may be prepared for any type of disaster. These responses should be practiced during the mock drills or exercises.

Disaster Drills

Disaster plans should be reviewed at least quarterly and practiced frequently. Landesman (2001) recommends that a community-wide emergency response plan be exercised at least once every 12 months. JCAHO standards require disaster drills and education.

Even though the people of Israel experience numerous disaster events and mass casualty incidents throughout the year, they still conduct approximately 20 drills per year. See Nursing Vignette 2–2. In addition, facilities mount cameras from the ceilings in emergency departments. The cameras record all actions and communication between the emergency department staff and emergency response personnel. These recordings are used to review all actions to make modifications to their disaster plans; the reviews are not used for finger pointing or to place blame. The personnel feel they can always perform better than they did in

---

NURSING VIGNETTE 2–2   Israeli Perspective on Preparing for Mass Casualty Events

Julie Benbenishty, RN

In order to educate staff effectively for mass casualty events, they must undergo drills and exercises. In Israel, a division of infantry soldiers plays the role of mass casualty victims. University students are invited to perform the role as well. Television makeup artists transform the foot soldiers into seriously wounded blast victims. Each soldier is given his own scenario to play out when he arrives at the hospital. Many are given secondary complications to act out, such as convulsions or nerve gas exposure symptoms. Only a select few are notified about the drill—the hospital administrator, chief of police, chief of emergency squad, and the nursing administrator. Before the drill occurs, the hospital staff, physicians, nurses, messengers, X ray technicians, social workers, admitting clerks, and

volunteers are given secondary jobs to do in times of mass casualties. All personnel are fully aware of where they must report when notified of a mass casualty event. A detailed network of telephone numbers is given out to all hospital staff. Every designated group leader is given 12 people for whom he or she is responsible, keeping the telephone numbers current. A systematic periodic telephone hotline is passed among all members of the network. This occurs four times each year. Drills are planned and implemented at least two to three times a year. All drills are videotaped at a number of locations. These locations include the entrance to the emergency department and throughout the entire trauma and emergency departments. After the drill is finished, all involved parties are recalled to the emergency department and the drill is rerun and critiqued.

the past. Through reviews and modifications, they are able to save more lives and use resources more efficiently.

Disaster plans can be exercised in one of three ways.

1. Desktop simulation exercises using paper or computer-based scenarios
2. Field exercises, which test the disaster plan in simulated field conditions
3. Disaster drills based on valid assumptions about what happens in disasters

Drills and training are most effective when many organizations, disciplines, and jurisdictions are involved. As Landesman (2001) sums up, "Coordination is also facilitated when participants are familiar with the skills, level of knowledge, and dependability of other responders on whom they may one day need to rely" (p. 118).

When all the agencies that will be expected to respond to a disaster participate in the plan development, implementation, and practice, there will be a greater likelihood that the needs of the community will be met. With a detailed preparation and involvement of all necessary agencies, the coordination of efforts will occur instead of chaos.

Mock disaster drills allow the participants to become educated to the plan, and the areas that need strengthening in the plan will become evident. Following the reviews of the mock disaster drills, the plans should be modified to make corrections and provide solutions to troublesome areas of response.

Perhaps the use of cameras in emergency departments in the United States is unrealistic. However, a means of reviewing actions and communication after a disaster event is necessary to improve the system. We can all agree that we need to consider more efficient means of delivering health care during chaotic and stressful events.

Casualty Distribution

The concept of casualty distribution needs to be addressed in the disaster plans with established protocols among emergency medical services and area hospitals. The significance of this plan is to ensure an even distribution of casualties. Another way to consider this concept is to assess the surge capacity of any given health care agency. One must ask, "If there should be a mass casualty event, how many victims could this agency safely admit for care?"

Contingency Plans

Advanced planning is required to care for patients when the health care infrastructure has been damaged. Many patients seek hospital care because of chronic medical conditions rather than trauma, due in part to damage or loss of access to usual sources of primary medical care. People may evacuate their homes without prescription medications or with a short supply as they may underestimate how long they will be kept from returning to their homes. Many injuries occur

during the rescue or cleanup activities following the disaster. All types of health care facilities including hospitals, ambulatory care centers, home health care agencies, pharmacies, and dialysis centers must have backup arrangements, such as special needs shelters, to care for their patients postimpact. This backup plan is not only for building locations, but also for human resources such as physicians, nurses, pharmacists, and radiologists. The patients will need to be visited in their new "home" sites where they have temporarily relocated.

Crowd Control

The management of volunteers and donations must be worked into the disaster plan. Frequently more resources are donated than are actually needed or requested. Unsolicited volunteers including survivors, family members, coworkers, and bystanders may show up at the disaster site. Procedures for managing large numbers of people and donations need to be established. A center should be planned outside the disaster area where public requests for aid can be managed as well as the collection, organization, and distribution of resources. In this way, ongoing emergency services will not be disrupted.

Expect the Unexpected

Regardless of the amount and extent of preplanning, disasters will require some unanticipated tasks. Public health officials must develop the capacity and training, and mutually agreed upon procedures, to participate in the community's coordinated, multiorganizational response to unexpected problems. Problem areas include shelters, utilities, communication systems, transportation, a huge influx of patients, expanding the morgue capability, and mental health needs. There have been instances when ice-skating rinks and caves were used as temporary morgues when other resources were exhausted.

Mental Health Component of Response

All disaster preparedness plans need to incorporate the mental health component of response. The importance of mental health services cannot be emphasized enough. The public, first responders, victims, and their families will have significant mental health needs during a bioterrorism or chemical terrorism event. It should also be noted that anxious members of the general public might seek unnecessary medical attention that could quickly overwhelm the health care system during a terrorism event. For example, in March 1995, in Aum Shinrikyo, the nerve agent sarin was released on a subway train. Twelve persons died, and 6,000 were reportedly injured. All of these people ran for help to the same hospital. Later, it was determined that approximately 1,300 were actually injured, the balance of those seeking medical attention were simply anxious about the threat of injury. This is a prime example of the "worried well" overwhelming the health care system during a terrorist event (B. Clements, personal communication, May 27, 2003). Mental health issues are covered extensively in Chapter 4.

SUMMARY

Because we will all be affected by disasters in our communities, the planning phase of disaster preparedness is extremely important. A disaster plan that is well thought out, practiced, evaluated, modified, and practiced again will best serve the community. Whether we are at home, school, work, or play, the implementation of the disaster plan must become automatic. The public looks to nurses and health care professionals for information and guidance. We have an obligation to become educated and prepared ourselves so that we may be ready to educate, prepare, and assist others.

CASE STUDY

Are You Prepared?

As the department manager of the emergency department of the community hospital, you are a member of your community's emergency preparedness team. You and your team are tasked with the duty of creating a mock disaster scenario to involve as many entities in the community, city, and state as possible. Your overall goal is to test the disaster preparedness plan in the community and, specifically, to test whether the correct communications are made to the appropriate authorities, employees, and disaster relief agencies.

1. What is the scenario you will create to involve the most agencies?
2. Will you require the assistance of the neighboring communities? The state?
3. Who are the key players for notification at specific agencies?
4. What kinds of communication devices will you be testing?
5. What is already in your disaster plan that will facilitate the "call in" of hospital personnel?

TEST YOUR KNOWLEDGE

1. The benefit of contingency plans is
   A. Performance of critical functions will be less disrupted if different scenarios are anticipated
   B. More committees can be involved in planning
   C. Those who implement the disaster plan will have more of a choice in plans
   D. All of the above
2. It is important for nurses to be knowledgeable about disaster planning and response because

1. Nurses will be tested on such knowledge during annual competency exams
2. Nurses have traditionally been sought out by neighbors, friends and communities for health care information and advice.
3. Nurses have the responsibility to teach emergency medical service workers.
4. Historically, professional nurses respond to the needs of society, including in times of disaster.
   A. 1 and 3
   B. 2 and 3
   C. 1 and 4
   D. 2 and 4
3. The key to effective disaster management is
   A. Having enough managers on the planning team
   B. predisaster planning and preparation
   C. postdisaster mitigation
   D. postdisaster reconstruction teams
4. Preassembled sets of supplies, pharmaceuticals and medical equipment ready for quick delivery are called
   A. 12-hour push packages
   B. Vendor managed inventory
   C. Hospital supply cart
   D. 24-hour response packages
5. Which of the following is *not* a federal agency?
   A. FEMA
   B. DOD
   C. VA
   D. SEMA
6. Which of the following is considered a Disaster Medical Assistance Team (DMAT)?
   A. DMORT
   B. VMAT
   C. NMRT
   D. All of the above
7. American Red Cross assistance is
   A. Free and is provided through funds donated by the American people
   B. Paid for by the recipients based on a sliding scale
   C. Provided for the American people by the federal government
   D. Free only to former ARC volunteers
8. Some of the items to be taken to the shelter in the event of a disaster include all of the following except
   A. Food
   B. Blankets and pillows
   C. Diversionary games
   D. The family pet

9. The approach communities take when they plan for threats most likely to occur in their region is called
   A. All-hazards approach to disaster planning
   B. Agent-specific planning
   C. Region-specific planning
   D. Agent-modified planning

10. The following principles of disaster preparedness are *true*
    1. Disasters and every day emergencies are the same
    2. Disaster plans need to be adjusted to people's needs
    3. Disaster planning is dynamic and changes as community needs change
    4. The lack of shared information causes community members to react inappropriately.
       A. 1, 2, 3
       B. 2, 3, 4
       C. 1, 2, 4
       D. 1, 3, 4

See Test Your Knowledge answers in Appendix B.

EXPLORE MediaLink

Interactive resources and an audio glossary for this chapter can be found on the Companion Website at http://www.prenhall.com/langan. Click on Chapter 2 to select the activities for this chapter.

REFERENCES

American Red Cross. (1991, November). *Emergency preparedness.* Washington, DC: Author.

American Red Cross. (1992, March). *Your family disaster supplies kit.* Washington, DC: Author.

American Red Cross. (2001, October). *Terrorism: Preparing for the unexpected.* Washington, DC: Author.

American Society for Healthcare Engineering. (n.d.). *Hazard vulnerability analysis chart directions for use.* Retrieved June 17, 2003 from www.ashe.org

APIC Bioterrorism Task Force and CDC Hospital Infections Program Bioterrorism Working Group. (1999, April 13). *Bioterrorism readiness plan: A template for healthcare facilities.* Retrieved January 23, 2003 from CD available from the Institute for Bio-Security at Saint Louis University School of Public Health at www.bioterrorism.slu.edu

Assessing facility bioterrorism preparedness: A guide for infection control professionals. (n.d.). Retrieved January 23, 2003 from www.bioterrorism.slu.edu

Association of State and Territorial Directors of Health Promotion and Public Health Education. (2000). *Model emergency response communication plan for infectious disease outbreaks and bioterrorist events.* Available on CD from Institute for Bio-Security at Saint Louis University School of Public Health.

Beachley, M. (2000). Nursing in a disaster. In C. M. Smith & F. A. Maurer (Eds.), *Community health nursing* (pp. 424–445). Philadelphia: W. B. Saunders.

Boyle, J. S. (2002). Emergency and disaster preparedness: Where is transcultural nursing? *Journal of Transcultural Nursing, 13(4),* 273.

Centers for Disease Control and Prevention. (2002). *National pharmaceutical stockpile.* Retrieved June 4, 2003 from http://www.bt.cdc.gov/stockpile

Centers for Disease Control and Prevention. (2003, August 11). *Strategic National Stockpile.* Retrieved September 23, 2003 from http://www.bt.cdc.gov/stockpile/index.asp

Clark, M. J. (2003). Care of clients in disaster settings. In M. Clark (Ed.), *Community health nursing* (pp. 623–653). Upper Saddle River, NJ: Pearson Education.

Department of Health and Human Services. (1996, June 21). *Health and medical services support plan for the federal response to acts of chemical and biological terrorism.* Available on CD from Institute for Bio-Security at Saint Louis University School of Public Health.

Department of Health and Human Services, Office of Inspector General. (2002, December). *State and local bioterrorism preparedness.* OEI-02-01-00550. Washington, DC: Author FEMA: *Federal Response Plan.* (2003, January 21). Retrieved January 26, 2003 from http://www.fema.gov/rrr/frp/frpfig1.shtm

Hayes, G., Goodwin, T., & Miars, B. (1990, February). After disaster: A crisis support team at work. *American Journal of Nursing, 90(2),* 61–64.

Institute for Bio-Security at Saint Louis University School of Public Health. (2002). *Public health preparedness toolkit: Key resources for public health departments.* Retrieved January 23, 2003 from www.bioterrorism.slu.edu

Institute for Bio-Security at Saint Louis University School of Public Health and APIC. (2002). *Mass casualty disaster plan checklist: A template for healthcare facilities.* Retrieved January 23, 2003 from http://www.bioterrorism.slu.edu/

Kater, V., Braverman, N., & Chowers, P. (1992). Would provision of child care for nurses with young children ensure response to call-up during a wartime disaster? An Israeli hospital nursing survey. *Journal of Emergency Nursing, 18(2),* 132–134.

Landesman, L. Y. (2001). Essentials of disaster planning. In L. Y. Landesman (Ed.), *Public health management of disasters* (pp. 109–119). Washington, DC: American Public Health Association.

Malilay, J. (1997). Floods. In E. K. Noji (Ed.). *The public health consequences of disasters* (pp. 287–301). New York: Oxford University Press.

Merchant, J. A. (1986). Preparing for disaster. *American Journal of Public Health, 76(3),* 233–235.

National Association of County and City Health Officials. (2001, January). Available on CD from Institute for Bio-Security at Saint Louis University School of Public Health.

National Disaster Medical System. (2004). *Welcome to NDMS.* Retrieved February 20, 2004 from http://www.ndms.dhhs.gov

Noji, E. K. (1997). The nature of disaster: General characteristics and public health effects. In E. K. Noji (Ed.), *The public health consequences of disasters* (pp. 3–20). New York: Oxford University Press.

Office of Emergency Preparedness. (n.d.). *NDMS catastrophic care for the nation: About teams.* Retrieved January 21, 2003 from http://www.ndms.dhhs.gov/NDMS/About_Teams/about_teams.html

Paris, J. (2000). Georgia inmates and staff coped with natural disaster–Lesson learned from Hurricane Floyd. *Correct Care, 14*(1), 8, 21.

Schwarz, T., & Kennedy, M. S. (2003). Disaster volunteer teams. *American Journal of Nursing, 103*(1), 64AA–64DD.

Smith, C. M., & Mauer, F. A. (2000). *Community health nursing: Theory and Practice* (2nd ed.). Philadelphia, PA: W. B. Saunders.

U.S. Department of Health and Human Services, Centers for Disease Control and Prevention. (2001, July). *The public health response to biological and chemical terrorism: Interim planning guidance for state public health officials.* On CD obtained from Institute for Bio-Security at Saint Louis University School of Public Health.

Willshire, L., & Hassmiller, S. B. (2002). *Disaster preparedness and response for nurses.* Retrieved January 23, 2003 from http://www.nursingsociety.org/education/case_studies/cases/SP0004.html

World Health Organization. (1989). *Coping with natural disasters: The role of local health personnel and the community.* Geneva: World Health Organization.

CHAPTER 3

Organization and Implementation of the Disaster Response

Dotti C. James

LEARNING OBJECTIVES

1. Describe and discuss the persons or agencies that must be notified when there is a suspicion of a terrorist event.
2. Define crisis versus consequence management and incident command system.
3. Discuss the optimal disaster response planning committee membership to plan a coordinated institutional response.
4. Discuss the necessary changes in the triage process during a mass casualty event (MCE).
5. Explore the possible methods of meeting the increased need for medications, equipment, and supplies during a mass casualty event.
6. Describe the role of the various search and rescue responding agencies.

MEDIALINK **www.prenhall.com/langan**

Resources for this chapter can be found on the Companion Website at http://www.prenhall.com/langan. Click on Chapter 3 to select the activities for this chapter.

CHAPTER OUTLINE

Know Your Terms
Audio Glossary
Web Links
    Bioterrorism Resources
    Disaster Response Resources
    Nursing Resources
MediaLink Applications
    Role Play: Chemical Explosion
    Essay Questions: Disaster Response

GLOSSARY

Chain of command. Delineation of authority

Consequence management. Second stage of a disaster, during which FEMA is the lead federal agency. The ultimate goal is to manage and minimize the impact of the event on the community and assist in returning to normal functioning

Crisis and management. First phase of a disaster during which the FBI is the lead federal agency. Crisis management involves either identifying perpetrators before an attack occurs or taking steps to identify the perpetrators after an attack has occurred with the ultimate goal of capturing the perpetrators and preventing additional attacks

Disaster response committee. Group responsible for developing the disaster response plan. In health care, it consists of administrators, management, ancillary support persons, nurses, physicians, and members of the community response agencies

Hospital Emergency Incident Command System (HEICS). A hospital-based incident command system used as a framework for reporting and communication, which entails assignment of specific roles to individuals in an effort to create a distinct chain of command that is temporarily enacted in response to a disaster situation

Incident Command System (ICS). A framework for reporting and communication, which entails assignment of specific roles to individuals in an effort to create a distinct chain of command that is temporarily enacted in response to a disaster situation

Presentation. Clusters or groups of symptoms causing patients to seek medical care. Presenting symptoms forming clinical picture.

Redundancy. Backup or alternate systems to provide needed services such as communication

Surge capacity. Estimation of the maximum patient load for which responding hospitals and agencies can provide care following a mass casualty event. It includes beds, staffing, equipment, and EMS systems. When considering needed beds, surge capacity is estimated to include a bed capacity of 500 acutely ill patients per million population for hospitalization and decontamination

Surveillance. The process of collecting and analyzing data to detect a change or trend in the health of the population

Universal identification card. Credentialing of health care worker as to qualifications, education, and skills

INTRODUCTION

The United States is facing a new era in warfare, a time when terrorism could strike at any moment, in any location, with little warning preceding an attack. The political environment in which we live has had a negative effect on people's feelings of safety and security. When these negative feelings couple with the current state of essential services in health care, hospitals and nurses face a serious challenge to prepare for the very real possibility of an event that results in large numbers of victims needing emergency care at the same time. Health care systems will be challenged to optimize their performance and their use of valuable resources. Nurses must rise to the challenge and assume a leadership role in preparing for the unexpected.

How prepared is the American health care system for a mass casualty event? The American Hospital Association (AHA) reports that 7 of 10 hospitals have added a bioterrorism response plan, with an additional 28% planning to add it in the following 6 to12 months (2002). Considering chemical terrorism, 76% have integrated this into their current plan, with 20% planning its addition. About half of the hospitals have added nuclear terrorism to the response plan, with an additional 27% to add it in the following 6 to12 months.

This chapter addresses the third and fourth stages of disaster, the impact stage and the emergency stage (Noji, 1997). The impact stage is the time when the disaster has occurred and efforts focus on minimizing the negative effects. The emergency stage focuses on aid to community members, initially from the members themselves, and later, from agencies outside of the affected area.

REPORTING AND NOTIFICATION

A disaster has occurred: What happens now? One of the initial steps in responding to a mass casualty event is notification of key agency personnel. The institutional readiness plan must address the reporting or communication system within the facility and other agencies. If this part of the plan is deficient, the agency cannot function in a coordinated manner, and personnel and the community are at increased risk for injury related to the particular agent or situation that has occurred. During a mass casualty event, Emergency Operations Centers (EOC) will open to coordinate local, regional, and national efforts (Figure 3–1). The communication patterns necessary may vary according to the type of incident that has occurred, for example, biologic, chemical, nuclear or radiation, and traditional events. Each institution should have a specific plan in place showing the required steps for properly reporting a suspicious incident.

Detailed information about specific biologic agents is included in Chapter 11, but some general communication principles can be applied to a bioterrorism event. If a bioterrorism-related event occurs, hospitals, clinics, and offices may be the first sites to recognize that something is happening and that the appropriate communication channels must be activated. Clinicians must remain vigilant to identify and react to clusters of patients with similar symp-

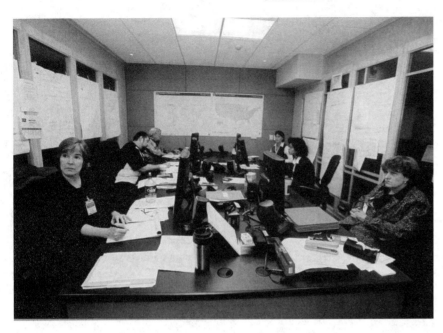

Figure 3–1. During a mass casualty event, Emergency Operations Centers (EOC) coordinate local, regional, and national efforts.

toms or unusual presentations. After the clinician becomes suspicious of the **presentation,** the diagnosis must be made. The laboratory diagnostic capability is critical to rapidly identifying the pathogen and making a correct diagnosis. The response to an infectious agent must be planned carefully in advance, with key personnel familiar with the infectious control procedures that need to be implemented. The initial person who becomes suspicious should contact his or her immediate supervisor. In a hospital situation, many of the appropriate personnel in the communication plan may be onsite. In a community-based incident, where care is delivered in multiple community agencies, a more aggressive response may be necessary, such as contacting suspected victims at home. It is important not to become lulled into a false sense of security. Because it has not happened in the past does not guarantee a problem-free future.

Departmental Notification

Some of the other key people or departments to be notified include the emergency department, emergency medical services, infection control staff, hospital administration, local and state health departments, the FBI, state and federal emergency management, and the CDC. The hospital is not responsible for notifying all of these agencies. The hospital notifies key within-hospital persons, as well as the local or state health department. In a community-based agency, the local health department is notified, and they contact other appropriate agencies. To ensure that this notification procedure proceeds smoothly, the emergency plans should be reviewed regularly and expanded to include multidisciplinary membership, as well as specific contact information. Communication is key to a successful response. Each agency or institution should answer each of these questions: Who should be notified of an event? Who

should be contacted for information? Who is in charge? Who should talk to the media? How should we communicate internally? How should we communicate with other agencies? Are any of these people in house? If not, who is the representative?

Specific agencies and personnel must also be notified if a potential bioterrorism event has been announced or suspicion has been raised by the presentation of symptoms. Some of these include the emergency department (if the contact has not occurred there), infection control staff, hospital administration, and the local health department. The local health department is responsible for notifying the state health departments. Once notified, the local health department has the responsibility to investigate and contact the state health department and SEMA, local law enforcement, EMS, and the FBI if the event is deemed credible. The state health department is responsible for contacting CDC and FEMA. In summary, the emergency department notifies the local health department, the local health department notifies appropriate state agencies and SEMA, the state health department contacts the federal governmental agencies that notify the president, who has the authority to send FEMA. When a known or suspected event occurs, health care professionals must be aware of the recommendations for reporting these known or potential bioterrorism incidents.

CDC Reporting Algorithm

The Centers for Disease Control and Prevention has formalized the reporting or notification procedure for when a bioterrorism-related incident is suspected (Figure 3–2). When health care agencies follow this reporting recommendation, all agencies that have a role in responding to an event are notified in a timely way and the governmental

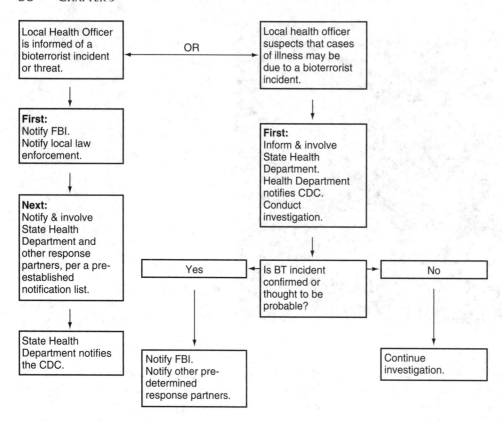

Figure 3–2. Notification algorithm for a bioterrorism event. *http://www.bt. cdc.gov/EmContact/Protocols.asp (CDC)*

response system is activated. This schematic provides definite guidelines for notification following a suspected biological incident. Specific names or phone numbers should be easily available to those designated within each institution. The reporting procedures should be reviewed and readily available to all members of the planning team, as well as professionals within the institution. When you look at the reporting algorithm, you can see that the order of who notifies whom is clearly delineated. This can become a template for names and telephone numbers that could be sized and laminated for attachment with the employee identification badge.

Agency Communication

Communication systems can become overloaded during a mass casualty event as many people attempt to use their cell phones to check on family members and friends. In September 2001, a communication system backup was in place in New York City. This communication plan was developed for first responders. However, the communication system backups and cell phone towers were based in the World Trade Center, so when the towers collapsed, all communication relying on the system was lost (Giorgianni, Grana, & Scipioni, 2002). This breakdown in communication systems is not an isolated incident. Other instances in hospitals, skyscrapers, and schools demonstrate similar system failures. The lesson is: the backup system should be

backed up also. Hospitals and health care agencies must not solely rely on telephone lines, cell phones, or satellite phones. Some facilities are backing up these traditional methods of communication with radio communication devices. Establishment of the communication system is only step one. Decisions must be made about how communication flows within and without the institution.

AUTHORITY DURING A DISASTER

Chain of Command

The chain of authority must be defined prior to a mass casualty event. According to the April 1999 Association for Professionals in Infection Control and Epidemiology (APIC) working group, the line of authority in an overt bioterrorism event places the FBI as the lead agency. Each major metropolitan area has a plan that can be implemented with the aid of the Metropolitan Medical Response System (MMRS). The key to success is coordination of efforts.

When large numbers of casualties are anticipated, all responding agencies should be aware of the role of other agencies and coordinate their efforts to avoid duplication of services or unnecessary use of resources. Communication among agencies and the community involves the adoption of the **Incident Command System (ICS)** that is present in the community to ensure effective communication and use of the same terminology. The ICS defines the chain of authority during the event, thus supporting a safe and coordinated response. It is the model for command, control, and coordination of the response. It is not the same authority structure that is in place on a day-to-day basis in the agency, but a method of interagency cooperation and promotion of a team response when team members come from multiple agencies. Responsibilities of the incident commander include:

- Assume command
- Assess situation or event
- Implement emergency management plan
- Determine response strategies
- Activate resources
- Order an evacuation
- Oversee activities
- Determine the end of the incident

(AHA, 2002, p.28)

Health care professionals should be familiar with the specialized terminology and processes associated with the ICS (FEMA, 1998). Each responder should know their role once the ICS is activated.

ICS was developed in the 1970s as an interdisciplinary agency coordination tool when responding to a series of forest fires in Southern California. The priorities of ICS are life safety, incident stability, and property conservation. When a situation involves hazardous materials, the Occupational Safety and Health Act of 1970 mandates the use of ICS. The incident commander is the first responder on the scene, although once a higher-ranking responder arrives, this person will likely assume command of the situation.

Hospital Emergency Command System

The specific management plan adopted by each facility should match the plan used by the area's civilian and military authorities. One such emergency management system is the **Hospital Emergency Incident Command System (HEICS).** For example, if the community is using HEICS, the hospital or agency should also adopt this system. If a traditional ICS plan is used, that system should be adopted by the hospital. If local, state, and regional planning is done, the chain of command is developed collaboratively and a smoother transition is made during an event.

The HEICS management system uses the logical management structure, defined responsibilities, clear reporting channels, and a common nomenclature that can help to unify hospitals and emergency responders. In this way, more cost-effective planning can occur and the accountability of each position is defined. Under HEICS, there is an incident commander with four chiefs reporting: logistics, operations, planning, and finance. These chiefs can contact their counterpart in other agencies and communicate effectively due to the common language. It is imperative that each agency and institution provides education to their responders so that they do not have to learn it during a crisis.

CRISIS AND CONSEQUENCE MANAGEMENT

Crisis management begins during the impact stage (Noji, 1997). The ultimate goal of crisis management is to investigate the incident to determine who did it and deal with the immediate crisis. In this instance, the FBI is always the lead agency, regardless of whether the agent is chemical, biological, or radiological. **Consequence management,** with FEMA as the lead agency, has the ultimate goal of dealing with the consequences from the incident, including handling the victims, resource management, and recovery efforts. The emergency and recovery stages occur during consequence management. While it is easy to divide the responsibilities on paper, in practice there are more gray areas.

Osterholm (Cole, 2000) states, "In practice, it will be impossible to divide these responsibilities. Whoever is trying to figure out who did it is going to be right in the middle of trying to respond to it. No one really knows who the hell is going to be in charge." Response is more efficient and effective if the planning occurs in advance. In addition, the effective use of community resources is enhanced during a coordinated effort.

In summary, certain agencies have the responsibility to organize or manage the response to a mass casualty event. In these events, crisis management is under the authority of the FBI, while management of the consequences or aftermath of the event is handled by FEMA. But we must remember that each federal agency has a plan, each state has a plan, each major metropolitan area has a plan, Metropolitan Medical Response System has a regional plan, and within regions or geographical areas, each facility has a plan. The most important question for you to ask is: *Are they coordinated?*

The agency or institution must also coordinate its efforts with the crisis and consequence management efforts occurring in the community. If the precise location of the incident can be identified during crisis management, that location becomes a crime scene, and care must be taken to avoid disturbing or destroying valuable evidence. During consequence management, each institution or agency charged with caring for victims must adhere to the response plan to avoid duplication of efforts, or ineffective use of resources.

INTERAGENCY COORDINATION

Within each city, health care agencies or institutions should begin planning how their roles will mesh with each other. Health care facilities (HCF) must develop their plan to mesh seamlessly with the state and regional plans so that resources are not wasted. State and regional authorities will be onsite before federal assistance is received and serve as a valuable resource for HCF operation during and following a disaster. Plans must be developed that cover specific instances in which victims, supplies, and personnel will be available to assist at collaborating institutions. Metropolitan areas and response organizations, such as the American Red Cross, are planning the implementation of a **universal identification card** for health care professionals. Ideally, prior to a mass casualty event, the credentials of health care providers are checked and recorded in a database. Each person is issued a card with a bar-coding system (similar to patient tracking systems). With this card, agencies and institutions will be able to *scan* the card and have instant verification of a person's credentials and qualifications. This will facilitate the organization and usage of volunteer professionals during times of increased need. Following a mass casualty event, as professionals and volunteers arrive, the cards are scanned and assignments matched with the skill set of each person. When the universal identification cards are unavailable, agencies must verify the credentials of each person who is not employed or known to that institution. Although volunteers cannot be the primary source of health care providers, they are an important component. More information on volunteers is available in Chapter 2.

When a disaster involves a search for victims, and possibly evidence, a coordinated effort is vital. Official agencies can provide sophisticated techniques and resources when responding to a mass casualty event. Nurses may want to become involved with one of these agencies, to become more involved during a disaster.

After completing the additional required education and training, nurses can be active participants in their efforts when disaster strikes. Each of these agencies has a mission and purpose when large numbers of casualties are expected.

Disaster Response Committee

A team effort is vital for a smooth implementation of the response plan. Acknowledging the efforts of all involved, and recognizing superior efforts, encourages others to contribute to the plan as well. Each person has a role during a disaster response. No one person can handle all the needed roles. Still, each must be aware of the contributions of others and be able to rely that those actions will be successfully completed during a disaster response. Finally, coalitions foster relationships before they are needed, when temperaments are cool and stress is reduced (Giorgianni, et al., 2002). Many areas are establishing regional response plans to maximize the resources of multiple hospitals and clinical agencies. The individual agency plan must be coordinated with the regional plan. For example, if the larger hospitals become filled and load balancing is necessary, where will the overflow victims be sent?

During a disaster response, the value of a diverse planning committee membership is apparent. These members contribute a fresh perspective on the system, as well as significant information about what can be expected from first responders. Those who work exclusively within the hospital or within the community may be unaware of what the other is doing, what constraints guide our practice, and what resources we can access. Working collaboratively enables understanding and provides a realistic perspective. It diminishes the constant "Why didn't they? . . . " that often accompanies the arrival of victims. Mutual support results in a smooth transition from ground zero to the acute care setting. This dialogue reduces the risk of miscommunications during a disaster. When large numbers of victims rely on the health care system, it is important that all responders are familiar with the role of other responders, to avoid conflicts or duplication of efforts and wasting of resources. Agreeing on what is possible in the field and how it will be continued in the acute care setting facilitates effective use of resources.

Disaster Response Plan

When an incident occurs and the plan is implemented, the questions to be answered include: What kinds of injuries can I expect? When can I expect the first victims? Who must come to the hospital for the most effective response? What types of communication networks must be activated?

Institutional Readiness

A key component in institutional readiness is getting involved in local planning. Several tools, such as "Mass Casualty Disaster Plan Checklist: A Template for Health Care Facilities" (Institute for Bio-Security at Saint Louis University School of Public Health & APIC, 1999) were described in detail in Chapter 2. During the implementation of the response plan, the value of using these templates is evident, as they aid in examining the appropriateness and adequacy of physical facilities, organizational structure, human resources, and communication systems.

Government funding has also supported adequate response efforts following a disaster. During 2002, the U.S. government allocated $135 million to assist hospitals in preparation efforts. By 2003, $514 million was appropriated to preparedness and improvements to the infrastructure (Austin, 2003).

A primary concern following a mass casualty event is the determination of **surge capacity.** Surge capacity is an estimation of the maximum patient load of responding hospitals and includes beds, staffing, equipment, and EMS systems. Each facility must be able to determine their ability to manage casualties quickly so that victims will be sent to the most appropriate facility. When considering needed beds, surge capacity is estimated to include a bed capacity of 500 acutely ill patients per million population for hospitalization and decontamination. In an urban area, there

---

BOX 3–1   Self-Assessment Questions

- Who is in charge?
- What will be expected of them?
- How many nurses and physicians are needed?
- How many nurses and physicians will actually be available?

- What working relationships with other agencies will be needed so that we can work together smoothly, wasting no precious resources?

Adapted from Assessing facility bioterrorism preparedness, www.bioterrorism.slu.edu

---

will be a need for 250 additional health care personnel per million population; in a rural area, 125 per million. There must be personal protective equipment for each of these (Austin, 2003).

Agency Self-Assessment

When the response plan is activated, each agency must prepare and organize for an efficient and effective response. The immediate self-assessment for mass casualty event response begins with questions about specific roles. See Box 3–1. These answers provide a starting point for any reorganization that is needed.

Management of Events

Before an incident, it is important to evaluate the physical plan of the institution or agency. Following an event, your response is based on the answers to several questions. Where does triage occur? Where does decontamination occur? What security is necessary? When examining a possible flow pattern during a mass casualty event, it is imperative that all responders are familiar with the flow pattern at your agency. If victims are being transported randomly to various departments, a traffic jam or bottleneck may result. A suggestion made during the training in Israel is that all victims go in one direction when leaving the ED; no victims return, rather they progress to the next area. Areas that are potential bottlenecks are X ray, CT, ultrasound, and laboratory areas. In addition, areas requiring intensive interventions, such as airway management, table thoracostomy, and blood transfusions, may also slow the flow of patients. Consider having someone oversee the event without having direct patient care assignments. Colleagues in Israel suggest that a physician remain on the roof of the hospital to observe for bottlenecks in the flow of victims, as this is difficult to determine from the midst of triage and decontamination. Directions for effectively managing patient flow issues can be transmitted from the roof to the ground via radio communicators.

In addition to decontamination procedures, an important response need when bioterrorism is suspected is the ability to quarantine or isolate suspected victims. In other disasters, such as bombings or earthquakes, a small percentage of victims are admitted to the hospital, typically about 15% (Levitin & Skidmore, 2003). Most are treated

and sent to their homes. Following the release of a biological agent, victims are sick and often require hospitalization. Without rapid identification of suspicious cases and isolation of these victims, the institution, professionals, and other patients are at risk. If the onset of a bioterrorism event is insidious, and community health care providers do not recognize the illness pattern or diagnostic clues, large numbers of casualties result, with widespread panic. Standard precautions include handwashing, gloves and masks, eye protection, face shields, gowns, isolation or cohort placement, management of equipment and environment, postmortem care, notification of pathology department, and decontamination of patients and environment.

Determining Capacity

Those in authority must be able to quickly determine hospitalization capacity, status of critical care beds, how many casualties they can handle, how many operating rooms are available, and how many ventilators are unused. Which patients can be discharged from the emergency room and inpatient floors quickly? Is it possible to internally relocate patients to provide additional space for victims? Nearby schools and hotels may provide efficient and necessary space for victims. How long will it take to prepare an appropriate triage area? How much time is needed to set up a decontamination area? How many staff can you rely on to come in quickly? One of the more impressive preparations of hospitals in Israel is the plan to empty the emergency department and set up outpatient surgery as an ED extension within 10 to 15 minutes. Nurses are categorized according to a tier system so that they know when they are required to come to the hospital in case of a mass casualty event.

In most instances, there will be no advance warning before an event occurs. On September 11, 2001, the public knew generally what had happened, and where it occurred. Health care professionals could anticipate what types of injuries could be expected from an explosion and building collapse. What was not known was why and who, and this, coupled with the suddenness, resulted in chaos during a time when response was critical.

During the past decades, hospitals were forced to downsize to meet the need to decrease operating costs. Consequently, there is little excess capacity to meet surges in demand. Every major U.S. city faces closed EDs daily and patients are diverted to facilities farther away. Sometimes this results from a slowdown in processing ED patients, but the effect is backups in accepting ambulances and long waits. Nurses must take an active role in preparations to meet the increased needs following a disaster and increase the surge capacity of health care agencies and institutions.

Surveillance

Surveillance is a concept usually associated with the public health department. There is, however, a form of surveillance that must occur within institutions and agencies to provide insurance that the early cases will be identified and reported in a timely manner. This surveillance is typically under the supervision of the infection control department. There is a process in place that regulates the types of information that is reported by the clinical laboratories as results are confirmed. Within the hospital, it is important to collect data related to the number of patients seen in the ER, and how many are admitted with specific symptoms. A syndromic surveillance process permits easy identification of trends or symptoms, presentations that are not typically seen in these numbers, or larger than normal numbers of

persons arriving at the ED, clinic, or physician office with similar symptoms or complaints. The first case identified is the **sentinel event,** the case or symptoms that first trigger an alarm. Many types of disasters will not be announced with an event as dramatic as those occurring on September 11, 2001. Careful observations and assessments by nurses and health care professionals will be a key component in identifying the occurrence of terrorism, and the specific type of event. Still, identification of suspicious illnesses or side effects of toxic agents within an institution cannot stop there. A thorough examination of the extent of the problem, number of occurrences, and disposition of the victims must be reported to the appropriate authorities so that the public can be protected, and so appropriate interventions can be provided to the victim and to the community as a whole.

As the facility becomes organized toward preparedness, consider providing written or computer resources for each area that may encounter victims of biological or chemical agents. Providing these in binders or CD-ROMs enables providers to quickly check on groups of symptoms or presentations during a disaster. The CDC provides these, as well as the Institute for Bio-Security at Saint Louis University School of Public Health (Table 3–1).

TABLE 3–1. ASSESSMENT AND TREATMENT OF CHEMICAL AGENTS

CHEMICAL AGENTS			
AGENT	SIGNS AND SYMPTOMS	DECONTAMINATION	PERSISTENCE
Nerve Agents			
Tabun (GA)	Salivation	Remove contaminated clothing	1–2 days if heavy concentration
Sarin (GB)	Lacrimation	Flush with a soap and water solution	1–2 days will evaporate with water
Soman (GD)	Urination	for patients	Moderate, 1–2 days
V Agents (VX)	Defecation	Flush with large amounts of a 5%	High, 1 week if heavy concentration
	Gastric disturbances	bleach and water solution for	As volatile as motor oil
	Emesis	objects	
Vesicants (Blister Agents)			
Sulfur Mustard (H)	Acts first as a cell irritant, then as a cell	Remove contaminated clothing	Very high, days to weeks
Distilled Mustard (HD)	poison.	Flush with soap and water solution for	
Nitrogen Mustard (HN 1,3)	Conjunctivitis, reddened skin, blisters,	patients	
Mustargen (HN2)	nasal irritation, inflammation of	Flush with large amounts of a 5%	Moderate
	throat and lungs	bleach and water solution for	
		objects	
Lewisite (L)	Immediate pain with blisters later		Days, rapid hydrolysis with humidity
Phosgene Oxime (CX)	Immediate pain with blisters later—		Low, 2 hours in soil
	necrosis equivalent to second and		
	third degree burns		
Chemical Asphyxiants (Blood agents)			
Hydrogen Cyanide (AC)	Cherry red skin or ~ 30% cyanosis.	Remove contaminated clothing.	Extremely volatile, 1–2 days
Cyanogen Chloride (CK)	Patients may appear to be gasping	Flush with a soap and water solution	Rapidly evaporates and disperses
Arsine (SA)	for air	for patients	Low
	Seizures prior to death	Flush with large amounts of 5% bleach	
	Effect is similar to asphyxiation, but is	and water solution for objects	
	more sudden		

Personal Protective Equipment Levels:
Level A: Fully encapsulated suit with SCBA
Level B: Non-encapsulated suit with SCBA
Level C: Splash Suit (tyvex coveralls) with an air purifying respirator (APR)
Contact Phone Numbers: CHEMTREC: 800-424-9300 National Response Center: 800-424-8802 Center for Disease Control: 888-232-3228 U.S. Public Health Service: 800-USA
Adapted from CDC & the Institute for Bio-Security at Saint Louis University School of Public Health.

Communication During a Disaster

Effective communication is vital during times of disaster. Those involved in the disaster response must be able to communicate with each other and coordinate their efforts. If utilities are disabled or destroyed, many forms of traditional communication are lost. These include telephone, FAX, and Internet access (Klitzman & Freudenberg, 2003). Today we are technology dependent, and this becomes critical when communication systems are disabled.

The communication system during a mass casualty event must be tested when lives are not depending on it. One method is to participate in your local planning bodies to answer two key questions: With whom should you communicate? What do they expect from you? During the collaborative exercises, potential problems can be identified in advance. Following a disaster, the communication system used may be different from the one used on a day-to-day basis. A multi-tiered plan is activated and the needed equipment is moved to the triage area.

Despite the intricacies and planning that accompanied an agency's communication plan, the situation can become complicated and direct communication difficult if the health care providers must use personal protective equipment (PPE). The easily recognizable colleague disappears into a cumbersome protective suit, accented with boots, heavy gloves, and a gas mask. Verbal communication may be difficult or impossible because of the responder's PPE and the noisy chaos surrounding the arrival of large numbers of casualties. Methods of easily identifying each professional must be used to avoid needless movement and searching for a specific type of worker. For example, fluorescent signs or vests can be color coded according to role, such as doctors, nurses, and administrators.

Each health care provider who may be an initial contact point for victims of bioterrorism should be familiar with their responsibility to report and the person identified as their next contact. It may be easier to provide the key personnel with a communication algorithm that can be carried at all times. Include appropriate telephone numbers. The entire communication plan should be easily available, but knowing the next step is a critical piece of information, and that simplicity may provide a smooth response when suspicious incidents occur.

CASUALTY MANAGEMENT

Preparations for Care

Certain types of injuries can be anticipated depending on the type of event. For example, conventional weapons result in blast injuries. It is more difficult to anticipate injuries with an unknown or unrecognized chemical or biological agent. For this reason, a high index of suspicion may alert health care providers of the risk of contamination from chemical or biological agents sooner, and decrease the overall number of injured. If this is an industrial accident, the chemical may be known. In a terrorist attack, there may be a period of time when the agent is unknown and the institutions must be prepared to provide care in this situation. A mass transportation accident, a building collapse, a natural disaster such as an earthquake or a tornado pose unique challenges to preparation and care. Maintaining contact with first responders on the scene of the event will enable the hospital or agency to prepare for the specific victims of that type of disaster.

Staff

A specific community's needs and resources will determine the use of paid professional nurses or volunteers following a disaster. The person in charge should plan for at least two shifts a day. In addition, plan for the protection of staff during decontamination and when caring for victims of biological agents. The Emergency Medical Services Authority (EMSA) of California (2003) has released recommendations for hospitals that provide practical information for staff protection, decontamination, and evidence collection, in addition to an algorithm for setting up a decontamination area.

Maintaining the chain of evidence is an important responsibility following a terrorist event. Although patient care is the primary function, management of evidence can typically be handled as well. If victims can undress without assistance, direct them to place their valuables in a clear plastic bag with a picture identification that is visible from the outside. Any assistance devices, such as glasses, canes, or hearing aids, should remain with the victim during decontamination. Clothing will be placed in a prelabeled paper bag. If there is a risk of secondary contamination due to the agent, place this paper bag in a clear plastic bag. The information to be placed on the bag should include the name, date of birth, medical record number, date, time, any decontamination done, and the geographical site where the incident or contamination occurred. The same procedure is followed if the staff removes the victim's clothing. If possible, it is helpful to take a Polaroid picture of the victim before undressing and place this within the bag. Ideally, the bags are stored without touching each other. Security or police officers should supervise this process if possible (EMSA, 2003).

Blood

Another issue to be addressed prior to need is the acquisition of adequate supplies of blood for the treatment of casualties. The American Association of Blood Banks (AABB) Interorganizational Task Force on Domestic Disasters and Acts of Terrorism has released a *Disaster Operations Handbook Hospital Supplement* (2003) to provide baseline information for meeting the need for blood following a disaster. In addition to outlining the process of obtaining blood supplies, they provide a formula for estimating the need. The recommendation is to determine the total anticipated admissions and the number of units of type O blood available. The estimation is that each victim could need three units of blood. Therefore, multiplying the anticipated admissions by three provides a rough estimate of the need. Subtracting what is available onsite provides an estimate of the number of units that must be acquired from another source.

Unit Organization

It is imperative that adequate supplies are available to handle large numbers of casualties. Following a terrorist event, the chaos and confusion will be heightened if necessary resources are not within easy reach. Each facility prepares to accept large numbers of casualties without depleting everyday supplies. This involves the placement of supply carts throughout the area near the emergency department. There are several types of supply carts that should be prepared. These include carts containing the supplies necessary to decontaminate the victims of chemical contamination, as well as medical supplies for treatments, such as dressings, tape, procedure-related items, intravenous needles, catheters, and syringes. In addition, there should be carts containing protective gear, such as clothing, boots, gas masks and gloves for providers, and carts containing pharmaceuticals. Unit organization includes daily assignment of personnel responsible for moving these carts to the designated areas if a disaster occurs.

Supplies on these carts are kept covered to decrease the opportunity for *raids* during normal busy periods. These supplies are mobile and moved to the triage and treatment areas following a mass casualty event. If professional nurses routinely check these carts, the staff can be confident that all supplies remain current. As supplies near their expiration dates they are moved to the regular hospital supply department to be used. Fresh supplies replace those removed, and supplies with older dates are rotated for routine use in hospitals or agencies. In addition to easily identified locations, such as hospitals and clinics, supplies may be kept in schools, hotels, or buildings near hospitals. This provides a fully functional area for those with minor injuries, freeing critical care areas within hospitals. These arrangements must be made carefully, paying attention to security issues, accessibility, and staffing needs when the plan is activated. It is important that the response plan incorporate the "walking well", or those who may not be injured physically, but are severely injured emotionally. Institutions should anticipate and plan for a possible panic in which people will attempt to crash the hospital, feeling that they will be safe once inside. If these persons are contaminated, they place the entire institution and personnel at risk. Adequate security, perhaps with support from law enforcement and the military, will be

needed. All agencies should activate a security system that implements the use of employee and physician identification cards, and possibly a visitor pass system. It is also important to **lock down** all entry points into the agency or hospital as quickly as possible.

Decontamination Basics

Protection of staff and agency may involve decontamination. If contamination is suspected, victims should not be brought into the hospital until they have been decontaminated. Decontamination is the physical process of removing harmful substances from personnel, equipment and supplies whenever there is a risk of secondary exposure from a hazardous substance. Immediate evacuation efforts should be undertaken to remove victims from the source of contamination. Those victims who are ambulatory must be directed towards the decontamination process. The personnel performing decontamination must be wearing Personal Protective Equipment (PPE). It is important for everyone to understand the level of PPE required (See Table 3–2).

Decontamination is primarily for chemical warfare. It is not needed for covert bioterrorism events. The only possible exception is an overt anthrax attack in which the toxins may mimic chemical exposures and warrant decontamination until the agent is known.

While water showers are frequently used, dry (powder form) decontamination supplies must also be available. The area for the decontamination procedures must have the availability of running water for showers and necessary ventilation. In addition, ideally the area should be 100 meters from the ER entrance and downwind from the hospital. Personnel should remain alert, moving up-

TABLE 3–2. PERSONAL PROTECTIVE EQUIPMENT LEVELS

LEVEL	EQUIPMENT
D (Minimum protection)	Liquid splash protection • Full face shield • Hood/gloves • Water repellent gown • Rubber boots
C (Preferred protection)	Liquid splash protection (above) Respiratory protection • Air purifying respirator/filter • Supplied air respirator with hood
B or A (Specialized protection)	Protective equipment • A: Vapor protective suit • B: Chemical resistant suit with hood • Both: Water/chemical resistant boots Respiratory protection • Atmosphere supplying respirator (ASR) • Supplied Air Respiratory (SAR) • Self-contained breathing apparatus (SCBA)

Adapted from California Emergency Medical Services Authority, 2003.

wind from source, evacuating the area or going to an upward room, closing windows and doors, covering mouth and nose, rinsing copiously if splashed with an agent, and reporting all suspicious situations and objects. Decontamination is described in detail in Chapter 6.

PATIENT TRACKING

Identification

One of the issues facing all health care facilities is the identification and tracking of patients. Pre-assembled medical records should be located throughout the Emergency Department. Staff must be able to identify people as soon as possible after they arrive for care, because patients must be moved rapidly and efficiently through the triage and decontamination areas, and into the facility for indicated treatments and procedures. The prepared medical records are opened using an identification system. The system does not need to be elaborate. A simple system such as each record containing adhesive number sheets is adequate, so that all treatment information, testing, and follow-up are documented using these numbers. As soon as possible after the patient enters the hospital, more traditional identification procedures can be enacted.

In some metropolitan areas, health care institutions and organizations are collaborating to implement a system that will use bar codes for tracking. These *bar code bracelets* are applied in the field and throughout the transport and treatment periods. As information about the victim is learned, it is entered into the computerized system and immediately available to all doctors and nurses. Some parts of it are familiar to those who have been involved in disaster response exercises or emergency services. The easily recognizable color coding has been included as well as the traditional information that can be entered manually on the reverse side. As first responders become more familiar with the new technology, the need to manually enter information may decrease.

Confidentiality

The Health Insurance Portability and Accountability Act (HIPAA) of 1996 protects health insurance coverage for workers and their families when they change or lose their jobs. It also addresses the security and privacy of health data. The HHS Office for Civil Rights (OCR) is charged with the enforcement of the HIPAA privacy standards such as the application of security standards.

This security of medical information is the challenge during an episode of mass casualties. Password protection of patient information will have to be incorporated within the identification and tracking systems. This may be increasingly difficult with larger numbers of casualties and victim information being entered at multiple points during care by multiple people with access to the scanning device. The need to link patient data and awareness of the need to protect the victim's privacy will become significant factors as decisions are made about patient records (Giorgianni, et al., 2002).

EXTERNAL SUPPORT

Governmental Support

The state emergency operations plan is developed and coordinated by state governments, which also establish a State Emergency Management Agency (SEMA) to coordinate the state response to a disaster event. Coordination of response services will be necessary if the disaster affects multiple areas (Beachley, 2000).

When a disaster occurs, the state governor will open the state's Emergency Operations Center where state agencies such as the police, National Guard, emergency medical services, and health, welfare, and social services agencies will work together at the same location to direct their specific agency's functions for disaster relief. A state coordinator will manage fire department resources and personnel in most states (Beachley, 2000).

When it is determined that the state *does not* have the resources to manage a disaster event, or the state has exhausted its resources, the state Emergency Management Agency advises the governor and requests assistance. The governor then notifies FEMA that federal disaster relief assistance is needed.

Because the government response and assistance time may be delayed, each area must be prepared to survive independently for up to 72 hours. This involves a five-day supply of needed resources. To accomplish this, negotiations with the vendors supplying medications and diesel fuel (for generators) must be conducted in advance. It is important to determine the vendor's current location of supplies. Is it in another part of the country? Airline transportation may be halted, requiring the movement of supplies over the highways. Some funding for preparation and response, for example, is available after the *Memorandum of Understanding* is signed and a needs assessment is completed. It can provide funds based on patients entering the ED, or a base amount for agencies without an ED.

Strategic National Stockpile

Most agencies know about the Strategic National Stockpile (SNS), formerly the National Pharmaceutical Stockpile. This source provides for things such as medications and vaccines. But these are traditionally transported on large airplanes that cannot land at smaller airports, so alternative methods for transporting these items to agencies is necessary.

The release of biological or chemical agents requires rapid access to large amounts of pharmaceuticals and medical supplies. The most effective way to disperse chemical or biological agents is through inhalation; therefore, protecting airways is the most important factor to address when a chemical or biological agent is suspected (U.S. Dept. of State, 2003). Supplies may not be readily available in the large amounts that would be needed unless special stockpiles are created. However, the location and type of terrorist events are unknown. This uncertainty, coupled with the inability of states and local governments to create sufficient stockpiles, resulted in the creation of national stockpiles of pharmaceuticals and medical supplies.

The Centers for Disease Control's (CDC) Strategic National Stockpile (SNS), ensures the availability and rapid deployment of necessary pharmaceuticals, antidotes, medical supplies, and equipment to adequately respond to events involving nerve agents, biological pathogens, and chemical agents. These stockpile packages are stored in strategic locations around the U.S., which enables rapid delivery anywhere in the country if the need arises. The stockpiles are designed to support local first response efforts, not as the primary first response tools, but rather to bolster the state's response over the time required to adequately respond. Once evidence shows that there has been an overt release of an agent that negatively affects public health, or subtle indications of a release are identified, the state requests deployment from the director of the CDC. The director, after consulting with the surgeon general, and the secretary of Health and Human Services, can then order the deployment of the Strategic National Stockpiles. These supplies can arrive by air or ground, depending on the circumstances of the event and the conditions of the roadways and airports. The supplies are sent in two phases, with each shipment accompanied by professionals to facilitate maximum use of the supplies (Table 3–3). In Phase I, the first shipment is called a **push pack.** The word *push* is used to indicate that the each state only needs to ask for the assistance. They are not required to request specific items.

The word *package* implies that the supplies sent are a complete package of medical supplies for responding to a broad range of threats. In Phase II, Vendor Managed Inventory or VMI is sent. These are tailored to provide pharmaceuticals, vaccines, medical supplies, and/or medical products specific to the suspected or confirmed agent. These packages and teams are evaluated at regular intervals to remain effective for new or current weapons (CDC, 2003a).

These supplies are not sent alone. The first shipment comes with a CDC team of five or six technical advisors known as the Technical Advisory Response Unit (TARU). This team includes pharmacists, emergency responders, and logistics experts who will help with receiving, distributing, dispensing, replenishing, and recovering SNS material.

Center for Emergency Response to Terror

One important source of information is the Center for Emergency Response to Terror (CERT). This agency is staffed 24/7. CERT is controlled by SEMA, and provides assistance and information about disaster response. This agency is helpful during the planning and response phase.

Each metropolitan area or region should have developed a collaborative plan with area hospitals and agencies for sharing information about supplies, available patient beds, nurses, physicians, and pharmacists. This vital information must be available to authorities when time is crucial. It is important to establish who is in charge of designating victims to specific hospitals, and that all involved know it.

Office of Emergency Preparedness

The Office of Emergency Preparedness (OEP), within the U.S. Department of Health and Human Services, has the departmental responsibility for managing and coordinating federal health, medical, and health-related social services and recovery to major emergencies and federally declared disasters including:

- Natural disasters
- Technological disasters
- Major transportation accidents
- Terrorism

Working in partnership with FEMA and the federal interagency community, OEP serves as the lead federal agency for health and medical services within the federal response plan. OEP also directs and manages the National Disaster Medical System (NDMS), a cooperative asset-sharing partnership between HHS, the Department of Defense (DoD), the Department of Veterans Affairs (VA), FEMA, state and local governments, private businesses, and civilian volunteers to ensure that resources are available to provide medical services following a disaster that overwhelms the local health care resources.

TABLE 3–3. STRATEGIC NATIONAL STOCKPILES: RESPONSE PHASES

PHASE	STAFF/SUPPLIES

I	• Medical supplies for broad range of incidents
	• 5–6 CDC technical advisors known as TARU (Technical Advisory Response Unit)
	  • Pharmacists
	  • Emergency responders
	  • Logistics experts
	  • Services: Receiving, dispensing, replenishing & recovering SNS supplies

II	• Pharmaceuticals • Vaccines • Medical supplies/products for confirmed or suspected agent

Adapted from website information CDC, 2003a

The OEP is also responsible for federal health and medical response to terrorist acts involving weapons of mass destruction (WMD). The OEP is developing a standardized training program for all field teams that will be described here.

National Disaster Medical System

The National Disaster Medical System (NDMS) was established in 1983 to assist in creating a system to effectively use civilian hospital beds during a disaster, and to create disaster medical assistance teams (DMATs) in 1984 to respond to disasters. Initially, the U. S. Public Health Service (USPHS) developed and equipped two DMAT prototypes that merged in 1992 to form the PHS-1 DMAT. The PHS-1 DMAT remains committed to respond rapidly, professionally, and compassionately in times of national disaster. Today, these teams receive specialized training in providing services necessary during a mass casualty event.

The Office of Emergency Planning/National Disaster Medical System (NDMS) is within the Department of Health and Human Services (DHHS). NDMS provides medical assistance in the form of medical assistance teams, medical supplies, and equipment. The NDMS will also assist in the evacuation of patients who cannot be cared for in the disaster area to other safe locations. Finally, NDMS also provides a national network of hospitals that are designated to accept patients in the event of a national emergency (Beachley, 2000).

There are many other federal agencies that support NDMS. Other agencies and programs involved in disaster relief include the National Guard, U.S. Department of Housing and Urban Development, and Small Business Administration.

Disaster Medical Assistance Team

The disaster medical assistance team (DMAT) is a regional group of volunteers and support personnel with the ability to quickly move into a disaster area and provide emergency medical care or augment the efforts of overloaded local health care organizations. The team consists of medical professionals and support staff organized, trained, and prepared to activate as a unit. Formerly under the control of the U.S. Public Health Service, DMATs are now under the Department of Homeland Security and can rapidly deploy for any type of disaster that requires an immediate medical response and function independently for 72 hours without any outside support. Conditions while on deployment can be particularly hazardous and uncomfortable. Typically the team members will find themselves in field hospitals consisting of tents or abandoned buildings (Anonymous, 1996; NDMS, 2004).

Their mission is the management of the medical response for mass casualty incidents with a goal of easing the pain and providing care for injured and ill patients. The three primary responsibilities of DMATs include triage, staging, and extended medical care. DMAT training concentrates on the skills that are unique to disaster situations. Each DMAT unit consists of approximately 35 individuals. DMAT may consist of more than 100 members to provide redundancy for each job role. This ensures that an adequate number of personnel are available each time.

Each team has a sponsoring organization, such as a major medical center, health or safety agency, non-profit, public, or private organization that signs a Memorandum of Understanding (MOU) with the Public Health Service. The DMAT sponsor organizes the team and recruits members, arranges training, and coordinates the dispatch of the team.

In addition to the standard DMATs, there are highly specialized DMATs trained to deal with specific medical conditions such as crush injury, burn, and mental health emergencies. The burn specialty teams (BSTs) are staffed by physicians and nurses with training and experience in treating severely burned patients (Schwarz & Kennedy, 2003).

DMATs can be grouped into four readiness levels. Level 1 DMATs are fully deployable within 8 hours of notification and can be self-sufficient for 72 hours. These DMATs are deployed with standardized equipment and supply sets to treat up to 250 patients per day. Level 2 DMATs are units that are not self-sufficient but are able to deploy and replace Level 1 teams utilizing and supplementing their equipment left onsite. Level 3 DMATs have local response capability only. Level 4 DMATs have a MOU executed in some stage of development but have no response capability (LADHS, 2004).

Hazardous Materials Team

The hazardous materials team (HAZMAT) is responsible for coordinating a national safety program for the transportation of hazardous materials by air, rail, highway, and water. The mission is to develop and provide a national safety program that will minimize the risks to life and property inherent in commercial transportation of hazardous materials. It is part of the Office of Hazardous Materials Safety (OHM). The functions of the OHM can be consolidated into five categories: regulatory development, enforcement, training and information dissemination, domestic and international standards, and inter-agency cooperative activities (Waeckerle, 2000). See Figure 3–3.

Disaster Mortuary Operation Response Team

The Disaster Mortuary Operation Response Team (DMORT) is a specialized unit whose function is the decontamination of human remains. The goal is the return of these remains to family members when possible for humanitarian and legal reasons (DMORT, 2004).

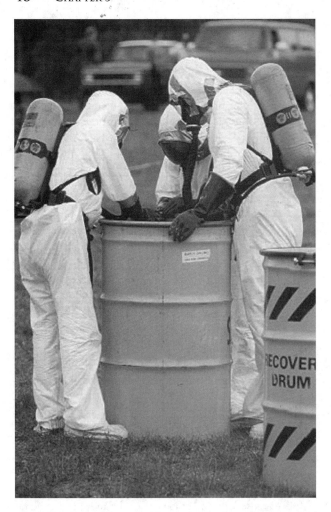

Figure 3–3. The hazardous materials team (HAZMAT) coordinates a national safety program for the transportation of hazardous materials by air, rail, highway, and water.

DMORTs can provide services such as the establishment of mobile morgue operations, forensic examination, DNA acquisition, remains identification, and search and recovery. In addition, DMORT teams can provide scene documentation, records data entry, embalming and casketing, antemortem data collection, and postmortem data collection. In relation to friends and families, they can establish family assistance centers; offer responders and families medical and psychology support, database administration, personal effects processing, and coordination of the release of remains; provide a liaison to the USPHS; provide communications equipment, and provide safety officers and specialists. The DMORT-WMD team works under the principles of the Incident Command System (DMORT, 2004).

In the early 1980s, the National Funeral Directors Association (NFDA) questioned its role during disaster situations and mass fatality incidents. No standardization existed at that time, so the organization began working toward creating a national protocol for a proper response. Initially, NFDA concentrated on the role of funeral di-

rectors, but no one profession could handle all aspects of an event. A multifaceted nonprofit organization open to all forensic practitioners was formed to support a national level response protocol for all related professions. This group purchased the first portable morgue unit in the country. The Family Assistance Act in October 1996 required all American based airlines to have a plan to assist families in the case of an accident. DMORT is one federal team that can help if needed. DMORT currently has over 1200 trained volunteers who respond to assist those in need.

One step in preparing for mass casualty events is determining where to keep the bodies of victims prior to identification or claiming by relatives. Although governmental agencies and systems will assist with this after the initial period, individual hospitals should include this in discussions with their local, state, and regional planning groups. It is important that agencies have explored options for the use of refrigerated trucks, commercial coolers, ice rinks, or other large, secure, refrigerated areas for at least the first 72 hours after a disaster. Most institutions do not have the capacity to handle mass casualties, and this planning cannot wait until the event. On average, hospitals can only house seven bodies in their morgues, which makes these negotiations for refrigerated space more imperative.

Veterinary Medical Assistance Team

The veterinary medical assistance team (VMAT) is comparable to the DMAT. VMATs are made up of highly trained veterinarians, veterinary technicians, and other support staff, who can be deployed to assist state or local governments in the event of a disaster when the local veterinary community is overburdened. Providing emergency care and treatment to ill or injured animals after the event of a disaster is the major role of VMAT. Though teams may also be activated to assist with food safety concerns, zoonotic disease, and toxicological problems.

VMATs provide nationwide coverage during times of disaster and can be deployed to any state or U. S. territory. VMATs triage and stabilize animals at a disaster site and provide veterinary medical care. The teams are mobile and can deploy within 12 to 24 hours. They carry a three-day supply of food, water, personal living necessities, and medical supplies and equipment. Members can provide any other needed veterinary services to support a complete disaster relief effort. The VMAT supplements the relief efforts of local veterinarians and emergency responders. The goal is a cooperative animal relief effort during times of disaster between VMAT, state and local officials, the state veterinarian, the local veterinary community, state and local veterinary medical associations, emergency management personnel, humane groups, Red Cross volunteers, and search and rescue groups (AVMA, 2004).

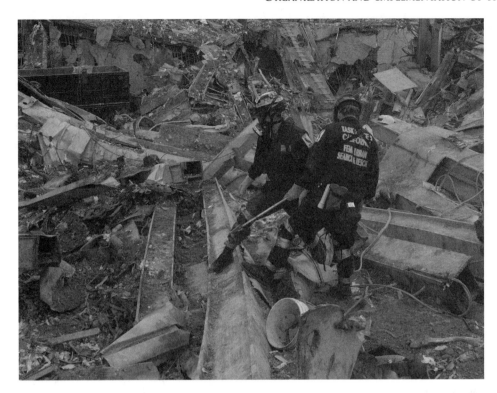

Figure 3–4. Although under the authority of FEMA, Urban Search and Rescue (US&R) is a partnership between local fire departments, law enforcement agencies, federal and local governmental agencies, and private companies.

Center for Sustainment of Trauma and Readiness Skills

The Center for Sustainment of Trauma and Readiness Skills (C-STARS) is capable of providing military aid to civilian hospitals. This agency is charged with getting the military medical people ready for disaster management, including physicians, nurses, nurse practitioners, physician assistants, respiratory therapy technicians, and medical technicians. Establishing proper channels prior to a need will permit areas affected by terrorist events to receive support from the military in the form of expeditionary medical packages (EMEDs) that provide an *instant "mini-hospital"* to assist with overflow. These contain up to 25 beds with electricity and oxygen. Other so called *packages* that may be needed are the critical care air transportation team (CCATT) that consists of a critical care RN, respiratory therapist, and two physicians; and the EMED + 25 that includes the previously mentioned services plus seven ICU beds and approximately 60 personnel to staff it. The same communication pattern discussed previously will permit you to access the hospital resources available through the government or military. This involves the hospital contacting those in the level above for assistance. If it is not available at that level, the hospital contacts the city, which can contact the state, which can contact the federal government that has the authority to initiate the military support. The plans must be made in advance, however. An individual hospital cannot directly contact these agencies. The chain of authority must be followed (M. Mandy, Personal Communication, March 2004).

Urban Search and Rescue

The Urban Search and Rescue (US&R), is a response system established under the authority of FEMA in 1989. It provides a framework for structuring local emergency services personnel into an integrated disaster response task force. For every US&R task force, there are 62 positions. To ensure that sufficient team members are available to respond to an emergency, they have more than 130 highly trained members. The US&R is a partnership between local fire departments, law enforcement agencies, federal and local governmental agencies and private companies. These task forces, complete with necessary tools, equipment, required skills, and techniques, can be deployed by FEMA for the rescue of victims of structural collapse and are totally self-sufficient for the first 72 hours of service. See Figure 3–4.

When a disaster involves a search for victims, and possibly evidence, a coordinated effort is vital. Official agencies such as US&R can provide sophisticated techniques and resources. The equipment necessary to support a task force weighs as much as 60,000 pounds and costs approximately $1.4 million. The equipment coupled with the members can completely fill a military C-141 transport. Some of the responsibilities of the US&R are conducting physical search and rescue in collapsed buildings, bringing emergency medical care to trapped victims; working with search-and-rescue dogs; assessing and controlling gas, electric service, and hazardous materials; and evaluating on and stabilizing damaged structures.

These federal resources are just a few of the more than 100 different federal level response teams or systems.

BOX 3–2   Eight Steps Toward Hospital Disaster Preparedness

- Assemble interdisciplinary team
- Review resources, strengths, weaknesses
- Develop written response plan
- Disseminate and practice the plan

- Evaluate adequacy of knowledge, skills, resources
- Review and re-engineer plan based on evaluation
- Modify training as needed to address weaknesses
- Repeat cycle continuously

(Adapted from Bioterrorism and Health System Preparedness: Part 3, National Bioterrorism Hospital Preparedness Program by B. Austin, 2003. http://www.ahrq.gov/news/ulp/ulpdistn.htm.)

Reviewing some of their potential roles during a mass casualty event may provide general guidelines for necessary services following a disaster and stimulate a discussion of the health care facility's (HCF) role during and following an event. The HCF disaster response committee can then determine the level of needed responses and the resources that are available after the first 72 hours, thus permitting better use of resources and personnel, as well as identifying areas that must be strengthened (FEMA, 2004).

Voluntary Agencies

The American Red Cross is very active in disaster relief, especially in shelters and minor first aid injury responses. Many nurses may choose to volunteer on more EMS-type response teams. The ARC supports five major programs to meet the human needs after a disaster.

1. **Damage assessment.** The gathering of information about the physical damage resulting from a disaster
2. **Mass care.** Providing shelter, food, and supplies
3. **Health services.** Trying to meet the emotional and medical needs of victims and disaster workers
4. **Family services.** An emergency assistance program to help families to return to some form of normalcy by providing food, clothing, shelter, and medical needs including eyeglasses, dentures, procurement of prescriptions, household furnishings, and occupational supplies and equipment
5. **Disaster welfare inquiry services.** Gathers information about the disaster area, what and who were affected, and individuals killed or injured, and makes this information available to concerned relatives through their local ARC chapter

All ARC assistance is free and provided through funds donated by the American people (ARC, 1975, 1985).

EXERCISES AND DRILLS

An effective method of developing and improving the ability to respond to a bioterrorism situation is to hold coordinated exercises with all responding agencies. This drill would also fulfill the JCAHO Environment of Care Standard EC 2.9.1, which requires annual emergency management exercises to evaluate the response plan (JCAHO, 2001b). During these times of increased risk, is an annual drill likely to be effective for all types of disasters? The hospital or clinic should also have collaborative plans for chemical, nuclear or radiological, and incidents involving blast or shrapnel injuries.

Johns Hopkins University Evidence-Based Practice Center (2002) reported the results of training and preparation programs for clinicians. This AHRQ sponsored report presented evidence about the current state of response preparedness in the United States. The report suggested that preparations provided a basic foundation that lacked a standardized language and practice definition, but which was improving through the use of realistic exercises. The report outlined eight steps toward hospital disaster preparedness (Box 3–2). The report further identified necessary responses during a bioterrorism incident. These include the use of a decontamination process, protection of workers, and containment and treatment of the infectious agent.

Regularly scheduled educational programs should be offered to all nurses and physicians. The programs can be in either traditional or nontraditional formats. Technology has permitted the addition of teleconferences, computer simulations, and mannequin simulations. Knowledge about disaster responses is continually changing. The most carefully developed plan is useless unless nurses and physicians are familiar with it and willing to work for its implementation. Disasters are not the time for creativity. Each member of the response team must respond almost automatically. This helps to use the available resources, both people and things, to their maximum level.

As frequent drills are held, the evaluation process must be seen as the final step in the drill. During the evaluation process, blame is not the focus. Each professional should look at the drill for areas where the system staggered, where slowdowns or mistakes occurred. Identification is followed by problem solving. How can we improve? What else is needed to enable the health care professional to provide competent and organized care?

National Nurses Response Team

Regularly scheduled educational programs should be offered to all nurses and physicians. Knowledge about disaster response is continually changing. There is no point at which you can say, "I am done. I know all there is to know about disaster response options." On a national level, the American Nurses Association (ANA) in conjunction with the Office of Emergency Response, U.S. Department of Health and Human Services, has established the National Nurses Response Team (NNRT). The NNRT consists of 10 regionally based teams of 200 registered nurses who can be called if assistance is needed in mass chemo prophylaxis or vaccinations, or other situations requiring large numbers of RNs (Schwarz & Kennedy, 2003). Responding as a team is safer, and facilitates assimilation into a response team. Each agency should examine their role and determine whether this group would be needed as part of their role in disaster response and contact the NNRT to determine the protocol for their participation in a response effort.

MEDIA RELATIONS

During mass casualty events, another role that must be considered is the management of the media. In the United States, media often arrive at the scene concurrently with first responders. Prior to an actual event, each agency should designate a competent, articulate media representative, and restrict all others from speaking to the media. Plan the early messages in advance, in writing if possible. To avoid confusion and misinterpretation, place written materials in the media's hands. In fairness, the media have a role during a disaster – that of announcing who, where, when, and how to obtain treatment and prophylaxis. The key is forming a team, rather than an adversarial relationship.

The media will demand information at all hours, day and night. Standard responses may be prepared for any type of disaster. These responses should be practiced during the mock drills or exercises. The spokesperson should remain calm, but be informed and articulate. Spokespersons should also remember to respect the patients' privacy and confidentiality and limit access to patient treatment areas.

The primary pitfalls of dealing with the media occur when variations or contradictions occur between broadcast and print media, which contributes to confusion. It is important to facilitate qualified individuals to interact to avoid a panic begun when sound bites replace facts. Be wary of off the record statements and speculation.

A lack of information, rather than too much information, can cause inappropriate response by community members. Some planners believe that providing the public with information may result in panic. However, if vital information is withheld, the public may respond with either no response or an inappropriate one (Clark, 2003). Boyle (2002) reminds us to "assure that plans for all major categories of emergencies respect the culture of the community and/or populations involved" (p. 273). This cultural awareness has major implications when disaster plans are developed regarding communication with the public. We must be cognizant of language barriers as well as cultural issues that may affect a community's ability to respond to a mass casualty event.

Following each exercise or actual event, the evaluation component of the response plan is important in the identification of deficits in the plan, or shortfalls in the implementation. Disaster managers refer to this as after-action analysis. How was the overall response? What is identified as a logjam? What changes are needed? If this process is conducted openly, without fear or punishment, new protocols or modified protocols are developed to improve the response process. It may be necessary to host an educational program to bring all staff to the same level of understanding. If educational materials do not cover information or interventions that are identified as helpful, collaboration with the health department may provide a head start to bring these to reality. Dr. Louis Goldfrank, Director of Emergency Medicine, Bellevue Medical Center, New York City, and a chair of the IOM Committee on Evaluation of the Metropolitan Medical Response System, summarized some of the conclusions reached following 9/11. "This disaster has taught us that decentralization of our resources is essential, that communications with rescue-and-hospital-based systems are fragile, that the psychological impact on the families, friends, coworkers, city, and county members cannot be overestimated" (Giorgianni, et al., 2002).

SUMMARY

It is important to remain current with knowledge about disaster response. Preparations for disasters are never complete. No institution can reach a state of total preparedness. As new information is gained, it will be disseminated rapidly to all significant parties. Some of the websites in the reference list are excellent resources for current information. Nurses become resource persons at your institution or agency and can post or provide in-services to update all responders. The American Public Health Association (APHA) website contains a 1-year report card on America following 9/11. There are areas of minimal improvement, and other areas in which progress has been made (APHA, 2002).

Professional nurses have been challenged to respond to a real threat facing the United States today. As the largest body of health care professionals, nurses are ready to accept this challenge and become leaders to face this threat to survival. The challenge is to become leaders in institutions or agencies, to actively seek answers to some of the questions raised, and to encourage colleagues to join in planning the response to a terrorist event. It is our hope, as it was the hope of our colleagues in Israel, that you will never have to use this knowledge or activate the response plan.

CASE STUDY

Release of a Biological Agent in a Domed Stadium

It is a Sunday afternoon at 3:00 p.m. The city's professional football team is playing and the domed stadium is filled to capacity (55,000). The EMS personnel onsite have called to report that they have seen 12 persons exhibiting symptoms of watery eyes, coughing, shortness of breath, hypotension, fever, and prostration. Family members of the victims have begun to talk with other spectators and people have begun to respond to the news of a possible biological release and are hurrying from the area. EMS suspects that many of these people will be coming to the hospital. You are the charge nurse in the Emergency Department.

- What is the first thing that you should do?
- Describe the process of activating the disaster response plan
- What departments/services should be notified?

TEST YOUR KNOWLEDGE

1. Identify three important members or groups to include when selecting for the Disaster Response Committee.

2. If a bioterrorism event is suspected, the correct order of notification is
   A. Emergency department → FEMA → CDC → American Red Cross
   B. Emergency department/infection control/administration → local health department → state health departments → CDC
   C. Emergency department → law enforcement → local health department → FEMA
   D. Emergency department → CDC → state health department → infection control specialists

3. List two tools or instruments that may be helpful in assessing and planning an agency response readiness.

4. Explain a method for tracking victims as they move through the health care agency following a mass casualty event.

5. Differentiate between crisis management and consequence managements.

6. During a mass casualty event, the central supply department has the responsibility of assembling and delivering appropriate supplies to the triage and treatment areas.
   A. True
   B. False

7. During triage and decontamination, it is most effective and efficient if the person who will care for the patient in the hospital performs the decontamination.
   A. True
   B. False

8. List three primary responsibilities of the disaster medical assistance teams (DMAT).

9. In order to receive assistance from the military (C-STARS), hospitals initiate the chain of authority, rather than contacting the military directly.
   A. True
   B. False

10. Following a mass casualty event or exercise, an evaluation team should meet to review the drill and determine which responder's performance was deficient and transfer that person to a less stressful area.
   A. True
   B. False

See Test Your Knowledge answers in Appendix B.

EXPLORE MEDIALINK

Interactive resources and an audio glossary for this chapter can be found on the Companion Website at http://www.prenhall.com/langan. Click on Chapter 3 to select the activities for this chapter.

REFERENCES

American Association of Blood Banks (AABB). International task force on domestic disasters and acts of Terrorism. (2003, February). *Disaster operations handbook hospital supplement. Coordinating the nation's blood supply during disasters and biological events.* Bethesda, MD: AABB.

American Hospital Association (AHA). (May, 2002). Disaster readiness: Where do you stand? *Proceedings from National Symposium on Hospital Disaster Readiness,* 37–38.

American Public Health Association (APHA). (2002). *One year after the terrorist attacks: Is public health prepared?* Retrieved May 15, 2003, from http://www.apha.org/

American Red Cross (ARC). (1975). *Disaster relief program, 2235.* Washington, DC: Author.

American Red Cross (ARC). (1985). *Disaster services, regulations and procedures, 3066.* Washington, DC: Author.

American Veterinary Medical Association (AVMA). (2004). Veterinary Medical Assistance Teams. Retrieved July 12, 2004 from http://www.avma.org/disaster/VMAT.

Anonymous. (1996). DMAT teams: There when disaster strikes. *Ed Management, 8*(9), 104–105.

Assessing facility preparedness: A guide for infection control professionals (n.d.). Retrieved July 23, 2003 from www.bioterrorism.slu.edu.

Association for Professionals in Infection Control and Epidemiology (APIC) Bioterrorism Task Force and CDC Hospital Infections Program Bioterrorism Working Group (BTWG). (1999). *Bioterrorism readiness plan: A template for healthcare facilities.* Retrieved May 15, 2003 from http://www.apic.org/educ/readinow.cfm.

Austin, B. (2003). National Bioterrorism Hospital Preparedness Program. *Bioterrorism and health system preparedness: Part 3.* Retrieved May 15, 2003 from http://www.ahrq.gov/news/ulp/ulpdistn.htm.

Beachley, M. (2000). Nursing in a disaster. In C. M. Smith & F. A. Maurer, (Eds.). Community health nursing. Philadelphia: WB Saunders.

Boyle, J. S. (2002). Emergency and disaster planning: Where is transcultural nursing. Journal of Transcultural Nursing, 13(4), 273.

Centers for Disease Control and Prevention (CDC). (2003a). *Notification Algorithm for Bioterrorism Event.* Retrieved May 30, 2003 from http://www.bt.cdc.gov/EmContact/Protocols.asp.

Centers for Disease Control and Prevention. (CDC). (2003b). *Decontamination following radiological or nuclear contamination.* Retrieved May 30, 2003 from http://www.bt.cdc.gov/radiation/index.asp#clinicians.

Clark, M. J. (2003). Care of clients in disaster settings. In M. Clark (Ed.), Community health nursing (pp. 623–653). Upper Saddle River, NJ: Pearson Education.

Cole, T. B. (2000). When a bioweapon strikes, who will be in charge? JAMA: Journal of the American Medical Association, 284(8), 944–948.

Department of Health and Human Services, Office of Inspector General. (2002, December). *State and local bioterrorism preparedness.* OEI-02-01-00550.

Disaster Mortuary Operational Response Teams (DMORT). (2004). DMORT. Retrieved July 12, 2004 from http://www.dmort.org.

DOD DFFUaE. (1998). *Domestic preparedness response workbook.* Retrieved May 10, 2003 from http://www.3gsoftwarellc.com/HCMH/Bioterrorism_Response_Plan.htm.

Emergency Medical Services Authority (EMSA). (2003). *Recommendations for hospitals: Chemical decontamination, staff protection, chemical decontamination equipment and medication list, evidence collection.* California Hospital and Health Disaster Interest Group. Retrieved May 15, 2003 from http://www.gnyha.org/eprc/general/nbc/general/Patient_Decontamination.pdf.

Environmental Protection Agency (EPA). (2000, July). *First responders' environmental liability due to mass decontamination runoff.* 550-F-00-009. Retrieved July 1, 2003 from www.epa.gov/ceppo/.

Federal Emergency Management Agency (FEMA). (1981). *Disaster operations: A handbook for local governments.* Washington, DC: U.S. Government Printing Office.

Federal Emergency Management Agency (FEMA). (1997). *Backgrounder: Terrorism.* Retrieved July 1, 2003 from http://www.fema.gov.

Federal Emergency Management Agency (FEMA). (1998). *Incident command system: independent study course.* Retrieved January 26, 2003 from http://www.slu.edu/colleges/sph/csbei/bioterrorism/key_references/FEMA/ICSSelfStudy.pdf.

Federal Emergency Management Agency (FEMA). (2003, January 21). *Federal Response Plan.* Retrieved January 26, 2003 from http://www.fema.gov/rrr/frp/frpfig1.shtm.

Federal Emergency Management Agency (FEMA). (2004). Urban Search and Rescue. Retrieved July 12, 2004 from http://fema.org/usr/about/.shtm.

Ganor, B. (1998). *Non-conventional terrorism: Chemical, nuclear, biological.* Retrieved August 1, 2003 from http://www.ict.org.il/articles/articledet.cfm?articleid=1.

Giorgianni, S. J., Grana, J., & Scipioni, L. (2002). Health system preparedness: Fine tuning communication, coordination, and care in a new era. *The Pfizer Journal, 6, 4.*

Hayes, G., Goodwin, T., & Miars, B. (1990, February). After disaster: A crisis support team at work. *American Journal of Nursing, 90,* 61–64.

Hudson, T. L., & Weichart, T. (2002). A method of transporting critical care mass casualties. *DMR: Disaster Management & Response, 9,* 1–5.

Human Resources and Services Administration (HRSA). (2003). National Bioterrorism Hospital Preparedness Program. Retrieved September 1, 2003 from http://www.hrsa.gov/bioterrorism.htm.

Institute for Bio-Security at Saint Louis University School of Public Health. (2002). *Public health preparedness toolkit: Key resources for public health departments.* Retrieved May 15, 2003 from http://www.bioterrorism.slu.edu.

Institute for Bio-Security at Saint Louis University School of Public Health and APIC. (2002). *Institute for Bio-Security at Saint Louis University School of Public Health Clinical Fact Sheets.* Retrieved July 1, 2003 from http://www.slu.edu/colleges/sph/csbei/bioterrorism/key_references/professional.htm.

Institute for Bio-Security at Saint Louis University School of Public Health and APIC. (2002). *Mass casualty disaster plan checklist: A template for healthcare facilities.* Retrived July 1, 2003 from http://www.slu.edu/colleges/sph/csbei/bioterrorism/key_references/professional.htm.

Joint Commission on Accreditation of Healthcare Organizations (JCAHO). (2001a). What the survey process expects of your organizations. *Joint Commission Perspectives, 21*(12), 6–7.

Joint Commission on Accreditation of Healthcare Organizations (JCAHO). (2001b). Using JCAHO standards as a starting point to prepare for an emergency. *Joint Commission Perspectives, 21*(12), 4–5.

Klitzman, S., & Freudenberg, N. (2003). Implications of the World Trade Center attack for public health and health care infrastructures. *American Journal of Public Health, 93*(3), 400–406.

Landesman, L. Y. (2001). *Public health management of disasters: The practice guide.* Washington, DC: American Public Health Association.

Levitin, H. W., & Skidmore, S. L. (2003). Emergency planning and preparedness. *Bioterrorism and health system preparedness: Part 2* (AHRQ-03-AV06A). Retrieved September 1, 2003 from http://www.ahrq.gov/news/ulp/ulpdistn.htm.

Los Angeles Department of Health Services (LA DHS). (2004). DMAT Overview. Retrieved July 12, 2004 from http://www.lahs.org/ems/DMAT.htm.

Levy, B. S., & Sidel, V. W. (2000). *War and public health*. Washington, DC: American Public Health Association.

Merchant, J. A. (1986). Preparing for disaster. *American Journal of Public Health, 76*(3), 233–235.

National Disaster Medical System (NDMS). (2004). Disaster Medical Assistance Team. Retrieved July 12, 2004 from http://www.ndms.dhhs.gov/dmat.html.

Newberry, L. (2002). Practical suggestions for helping emergency nurses handle mass casualties. *DMR: Disaster Management & Response, 9*, 1–5.

Noji, E. K. (1997). The nature of disaster: General characteristics and public health effects. In E. K. Noji (Ed.), The public health consequences of disasters. New York: Oxford University Press.

Office of Emergency Preparedness (OEP). *NDMS Catastrophic care for the nation: About teams*. Retrieved May 15, 2003 from http://www.ndms.dhhs.gov/.

Office of Inspector General. (2002). *Executive summary*. OEI-02-01-00550. Retrieved September 1, 2003 from http://www.oig.hhs.gov.

Paris, J. (2000). Georgia inmates and staff coped with natural disaster–Lesson learned from Hurricane Floyd. *Correct Care, 14*(1), 8, 21.

Schwarz, T., & Kennedy, M. S. (2003). Disaster volunteer teams: Where to go when you want to help. *American Journal of Nursing, 103*(1), 64AA–64DD.

Tucker, J. B. (1997). National health and medical services response to incidents of chemical and biological terrorism. *Journal of the American Medical Association, 278*, 362–368.

U.S. Department of Health and Human Services, Centers for Disease Control and Prevention. (2001). *Responding to a biological or chemical threat: A practical guide*.

U.S. Department of Health and Human Services, Centers for Disease Control and Prevention. (2001, July). *The public health response to biological and chemical terrorism: Interim planning guidance for state public health officials*. Retrieved May 15, 2003 from http://www.bt.cdc.gov/Documents/Planning/PlanningGuidance.PDF

Waeckerle, J. F. (2000). Domestic preparedness for events involving weapons of mass destruction. *Journal of the American Medical Association, 283*(2), 1–7.

Willshire, L., & Hassmiller, S. B. (2002). *Disaster preparedness and response for nurses: Case Study*. Retrieved May 15, 2003 from http://www.nursingsociety.org/education/case_studies/cases/SP0004.html

World Health Organization (WHO). (1989). *Coping with natural disasters: The role of local health personnel and the community*. Geneva: World Health Organization.

CHAPTER 4

Promoting Mental Health: Predisaster and Postdisaster

Dorcas E. McLaughlin, Ruth B. Murray, and Julie Benbenishty

LEARNING OBJECTIVES

1. Compare and contrast psychological responses of survivors in each phase of a disaster and various intervention methods.
2. Examine ways to promote mental health both predisaster and postdisaster, including prevention, psychological first aid, triage, crisis assessment and intervention, and followup.
3. Discuss ways to help survivors cope with loss.
4. Describe adverse mental health outcomes postdisaster among individuals and families.
5. Identify vulnerable or at-risk groups for adverse mental health outcomes.
6. Explore modalities to treat adverse mental health outcomes following disasters.
7. Describe vicarious traumatization and methods to prevent and alleviate symptoms.

MEDIALINK www.prenhall.com/langan

Resources for this chapter can be found on the Companion Website at http://www.prenhall.com/langan. Click on Chapter 4 to select the activities for this chapter.

CHAPTER OUTLINE

Know Your Terms
Audio Glossary
Web Links
    Government Mental Health Resources
    Professional Mental Health Resources
MediaLink Applications

GLOSSARY

Acute Stress Disorder (ASD). An anxiety disorder that describes the acute stress reactions that occur in the first 4 weeks following trauma

Bereavement. Response to loss, leading to distress and the complex effects referred to as grief

Comprehensibility. The person's ability to make sense of or understand the situation and a confidence that the world as a whole, and the current disaster, is basically predictable

Crisis intervention. Short-term, action-oriented intervention with the goals of restoring the individual's equilibrium, reducing distress, restoring the person to the predisaster level of functioning, and preventing adverse mental health outcomes

Dissociation. A defense mechanism in which a person's thought processes and feelings associated with the trauma are pushed aside or repressed. The person feels completely unreal or outside of self and has periods of amnesia

Flashback. Reliving of the trauma event during the early postimpact phase or even later. This can happen visually in images, or it can be reexperienced with sounds, smells, feelings, or other such bodily memories when someone is reminded of the disaster

Manageability. Ability to find and utilize resources to meet the demands of the situation

Meaningfulness. Ability to integrate cognitive, emotional, and realistic issues and to find sense or meaning in the situation, and thus be motivated to act and to cope effectively

Natural debriefing. The spontaneous formation of groups in which survivors and rescue workers share their experiences with others, which fosters an experience of empathy, normalization, and validation and promotes healing and recovery

Post-Traumatic Stress Disorder (PTSD). Disorder characterized by the development of a persistent anxiety response following a traumatic event. The individual's subjective response to the traumatic experience must involve helplessness, intense fear, or horror. Symptoms are grouped into three categories: (1) a reexperiencing of the traumatic event; (2) avoidance of activities, places, or things related to the trauma; and (3) hyperarousal. Symptom duration must be at least 1 month following the trauma and symptoms must be severe enough to impair functioning. Symptoms may be acute and occur following the trauma or be delayed

Psychological Debriefing (PD). An in-the-field, early intervention developed to help soldiers and rescue workers to cope with stressful events and assist them to return to their duties as quickly as possible

Sense Of Coherence (SOC). Ability for the survivor to make sense out of the situation or find meaning in the experience, regardless of the reality. Global orientation in which one has a pervasive, dynamic feeling of confidence that one's internal and external environments are predictable and that the probability is high that events will turn out as reasonably as can be expected

INTRODUCTION

Every year people all over the world are affected by a variety of disasters generated by human or natural forces. Any disaster results in extensive damage and suffering, seriously disrupts the functioning of those affected, and exceeds usual coping resources. In the immediate aftermath of a disaster, most people manifest stress reactions; however even when these stress reactions are extreme they are not considered pathological. Although some have immediate mental health needs, the vast majority of disaster survivors show considerable strength and resilience. Nurses are instrumental in promoting mental health and the recovery process in each stage of disaster.

Nurses, because of their presence in community and acute care settings, are in a unique position to intervene in disasters. Nurses care for physical injuries and have interpersonal skills to provide psychological intervention. Nurses can play an integral role in assisting with the normal recovery process and in assisting those with specific mental health needs. To effectively promote mental health, nurses must increase their understanding of the personal, emotional, and social dynamics associated with disasters; further develop their skills to assist survivors to cope; and be aware of their own risk for psychological trauma as they care for others.

LEVELS OF VICTIMS

People are affected by disasters in many ways. Some are minimally affected; others are devastated. In general, it is believed that the more direct the exposure to the disaster, the higher the risk for psychological trauma. Families, friends, rescue workers, health care professionals, even bystanders may experience psychological trauma.

Taylor and Frazer (1981) have identified six levels of victims. See Box 4–1 for definitions and examples.

FRAMEWORKS FOR UNDERSTANDING RESPONSES TO DISASTERS

This chapter explores frameworks for understanding phases of disasters, stress responses to disasters, guidelines for assessment, and a variety of psychosocial nursing interventions to promote mental health both predisaster and postdisaster. Assessment and planning pertinent to interventions will be integrated throughout since these steps of the nursing process proceed quickly and together in times of disasters. The final section will focus on the assessment in adverse mental health outcomes and interventions used to promote recovery.

BOX 4–1   Taylor and Frazer's Six Levels of Victims

---

1. **Primary victims.** Individuals who experience maximum exposure to the disaster
   "When we finally reached the scene, there was so much debris and dust. I heard that there were dead bodies and body parts, but I didn't look. I had already been through so much. In the past three days, I've slept less than ten hours because of the nightmares. I'm still in shock."
   School children, following an earthquake of 6.7 on the Richter scale, cried and described memories of the house falling down, objects hitting family members, parents screaming, furniture and toys crushed, and everyone crying as the family scrambled to get outdoors.

2. **Secondary victims.** Relatives and friends of the primary victims
   "My granddaughter asked, 'If I pray really hard will Mommy come back?' Trying to hold back my tears, I told her that I didn't know. I feel so helpless. There is no closure when they can't even find the bodies. There is no moving on, but time still passes."

3. **Third-level victims.** First responders and health care personnel who participate in rescue and recovery activities
   "Like many others I had been up for more than 24 hours. We were tired, exhausted, stressed to the max physically, emotionally, and professionally. I was ordered to go sleep. On my way home, still

dressed in my scrubs, I stopped for a cup of coffee. A police officer tapped me on the shoulder and said, 'Thank you.' For a few minutes, I lost my composure and started sobbing."

4. **Fourth-level victims.** The community, including those who converge, who altruistically offer help, who share the grief and loss or are in some way involved
   "I watched the first jet as it flew directly into the World Trade Center. I gasped and yelled to persons on the street. Run! Run for your life!!! People looked at me as though I was a madman. Then we all ran as fast as we could. Later, I went back to help. There is a part of me that doesn't want to remember this. I'm still traumatized."

5. **Fifth-level victims.** Individuals who are upset or psychologically distressed but not directly involved in the disaster
   "When I heard the news about another suicide bombing, I felt true shock again. The mood at the hospital was very somber. We had to go on with our work. I get nervous thinking something else terrible is going to happen."

6. **Sixth-level victims.** Those individuals indirectly or vicariously affected by the disaster
   "I know nurses in Israel who take care of survivors every day. I can't imagine how they keep facing one disaster after another."

Phases of Response to Disasters

A disaster may be described as a sequence of phases in which various psychological responses are manifested, both in individuals and in the community as a totality. The first two phases occur in the predisaster period and the last three phases in the postdisaster period (Raphael, 1993). The normality or predictability of the response of individuals, groups, and the whole community are discussed in the following pages.

Predisaster Period

Preparation and Planning Phase. Although disasters are unexpected, sudden, and chaotic, they can be anticipated to varying degrees. The recent terrorist attacks have mandated more attention to disaster planning in the United States; some countries have well-developed plans. The goals of disaster planning are to (a) educate people to understand responses and intervene effectively, (b) prevent or minimize injuries and deaths, (c) minimize property damage, (d) effectively triage, and (e) facilitate return to predisaster individual and community functioning. Studies have examined the effect of disaster preparation on out-

come and have shown that education and training facilitate postdisaster adjustment (McFarlane, 1995). Accurate information conveyed through educational programs, written materials, and the media can help people take effective action in response to potential disasters and lessen the consequences of adverse mental health outcomes. In order for nurses to promote psychological recovery and prevent adverse mental health outcomes, knowledge and skills are needed and must be developed (National Institute of Mental Health, 2002).

Planning must consider the needs and responses of different cultural groups in the community. Representatives of diverse groups should be included in the planning. Cultural traditions, rituals, and norms should be acknowledged in relation to resolving conflict and negotiation methods, group education, use of resources, and ethical issues (Antai-Otong, 2002; Boyle, 2002; Spector, 2000; Weaver, 1995).

Threat and Warning Phase. This phase consists of recognizing that a disaster could occur (threat) or that a disaster is approaching (warning). Responses among those at risk for disaster may range from active planning and protective measures to denial of the reality of a threat. There has been a dramatic surge of interest in the psychological impact of disasters on people, especially in the wake of the recent terrorist attacks and mass violence. The destruction of the World Trade Center, the bombing of the federal building in Oklahoma City, the school shootings at Columbine High School in Colorado, and terrorist actions in other communities make us acutely aware of our own vulnerability. These atrocities shatter our belief that the world is a predictable, safe place. The unpredictability, lack of control, and malevolence associated with terrorist attacks and mass violence are more disturbing to mental health than natural disasters related to weather changes or geophysical forces are likely to be (Weisaeth, 1994). The increased media attention to these tragedies has increased our awareness of their far-reaching psychological effects and the need for psychological preparedness.

Postdisaster Period

Impact Phase; Rescue (the First Hours or Days Following a Disaster). The impact of a disaster is the period of greatest damage and disorganization. This phase is variable, depending on the degree of life threat, number of deaths and injuries, and the extent of destruction to the community (Figley, Giel, Borgo, Briggs, & Harotis-Fatouros, 1995). The person is hit with the event; behavior is automatic; concern is with the immediate present. These stressors precipitate a physiologic response. Stress responses occur when information enters the brain through the senses. The cerebral cortex analyzes data, appraises their relevance, and mediates with the limbic system. The limbic system ascribes emotional meaning to the information, such as anxiety, fear, rage, or anger. The hypothalamic-pituitary-adrenal (HPA) axis is activated. The corticotropin-releasing hormone (CRH) is released by the hypothalamus, which activates the pituitary production of adrenocorticotropic hormone (ACTH) and the autonomic nervous system response. The sympathetic nervous system releases epinephrine and norepinephrine into the body in preparation for "fight or flight," the response to danger. The locus coeruleus-norepinephrine (LC-NE) system releases norepinephrine from neurons throughout the brain. Together, the HPA and LC-NE involve the central nervous system in neutralizing the perceived threat and restoring homeostasis. Physically and emotionally the person is in the Alarm Stage of the General Adaptation Syndrome (Selye, 1965; 1980). Table 4–1 summarizes the normal initial responses aimed at survival (Ganong, 1999; Murray & Zentner, 2001; Selye, 1965; 1980).

People respond with a variety of psychological effects that vary in severity and type. These responses include emotional, cognitive, and behavioral reactions. Table 4–2 summarizes these reactions (Fink, 1967; Murray & Zentner, 2001). Reactions are influenced by developmental level and maturity, prior experiences, and cultural background. The range of responses is a way for individuals to protect themselves from overwhelming emotion. The

stress associated with disaster may intensify existing psychological problems, causing psychotic symptoms such as delusions or hallucinations. For example, a survivor with a history of mental illness who suffers from delusions may feel responsible for the disaster or that someone intended the disaster only for the self.

However, most people show a great deal of strength and resilience in disasters. Positive responses include efforts to cope physically and emotionally and altruistic efforts to help others. Following impact, natural leaders and rescue workers from the affected community begin to appear and attend to the physical and psychological needs of others (Raphael, 1993). Rescuers do everything possible to prevent loss of life and property; efforts are focused on stabilizing the situation.

Early Postimpact Phase; Inventory and Recoil (Day After the Disaster to 2 or 3 Months). This is the phase where people begin to take inventory and comprehend what has occurred as a result of the disaster. Survivors become fully aware of the losses sustained. Grief reactions occur; both women and men may weep as they focus on the immediate past and how they managed to survive, and become aware of the full impact of the event. Masses of people converge on the disaster site and may inadvertently create additional problems. Some wish to help; others search for loved ones, and many are curious. The media also bring in crews to report on the event. Survivors attempt to reestablish contact with family and community. Generally, people naturally gather to demonstrate mutual support, share experiences, and make meaning out of what has happened (Raphael, 1993). Psychological and physical first aid must be implemented, which aims at meeting basic needs for food, shelter, safety, and connection with others, while also attending to physical injuries. The person may experience shock, defensive retreat, and beginning acknowledgment and grief typical of the phases of crisis described in Table 4–2 (Fink, 1967; Murray & Zentner, 2001). During this period a number of crises may arise, affecting physical or emotional health, employment, or financial stability. Survivors may suffer from a wide variety of symptoms, such as depression, post-traumatic stress disorder, generalized anxiety disorder, dissociative disorder, or various physical problems. Most survivors and disaster rescue workers experience normal stress responses, but generally do not develop long-term, chronic mental health problems (Freedy & Kilpatrick, 1994; Freedy, Saladin, Kilpatrick, Resnick, & Saunders, 1994). Studies indicate that most of these reactions subside in a few days or weeks(Aguilera, 1998; Hoff, 2001; Raphael, 1993). The helping response at this time should be supportive counseling and, if necessary, referral and treatment.

During the first few weeks following impact, survivors may go through a "honeymoon" phase. Survivors are grateful to be alive. The outpouring of community support lifts spirits and optimism is high concerning the promise of government aid. However, in the weeks that follow, disillusionment may

TABLE 4–1. RESPONSES TO STRESS: GENERAL ADAPTATION SYNDROME (GAS) AND LEVELS OF ANXIETY

GAS STAGE	PHYSICAL RESPONSE	BEHAVIORS RELATED TO ANXIETY
Alarm Stage	Pupils dilate; blurred vision. Hearing sharper or diminished.	Misinterpret stimuli. Confusion. Poor concentration. Selective inattention. Need for assistance.
Severe Anxiety or Panic	Stronger, faster heart rate and respirations. Palpitations, arrhythmias, elevated blood pressure.	Feeling of impending doom. Terror. Fearful. Agitation. Irritability. Demanding. Impulsive. Paresthesias.
	Muscle tone increased. Headaches.	Muscle tension. Excitable, restless movements. Tremors. Rigidity. Weakness.
	Basal metabolism rate increased. Body temperature elevated. Perspiration. Altered glucose, protein, and lipid metabolism. Increased startle response.	Insomnia. Urgency of speech and movement. Fatigue. Dehydration. Weight loss. Appetite changes. Smooth muscle of gastrointestinal and urinary tracts less motile, interfering with digestion and elimination of wastes.
	Hypoglycemia from glycogenolysis due to high energy demands.	Blood glucose increase. Appetite changes. Dehydration. Fatigue. Poor concentration.
	Increased blood clotting and suppressed immune response if Stage persists.	Blood stasis; thrombus formation. Resistance to infection and disease reduced.

TABLE 4–2. INDIVIDUAL RESPONSES IN THE CRISIS PHASES

PHASE AND DURATION	EMOTIONAL RESPONSE	COGNITIVE RESPONSE	BEHAVIORAL RESPONSE
Initial Impact; Shock (duration of 1 to 24–48 hours)	Anxiety. Helplessness. Overwhelmed. Detached. Hopelessness. Despair. Panic. Self-concept threatened. Self-esteem low. Anguish may be expressed by silent, audible, or uncontrollable crying	Disorganized thinking. Unable to plan, reason logically, or understand situation. Impaired judgment. Confusion. Disoriented. Preoccupation with image of lost object/person. Hallucinations. May ignore physical symptoms or describe physical distress.	Disorganized. Aimless wandering. Habitual behaviors used unsuccessfully. Withdrawn. Docile. Hyperactive. May appear overtly as if nothing happened or may be unable to carry out routine behavior. Lacks initiative for daily tasks. May need assistance meeting basic needs. Very suggestible, even if contrary to values or well-being.
Defensive Retreat (duration of hours to weeks)*	Superficial calm. Usually feels as if nothing is wrong because of use of repression or dissociation. Apathetic or euphoric. Feelings displaced onto other objects or people.	Tries habitual coping mechanisms unsuccessfully. States nothing is wrong. Avoids thinking about event. Denies physical injuries. May try to redefine problem unrealistically. May be disoriented. States same ideas repetitively. May be unable to plan alternate courses of action. Memory loss.	Tries habitual behaviors unsuccessfully. May seek support of others indirectly. Usually withdraws. Superficial responses. May avoid reality with overactivity. Resistant to change suggested by others. Unwilling to initiate new behavior. Ineffective, disorganized behavior. Denies through demands, complaints, or projections of inadequacy.
Acknowledgment of Reality (duration varies)	Tension and anxiety rise. Loneliness. Irritable. Depressed. Agitated. Apathetic. Self-hate. Low self-esteem. Grief – mourning occurs. Gradually self-concept becomes more positive. Gains self-confidence in ability to cope.	Becomes aware of facts about change, loss, event, and physical status. Asks questions. Attempts problem solving. May be disorganized in thinking. Trial-and-error approach to problems. Gradually perceives alternatives. Makes appropriate plans. Gives up unattainable goals. Validates personal experiences and feelings.	Exhibits mourning behaviors. Gradually demonstrates appropriate behaviors and resumes roles. Uses suggestions. Tries new approaches. Greater maturity demonstrated. Coping skills improved.
Resolution Adaptation, Change (duration of mourning and crisis work may be 6–12 months)	Painful feelings and memories integrated into self-concept and sense of maturity. New sense of worth. Firm identity. Gradual increase in self-satisfaction about mastery of situation. Gradual lowering of anxiety. Does not feel bitter, guilty, or ashamed.	Perceives meaning in situation. Integrates crisis event into self. Problem solving successful. Discusses feelings about event. Organized thinking and planning. Redefines priorities. Does not blame self or others. Remembers realistically.	Discovers new resources. Uses support systems and resources appropriately. Resumes status and roles. Strengthens relations with others. Adaptive in relationships. Lifestyle may be changed. Initiates measures to prevent similar disaster if at all possible.

*Note: Temporary retreat emotionally, mentally, and socially is adaptive and protective from perceived stress and loss and overwhelming anxiety. Allows time to gradually realize what has happened, avoids debilitating effects of high anxiety or panic. Initially person fluctuates between the phrases of defensive retreat and acknowledgement of reality.

occur when survivors make a more realistic appraisal of the full extent of loss, financial resources needed to rebuild, and the likelihood that things will never completely return to the way they were prior to the disaster. Disillusionment may last from several months to a year or longer and is characterized by disorganization and withdrawal of services and support. If disillusionment becomes entrenched, it may be considered a second disaster to the individual and to the community.

Recovery Phase: The Implementation of Long-Term Recovery Programs (Beginning 2 to 3 Months Following the Disaster). The recovery phase is the prolonged period of return to the predisaster level of functioning. Individuals and communities attempt to bring their lives and activities back to normal (Raphael, 1993). Cleanup of debris and rebuilding of physical structures occur. Survivors begin to solve their own problems and work to rebuild the community. During this phase, survivors work through the grief related to the crisis, become more realistic in acknowledging the realities and implications of the crisis, and move through the resolution or adaptation phase of crisis (see Table 4–2) (Fink, 1967; Murray & Zentner, 2001). The emotional, cognitive, behavioral, and spiritual effects of devastation and implications for the future must be dealt with through interventions with individuals, families, and community groups. The recovery phase may last for several years.

Explanation for Resiliency Response: Salutogenic Model

The Salutogenic Model can be useful for understanding why some people manage to endure, remain emotionally stable, and continue to function, especially after experiencing repeated natural or man-made disasters or terrorist attacks. Antonovsky (1979; 1987), in his studies of holocaust survivors, developed the Salutogenic Model, which focuses on the origins of health and on health-enhancing properties in contrast to models that focus on disease. Whether the outcome to stressful situations will be pathological, neutral, or maturing depends on how adequately tension is managed. He described a variety of generalized resistance resources (GRRs), such as ego strength, cultural stability, social supports, physical health, and financial stability, that help to manage stress. See Box 4–2 for factors that influence an individual's response to a disaster.

However, he found what was common to all GRRs was the **sense of coherence** (SOC), the ability for the survivor to make sense out of the situation or find meaning in the experience, regardless of the reality. Antonovsky further defines sense of coherence as a global orientation in which one has a pervasive, dynamic feeling of confidence that one's internal and external environments are predictable and that the probability is high that events will turn out as reasonably as can be expected. There are three components to developing a sense of coherence: comprehensibility, manageability, and meaningfulness. **Comprehensibility** is described as the person's ability to make sense of or understand the situation and a confidence that the world as a whole, and the current disaster, is basically predictable. The person has an attitude or perspective for dealing with distressing situations and a belief that the self can actively influence and control the environment and cope with stressors. **Manageability** refers to the ability to find and utilize resources to meet the demands of the situation. The person feels competent about seeking and accepting help and doing what is necessary to maintain self. **Meaningfulness** refers to integrating cognitive, emotional, and realistic issues and to find sense or meaning in the situation, and thus be motivated to act and to cope effectively. The person cares about self and life. The demands and problems are worth investment of energy; the situation, self, and family are worthy of commitment to goals and engagement with life and others. Stressors associated with the disaster are viewed as challenges rather than burdens. There is also a sense of boundaries; the person does not believe everything is comprehensible, manageable, and meaningful (Antonovsky, 1979, 1987).

ASSESSMENT AND INTERVENTION WITH SURVIVORS

Stress Responses to Disasters

Various responses to the stressors and crises of a disaster were discussed in the preceding pages. It is important for nurses who care for survivors to expect recovery and convey a sense of hope. People vary enormously in the ways they respond to disasters. Survivors are often confused by their reactions and are uncertain about the best way of adapting to their distress. It is essential to communicate that trauma reactions in the immediate aftermath of a

---

BOX 4–2   Factors that Influence Response to and Outcome of Disasters

1. Perception of the event (The perception of the event is reality regardless of how others might define reality.)
2. Physical and emotional status
3. Coping mechanisms and level of personal maturity
4. Previous experiences with similar situations
5. Realistic aspects of the current situation
6. Cultural influences
7. Availability and response of family and close friends, community groups, or other helping resources

disaster—such as anxiety, sadness, irritability, intrusive thoughts, memory problems, relationship difficulties, sleep disturbances, and appetite changes—are highly prevalent. These are normal stress responses to abnormal events. These responses are usually time-limited and most resolve completely (Green & Lindy, 1994).

Experts agree that early intervention following disasters can reduce psychological distress and prevent chronic mental health problems (National Institute of Mental Health, 2002). Interventions include (a) acknowledgment of perceptions and the reality of the experiences; (b) assurance about perceived strengths; (c) validation of ability to survive and manage; (d) education about normal stress reactions, behaviors that may indicate adverse mental health problems, and ways to increase self-care and coping skills; and (e) linkage with or referral to services. Frequently, survivors do not see themselves as needing mental health services. Often they turn to family members or significant others for assistance in coping with the psychological distress following disasters.

Mental Health Triage

Nurses must triage for the mental health needs of survivors. While most survivors experience normal stress reactions, some may need immediate mental health intervention to manage feelings of panic or intense grief. Signs of panic include palpitations, trembling, rapid speech, difficulty breathing, agitation, erratic behavior and concerns about survival. Signs of intense grief include sobbing, numbness, immobilization, and rage.

Interventions include establishing trust and rapport and being firm and positive to ensure that the person does not injure self further. Demonstrate empathy. "You're hurting a lot." Offer presence. Acknowledge and validate the survivor's experience: "I'm sorry this happened to you." "You are alive." "I'm here to help you." The triage process can link those affected with either supportive counseling, or if necessary, to emergency mental health care. Identify and refer those who are particularly stressed or at risk for adverse mental health outcomes to a mental health professional. Medications may be appropriate and necessary. Triage can also ensure that those likely to be at higher risk are linked to follow-up care.

Psychological First Aid or Emergency Care

The initial intervention following a disaster should be psychological first aid, which can be combined with physical care to individuals. Psychological first aid includes the following: (a) comforting and consoling; (b) protecting from further threat or distress, as much as possible; (c) providing care for physical needs and shelter; (d) supporting goal-oriented, reality-based tasks; (e) reuniting with loved ones; (f) facilitating ventilation of feelings about the experience as appropriate for the individual or group; (g) facilitating linkage to systems of support;

(h) fostering some sense of mastery; and (i) identifying and referring those who need additional counseling (Aguilera, 1998; Hoff, 2001; Raphael, 1986). Psychological first aid, like Maslow's theory on hierarchy of needs (Maslow, 1968, 1971), involves providing for physical needs, establishing safety and protection, facilitating a sense of belonging by connecting individuals with others, and helping survivors regain a sense of positive self-esteem and control.

Providing for Physical Needs

Providing for physical needs plays an important role in containing the distress of those affected by disaster. Approach survivors in a calm, gentle manner and demonstrate support and empathy. Provide them with food, water, shelter, clothing, and blankets. Facilitate rest and restorative sleep. Provide care for immediate health care problems as soon as possible.

Establishing Safety and Protection

To ensure physical safety, survivors should be moved away from the site of the disaster. To promote feelings of safety, create a calm and stable environment and provide reassurance by verbally telling the survivors that they are in a safe place. To the extent possible, provide personal space and privacy and help survivors secure personal belongings they have brought with them. Protect survivors from disturbing stimuli as much as possible. Greater sensory exposure, such as seeing, smelling, or hearing distressing things, increases the likelihood of adverse mental health outcomes. To avoid secondary traumatization, protect survivors, especially children, from onlookers and interviews by the media.

Facilitating a Sense of Belonging and Connection with Others

Connecting survivors with family members, natural support systems, and community resources is essential to promote healing and recovery. Survivors of a disaster may have lost connection with everything familiar to them. Families will be concerned with safety of their members and a desperate searching for missing family members is likely. Set up an information center to assist with the registration of those affected by the disaster and to facilitate locating and verifying the personal safety of family members and friends. Children should be reunited with their parents as soon as possible to avoid adverse mental health outcomes (McFarlane, 1987).

Provide opportunities to grieve losses. Use active listening. Allow time for ventilation of feelings. If the survivor begins to cry, remain with the person, and offer tissues. Avoid attempting to get the person to stop crying or regain immediate composure. Touching or giving a hug has often been a part of consoling and comforting. Sometimes touch is appropriate, other times it may violate a person's personal or cultural boundaries. Before you touch someone ask, "Would it be alright if I gave you a hug or touched your shoulder?"

People may need to share their experience with others. As natural groups form, support sharing that occurs spontaneously. This natural sharing of experiences with others in a caring and supportive setting (a) promotes psychological recovery, (b) begins the process of making meaning of the disaster, (c) gives testimony to those affected by the disaster, (d) validates feelings, and (e) generates support from others. However, others may choose not to talk about the disaster because they do not feel ready to face the emotions brought on by discussing their experiences. Avoid probing or forcing survivors to talk about the disaster. Some survivors may not be able to attend to emotional needs because they are busy coping with other consequences of the disaster; therefore, link survivors to support systems and services that they may access at a later time.

Fostering Positive Self-Esteem; Facilitating Sense of Mastery and Empowerment

Help each person feel a sense of importance and uniqueness. Counteract feelings of powerlessness by helping survivors gain some sense of control over their situation. As soon as possible, encourage survivors to resume daily activities, reestablish social support systems, and participate in resolving problems caused by the disaster. Providing structure can assist the person to shape the stressful trajectory and facilitate a sense of meaning and stronger sense of coherence (Motzer & Stewart, 1996). It is important to help survivors progress from a sense of helpless victim to a sense of being a survivor. Promoting a sense of self-esteem, mastery, and ability to reintegrate into the social community enhances the subjective quality of life and increases global sense of well-being and overall psychosocial functioning (Bengtsson-Tops & Hansson, 2001).

Impact on the Family Unit

The devastating effects of disasters may have considerable implications for family dynamics and stability. Disasters often cause family separations, disabilities, or deaths. Relationships may be strained. Children's ability to cope with disaster is affected by the capacity of parents and other adults to handle their own distress and support the child. Flick and Homan (1994) found a relationship between the mother's sense of coherence and her ability to nurture her children in extreme circumstances of homelessness. The stress of the disaster may increase the sense of closeness as family members turn to one another for emotional support. For others, as distress increases, marital conflict and parental-child conflicts become more intense and disruptive. Family members need the psychological first aid previously discussed, reassurance and support, information about normal stress responses, and referral to community services. Education following an extreme situation has been found to improve

the sense of coherence and quality of life in individuals as diverse as those diagnosed with schizophrenia (Landsverk & Kane, 1998) or who experienced cardiac arrest (Motzer & Stewart, 1996). Family members would likewise benefit.

Impact on the Community

Several groups of people in a community are particularly vulnerable to the impact of a disaster (Hoff, 2001).

- People who are poor, homeless, or elderly, or have few physical resources
- People who have reduced capacity to adapt to rapid change, such as the elderly, single-parent families, refugees, or the physically ill
- People who are "loners" or friendless, or recent immigrants, who lack physical and social resources that they can rely on in an emergency

Displacement, relocation, property loss, and unemployment following a disaster are just a few of the factors that disrupt the functioning of the community. This social disruption is an enormous source of stress, especially for those with few physical or social resources, the physically or mentally ill, or recent immigrants or refugees (Hoff, 2001). Each community responds to the disruptions differently and is influenced by its cultural perspectives. Only by understanding the culture of the community can the nurse effectively intervene. Community structure is also altered with the convergence of rescue workers and the media following the disaster and apparent lack of continued interest and abandonment as workers and media move on in a few days or weeks. Strong leadership is critical.

Community groups may develop to facilitate support and they should be encouraged. Cultural groups within the community may vary in their response; stoicism and resilience may be strong values (Lowe, 2002; Murray & Zentner, 2001; Nagata & Takeshita, 1998; Spector, 2000). Rituals are also an important step in the healing process. Spiritual services, restoration projects, and establishing memorials are ways of providing closure, paying tribute to the courage and suffering, and making meaning out of the disaster. Supportive networks help people in the ongoing recovery process, both through the exchange of resources and practical assistance, and emotional support.

Psychological Debriefing

Psychological debriefing (PD) developed as an in-the-field, early intervention to help soldiers (Solomon & Benbenishty, 1986) and rescue workers (Mitchell & Everly, 2000) to cope with stressful events and assist them to return to their duties as quickly as possible. Because PD was thought to have beneficial effects on participants, pervasive and routine application of PD to survivors exposed to traumatic events occurred. Empirical studies to date, however, fail to document its effectiveness (Rose & Bisson, 1998; Bisson, McFarlane, & Rose, 2000). PD presupposes that sharing experience about the disaster provides emotional release, which prevents long-term psychological effects (Solomon, 1999). PD has often been mandatory and included talking about the disaster experience, emotional catharsis, and group support. Participants were given information about psychological responses to disasters and available counseling services. Recent studies suggest that psychological debriefing is not always an appropriate mental health intervention following disasters, and in some instances may add to distress and interfere with recovery depending on the group members, the situation, and methods used (Raphael & Wilson, 2000; Rose & Bisson, 1998), especially if the person is from a culture that values stoicism and talking about feelings is considered immature or embarrassing (Lowe, 2002; Murray & Zentner, 2001; Nagata & Takeshita, 1998; Spector, 2002).

Natural debriefing refers to the spontaneous formation of groups in which individuals share their experiences with others. When survivors and rescue workers have opportunities to tell their stories, empathy, normalization, and validation are experienced, which promotes healing and recovery. Mutual support and opportunities to identify further needs can also be provided in supportive or natural debriefing (Ursano, Fullerton, Vance, & Wang, 2000). An example is defusing, an informal, unstructured strategy of providing psychological first aid to individuals, or small groups in active combat settings, often utilized by the military to prevent need for formalized intervention. Talking with peers is encouraged as a way to effectively defuse stressors (Fillion, Clements, Averill, & Vigil, 2002).

If psychological debriefing is used, incorporate the practice guidelines developed by The International Society for Traumatic Stress Studies, which include (a) facilitation by a well-trained, experienced therapist, (b) clearly stated objectives, (c) clinical assessment of potential participants, and (d) evaluation procedures. PD should not be mandatory nor should participants be required to disclose their experiences and feelings (Bisson, McFarlane, & Rose, 2000; Fillion et al., 2002). Survivors who talk about vivid accounts of intense trauma may potentially traumatize others who were minimally exposed. If the debriefing occurs in a group setting, it should consist of participants with similar experiences. Debriefing is recognized as one form of support and does not replace individual treatment programs. While it is perceived as helpful to some survivors, it is not helpful to everyone (Raphael & Wilson, 2000).

Crisis Intervention

Initial interventions after a disaster builds on the model developed by Gerald Caplan (1964), who proposed crisis intervention as a preventive method to decrease the likelihood of psychological disorders. A crisis occurs when stressors are overwhelming and usual problem solving and coping skills are inadequate (see Table 4–2). Disasters by their very nature precipitate crises. Crisis intervention is a short-term, action-oriented intervention with the goals of restoring the individual's equilibrium, reducing distress, restoring the person to the predisaster level of functioning, and preventing adverse mental health outcomes. Crisis intervention encourages expression of feelings, review of the disaster experience, and working through psychological responses. Several balancing factors are important to the successful resolution of crisis, as explained in Box 4–2 (Aguilera, 1998; Caplan, 1964; Hoff, 2001; Murray & Zentner, 2001).

Six-Step Model of Crisis Intervention

The six-step model of crisis intervention has been used to help individuals who are experiencing various kinds of crises (James & Gilliland, 2001). The six steps also reflect the descriptions presented by Aguilera (1998), Caplan (1964), Hoff (2001), and Murray & Zentner (2001).

1. **Defining the problem.** Define the problem from the individual's perspective.
2. **Ensuring safety.** Assess dangerousness to self or others, including a lethality (suicide) assessment.
3. **Providing support.** Approach the individual and establish rapport. Demonstrate support and caring.
4. **Examining alternatives.** Explore choices and options available to the individual. Identify coping skills and support systems that can be used immediately.
5. **Making plans.** Collaborate with the individual in making a short-term, realistic plan. Identify specific action steps to solve the problem.
6. **Obtaining commitment.** Assist client in committing to specific action steps that can realistically be accomplished.

The nursing process corresponds closely to the steps of crisis intervention.

Assessment: A Component of Crisis Intervention

Assessment is the first step; a therapeutic approach is essential and needs to be performed simultaneously with intervention. Both components of this process are explained together.

Focus on the immediate problem and the person's feelings. Ask: "What happened?" Expect to hear about the person's feelings as well as about the event. Remain calm. Take time to listen and convey that even amid the hurry and task demands of the impact, the person is important. Be genuine; show unconditional positive regard and empathy. Assess the level of anxiety and affect. Understand the problem from the survivor's perspective. "What does this event mean to you?" Is the trauma perceived accurately or is it distorted? The perception is the reality for the person. Do not argue or try to persuade the person differently if the perception is greatly distorted, but assure safety.

Determine situational supports. Ask: "Who are the people you are particularly close to?" or "Who can be called to help you?" The survivor may not have identifying information and may be unable to think of whom to notify. Let the person rest. Often, with a little time, the person can recall who could be contacted.

Observe the person to give you a sense of the survivor's ability to handle problems and cope. Ask: "How have you coped with tough times in the past? Has anything like this ever happened before? How do you deal with stress? What works?" Disorganized thought or speech may not be an indication of the usual pattern of functioning. As anxiety lowers, the person can usually answer questions more accurately.

Another aspect of the assessment process is to assess the client's safety. Ask if the client is suicidal or homicidal. Be specific. "Do you have any thoughts of hurting yourself or others? Have you thought about ending your life? Do you have a specific plan?" Convey what you observe: "You sound really angry about _____. What have you thought about doing?" Asking these questions will not precipitate suicide, but rather give an opportunity to talk about feelings and convey the importance of continuing to strive for life.

Mental state assessment should include potential organic factors, such as head injury or toxic effects. Refer the person to appropriate medical care resources and link the person to ongoing systems of social support.

Impact of Assessment

Be sensitive to the impact of the assessment on the acutely traumatized person. When someone has suffered a severe trauma, panic attacks, dissociative reactions, or flashbacks may occur. In a panic attack, the person may feel like he or she is having a heart attack and a fear of death is expressed. Palpitations, difficulty breathing, and a desire to escape are common. Panic attacks require a direct and structured intervention. Remain with the person and assure his or her safety. Maintain a calm, serene manner. Encourage the person to use deep abdominal breathing and to focus on the breathing, a sound, or counting to 10.

Survivors may experience episodes of dissociation and flashbacks when they recall details of the traumatic event. **Dissociation** is a defense mechanism in which a person's thought processes and feelings associated with the trauma are pushed aside or repressed. The person feels completely unreal or outside of self and has periods of amnesia. If the person dissociates during the assessment process, one of the observable behaviors is a blank stare. Eyelashes may flutter and even close. A quick shift in consciousness may happen, in which the person appears to have changed mood or to be asleep. Gently address the person by name, until the eyes open and the person reconnects with the interviewer. The person may make the comment, "I must have dozed off." Shift the conversation to a less anxiety-laden topic.

As trust and rapport develop, the individual may be able to share more details of the traumatic event. If the survivor has been severely traumatized or experienced other violent events, especially if the trauma history indicates severe childhood sexual, physical, and psychological abuse, behaviors associated with dissociative identity disorder (DID) may appear (American Psychiatric Association, 2000). This disorder is characterized by the existence of two or more personalities in a single individual. The transition from one personality to another is sudden and generally precipitated by stress. As the person talks about the disaster, past events may be interwoven. The person may dissociate and appear confused and may ask, "Who are you and where am I?" Reintroduce yourself and answer the question. Ask: "Who am I speaking to?" If the person identifies self as someone else, ask: "Do you know _____?" (the core personality, the survivor who has presented for the assessment). The dissociated or alternate personality generally will be aware of the core personality. Ask: "Is there something that you would like to share with me?" Remain calm and listen to the dissociated or alternate personality. Demonstrate respect, caring, and support. Eventually, thank them for sharing with you and ask to speak to _____" (the core personality). As anxiety decreases and the person feels safe, the alternate personality will allow the core personality to reemerge.

A **flashback** is reliving of the trauma event during the early postimpact phase or even later. This can happen visually in images, or it can be reexperienced with sounds, smells, feelings, or other such bodily memories when someone is reminded of the disaster. Not everyone realizes that they are suffering from a flashback. Tell the survivor, "It feels real, but it actually isn't happening again." If someone is in the middle of a flashback help him or her to "become grounded." Remain calm and speak in a gentle, confident manner. Encourage the person to keep eyes open, focus on your voice, take slow gentle breaths, put feet firmly on the ground, and slowly look around the room to establish location and safety. Attempt to differentiate the present environment from the past by noting details or objects that could not have been around when the prior trauma event occurred. For example, remind the person that you were not present when the trauma occurred. Offer your hand to show support; however, allow the survivor to decide whether to reciprocate.

Crisis Intervention

Crisis intervention aims to help people come to terms with the disaster, loss, and other distressing events they have suffered throughout the disaster, with an emphasis on enhancing positive coping and facilitating active mastery and involvement in the recovery process. In-depth counseling is not appropriate in the earliest stages, but should be available for those considered at higher risk of adverse mental health outcomes.

Provide support, reinforce adaptive behaviors, and help the person identify strengths. Communicate caring and empathy. Some people in crisis believe there are no options. Immediate social support may counteract long-term adverse effects (Davidhizar & Shearer, 2002). Assist survivors to recognize that alternatives are available. Alternatives may include situational supports, such as people known to the survivor who care and would want to help. Assist the individual to develop some plan of action for possible solutions to the problem. If the solutions are not effective, the nurse and survivor work toward finding other solutions. Restore a sense of control and power by using collaboration in planning. Individuals often feel totally out of control. Active roles are important for those affected by disasters, because activity counteracts feelings of powerlessness and helplessness that may have occurred during the impact (Aguilera, 1998; Hoff, 2001; Raphael, 1993).

For many types of trauma, experience indicates that relatively few survivors make use of available mental health services postdisaster. This may be due to a lack of awareness of the availability of such services, low perceived need for them, lack of confidence in their utility, or negative attitudes toward mental health care. Thus, crisis intervention on location at the time of disaster is important.

ADVERSE MENTAL HEALTH OUTCOMES: ASSESSMENT AND INTERVENTION

Importance of Timing

The majority of disaster-affected persons spontaneously recover. There is evidence that many acute stress symptoms may subside in the initial days after a disaster. Most of the recovery takes place in the first three months (Koren,

Arnon, & Klein, 1999; Riggs, Rothbaum, & Foa, 1995). Most survivors experience full psychological recovery in 12 to 24 months (Aguilera, 1998; Freedy & Kilpatrick, 1994; Freedy et al., 1994; Hoff, 2001). Consequently, assessing a trauma survivor in the first few days after an event may result in a diagnostic decision that would not be made if the assessment were conducted several weeks later. Trauma survivors may need a period of time to integrate the effects of a traumatic experience. Survivors are usually reluctant to seek mental health services in the aftermath of a disaster. Relief efforts for disaster victims are based on the observation that individuals in need of any type of help typically do not contact formal service agencies, except as a last resort. Instead, survivors prefer to turn to family and friends (Solomon, 1999). For a small number of survivors, stress reactions will be more long term and may lead to mental illness or changes in physical health (Burkle, 1996). Ongoing assessment and intervention are essential.

Risk for Adverse Mental Health Outcomes

Protective factors may moderate adverse mental health outcomes. These include (a) social support, (b) coping style, (c) community response, (d) higher income and education, (e) successful mastery of past disasters and traumatic events, and (f) limited exposure to any of the aggravating factors listed above. Information about positive coping strategies (Zook, 1998), such as humor or assertiveness, and availability of recovery services, along with expressions of care, concern, and understanding, on the part of the recovery services personnel are also protective factors.

Many people show resilience and adaptation following disasters. Certain factors both predisaster and postdisaster contribute to a greater risk for difficulty with recovery postdisaster. Box 4–3 summarizes these risk factors (Antonovsky,

---

BOX 4–3   Risk Factors for Difficulty with Postdisaster Recovery

- Lack of preparation for disasters
- Severity and duration of exposure, and perceived life threat, loss, injury
- Exposure to gruesome or massive death, combat, violence, destruction, bodily injury, or dead or maimed bodies, or intentional violence to loved ones
- Death of loved ones—family or friends; recent divorce
- Extreme environmental destruction, loss of home, valued possessions, or community structures
- Intense emotional demands; loss of communication with or isolation from support systems, stigma, or discrimination experiences
- Extreme fatigue, sleep deprivation, or exposure to other traumas
- Poverty, homelessness, unemployment, marital stress; family instability

- Guilt feelings that one could or should have done more; feelings of helplessness, powerlessness
- Gender; females may be more at risk or may be more likely to express feelings of severe stress
- Age, such as elderly or children, especially if separated from loved ones or parents
- Existing or preexisting psychopathology; developmental disabilities
- History of childhood trauma or abuse
- Relationship status; married women or single parents are more vulnerable, possibly because others rely on them for support which increases stress
- Exposure to toxic contamination
- Occupations of rescue worker or body handler

1979, 1987; Ardta, 1999; Asaro, 2001a, 2001b; Bryant & Harvey, 2000; Burgess, Hartman, & Baker, 1995; Carr, Lewin, Webster, & Kenardy, 1997; Clark, 1997; Fillion et al., 2002; Glaister & Abel, 2001; Green & Lindy, 1994; Hoff, 2001; Ignacio & Perlas, 1994; Ludin, 1994; North, Smith, & Spitznagel, 1997; Raphael, 1996; Ursano et al., 2000). However, studies have also reported on the stress inoculation effect of prior exposure and a strengthening of protective factors through successful mastery of previous traumatic events (Ursano, Grieger, & McCarroll, 1996). Assess for these risks. Listen carefully to expressions of feelings of anger, shame, and survivor's guilt that arise from these risks.

Anger

Anger is a common and normal feeling during the acknowldgement phase of crisis (see Table 4–2), in response to experiencing any of the aforementioned risks. The person may cry, blame others, be irritable, curse, pound fists, and proclaim, "The world is unfair" or "You are no help." Sometimes anger is internalized, and may express itself with headaches, sleep disturbances, eating problems, and weight loss. Other signs of depression may be present and also indicative of anger, including hopeless statements, "Why try? It won't make any difference," or despair, such as decreased interest in daily activities or other events. Panic attacks may continue, but normally they will lessen over time. Interpersonal relations may be strained or erratic. The person may blame others who are not responsible for what has happened. Severe anger may also result in violence toward self (suicide) or others (homicide).

Shame

Survivors may feel shame about their behavior during the event or when others blame them for the event, the trauma, or the consequences. Tragedies amplify our awareness that the world is ambiguous and unpredictable. Researchers have found that people naturally search for the meanings of traumatic events in order to maintain the belief that the world is predictable and just (Janoff-Bulman, 1992). It is difficult to find meaning in traumatic events, especially those involving human malevolence. Because of this desperate need to understand traumatic events, which may not have any real meaning, people tend to come up with a reason based on irrational thinking (Pennebaker, 1997). For example, when something bad happens to someone, people often conclude that the victim must have deserved what happened. Likewise, victims, in an attempt to find meaning to a meaningless tragedy, may blame themselves. Although victim blaming or self-blaming explanations may be inaccurate and personally devastating, it meets the need for understanding of the event and maintains the belief that the world is safe and predictable (Janoff-Bulman, 1992).

Survivors' Guilt

Individuals, both children and adults, may feel guilty for surviving or being uninjured when others were killed or injured, when they were unable to rescue someone, or when they had to leave someone dying in the disaster. During a disaster, individuals often have to act quickly in order to survive. Studies suggest that after a disaster, people overestimate their preexisting predictive knowledge of the event (Fischhoff, Crowell, & Kipke, 1999). This overestimation can lead to an inaccurate assessment of responsibility for the results of actions taken or not taken during a disaster. Survivors are often more self-critical than self-supporting (Schiraldi, 1999). Often they are particularly troubled by the fact that they were unable to exert control over what was happening (Carlson & Dalenberg, 2000). They may ruminate over their own activities or be preoccupied by thoughts about what they feel they should have done. Survivors are often unable to function or to address other issues until they process their guilt feelings. It is therapeutic to repeatedly say, "Whatever decisions you made at the time of the disaster were the right ones because you are alive." Individuals who experience the risks previously listed or repeatedly express anger, shame, or survivor's guilt are at risk for developing acute stress disorder or posttraumatic stress disorder. Linking survivors to support networks and identifying those at risk who may need follow-up services is important. Offering interventions previously described has been shown to be effective. Anger, shame, and guilt can be diminished over time by supportive counseling, which involves comforting, reassurance, information giving, and allowing people to discuss their experience, if they feel the need.

Early identification of those at risk for negative outcomes following a disaster can facilitate prevention, referral, and treatment. Screening can be accomplished by brief semistructured interviews and standardized assessment questionnaires. Screening should address the crisis assessment points and risk factors previously discussed. Especially important are acute levels of traumatic stress symptoms, which predict chronic problems.

Even when those who might benefit from mental health services have been adequately identified, factors such as embarrassment, fear of stigmatization, and cultural norms may limit motivation to seek help or pursue a referral. Those making referrals can address these attitudes and attempt to prevent avoidance of needed services. Therapeutic interviewing techniques can motivate the person to accept referral (Aguilera, 1998; Hoff, 2001).

Postdisaster Mental Disorders

Disaster survivors may display a wide range of stress reactions and symptoms. There is typically a dose-response relationship between degree of exposure and outcome. Women and men seem to be about equally at risk for symptoms following disaster, but they may present different complaints. Women tend to report more anxiety, depression, and post-traumatic stress disorder, whereas men are more likely to abuse alcohol, have physical or somatic complaints, or have symptoms associated with hostility or acting out (Green, 1993). The most commonly reported mental disorders include Acute

Stress Disorder, Post-Traumatic Stress Disorder, grief and bereavement complications, depression, Generalized Anxiety Disorder, substance abuse, prolonged disturbances in interpersonal relationships, and physical illness arising from psychological factors (American Psychiatric Association, 2000). It is essential to treat survivors for all presenting problems with a variety of counseling strategies and medications as needed. These conditions are discussed in the following pages.

Acute Stress Disorder

Acute Stress Disorder (ASD) is an anxiety disorder that describes the acute stress reactions that occur in the first 4 weeks following trauma. Diagnostic criteria include dissociative, reexperiencing, avoidance, and arousal symptoms. Symptom duration must be at a minimum 2 days or maximum of 4 weeks, and there must be significant impairment in functioning. ASD and Post-Traumatic Stress Disorder (PTSD) share many of the same symptoms (American Psychiatric Association, 2000). Most of those who experience these symptoms recover without treatment (Bryant & Harvey, 2000). Studies support that ASD, especially dissociative symptoms, predict the development of PTSD (Koopman, Classen, Cardena, & Spiegel, 1995). Use of interventions described in a later section can help the person overcome ASD and prevent PTSD.

Post-Traumatic Stress Disorder

Post-Traumatic Stress Disorder (PTSD) is characterized by the development of a persistent anxiety response following a traumatic event, and differs from ASD with a later onset and less emphasis on dissociation. The individual experiences or witnesses a traumatic event, such as actual or threatened death, serious injury to oneself or another person, a threat to the personal integrity of oneself or others, or violence to a loved one, such as homicide. To meet the stressor criteria of PTSD, the individual's subjective response to the traumatic experience must involve helplessness, intense fear, or horror. Symptoms are grouped into three categories: (1) reexperiencing of the traumatic event as indicated by intrusive thoughts, nightmares, or flashbacks; (2) avoidance, as indicated by marked efforts to stay away from activities, places or things related to the trauma; and (3) hyperarousal, as indicated by difficulty concentrating, insomnia, and exaggerated startle reactions. Symptom duration must be at least 1 month following the trauma and symptoms must be severe enough to impair functioning. Symptoms may be acute and occur following the trauma or be delayed (American Psychiatric Association, 2000). Some people who display PTSD symptoms in the immediate aftermath of a traumatic event recover in the following few months without formal intervention (Riggs, et al., 1995).

Disorders of Extreme Stress Not Otherwise Specified

Recent studies suggest that more complex syndromes of Post-Traumatic Stress Disorder or Disorders of Extreme Stress Not Otherwise Specified (DESNOS) may appear in survivors of prolonged, repeated, intense trauma, such as those who have been held hostage; who have been repeatedly tortured or exposed to chronic personal physical or sexual abuse; who have been in concentration camps, or who have lived for months or years in a society in a chronic state of war. Symptoms of DESNOS include (a) difficulties in regulating affect (e.g., persistent depression, suicidal preoccupation, self-injury, explosive anger), (b) alterations in self-perception (e.g., shame, guilt, sense of defilement, a sense of difference from others or helplessness), (c) alterations in consciousness (e.g., amnesia; transient dissociative states, intrusive thoughts, ruminative preoccupations); (d) difficulties in relations with others (e.g., isolation, disruptions in intimate relationships, persistent distrust), (e) alterations in perceptions of the perpetrator of the atrocities (e.g., a preoccupation with revenge, unrealistic attributions of total power to the perpetrator, or, paradoxically, gratitude toward or identification with the perpetrator) (Roth, Newman, Pelcovitz, van der Kolk, & Mandel, 1997).

Grief and Bereavement Complications

Bereavement is the response to loss, leading to distress and the complex effects referred to as grief. In situations of traumatic or catastrophic loss, the bereaved person may demonstrate both traumatic stress and bereavement reactions (Raphael & Martinek, 1997). Symptoms of grief include a longing for the loved one, a sense of emptiness, pain or heaviness in the chest, and hopelessness about the future. Individuals may cry easily, lose appetite, feel restless, and complain of stomach upset or headache.

Initially there may be a period of shock, numbness and disbelief, and to a degree, denial. This initial period usually gives way to intense separation distress or anxiety. The bereaved person is highly aroused, seeking for the lost person, particularly if it is not certain that the person is dead, or the body has not been identified. Anger may be expressed toward the deceased for being among those who died. Anger is also directed toward those who may be perceived as having caused or been associated with the death, who are alive when the deceased is not.

Rando (1984) described emotional, cognitive, behavioral, physical, and spiritual assessment components or factors. Risk factors for complications of bereavement have been identified (Parkes & Weiss, 1983; Raphael & Minkov, 1999), and they include (a) a high level of ambivalence in relation to the deceased, (b) an extremely dependent relationship, (c) perceived lack of social support, (d) other concurrent crises or stressors, (e) circumstances of death which are unexpected, untimely, sudden, or horrific and shocking, (f) past history of losses, and (g) prolonged denial of the death and acting as if the deceased person is still alive. These risk factors, along with emotional and cognitive reactions, behavior, physical status, and spiritual beliefs, should be assessed.

Survivors must come to terms with the loss of their loved one, as well as the manner in which it occurred.

Traumatic deaths are particularly likely to result in intense and prolonged grief if the death was violent or if the death was brought about by a malevolent act or homicide. It is common for survivors to agonize about what their loved ones experienced during their final moments of life. Survivors may experience feelings of rage toward the perpetrator (Asaro, 2001a, 2001b; Raphael & Martinek, 1997). The death of a child is particularly difficult because parents expect to die before their children.

Trauma may interfere with the ability to go through the process of bereavement. Concerns about the bereaved seeing the body of the deceased due to injuries sustained in the disaster may prevent the bereaved from viewing the body. Seeing the body, even when it is disfigured, is not inherently damaging. Inability to see the body of the dead person may further contribute to risk of adverse outcome because it interferes with opportunities to say goodbye (Singh & Raphael, 1981). Obstacles to a normal response to the death of a loved one may contribute to a feeling of lack of closure or permit fantasies that the deceased person has not died. Legal processes may delay funeral proceedings. Both bereaved and traumatized individuals are likely to experience similar symptoms in terms of intrusive thoughts, avoidance responses, and high levels of arousal.

The psychotherapeutic aim is to facilitate the normal grieving process. See Box 4–4. This involves dealing with the circumstances of the death, reviewing the lost relationship, expressing feelings, mourning the deceased, accepting the new realities that result from the loss including any role or status changes, and dealing with simultaneous life stressors (NSWHealth, 2000).

Effects of Disasters on Special Populations

Populations at special risk for adverse mental health conditions include children and adolescents; the elderly, especially the frail elderly; refugee and migrant groups; and the developmentally or mentally disabled. These individuals may perceive the stress associated with a disaster quite differently from others, and may be in particular need of help and support. People from diverse cultural background may also respond differently.

Children and Adolescents

The clinical presentation of PTSD approaches the adult pattern with increasing age, for example, in adolescents. However, PTSD in children is manifested with the following variances (American Psychiatric Association, 2000; Clark, 1997; Drell, Siegel, & Gaensbauer, 1993).

1. Disorganized, agitated behavior.
2. Range of behavior from quiet, anxious, vigilant, fearful of adults, and despair, to panic and fury
3. Reexperiencing the traumatic event through nightmares, repetitive play, unusual preoccupations, in which aspects of the trauma event or same themes are expressed

Rand (2001) reported that the limbic system and prefrontal cortex appear to not develop normally and that there are fewer neural networks formed if the child is repeatedly abused. MRI studies have shown altered brain development in children who suffered abuse and terror and the consequent PTSD in contrast to normal controls, including smaller corpus collosium and larger lateral ventricles. Brain volume correlated with severity of intrusive thoughts, hyperarousal, avoidance, and dissociation. Apparently, the increased catebolaminergic neurotransmitter production and steroid activity during the trauma experienced in childhood affects brain development (DeBellis et al., 1999).

Studies about the effects on children of repeated physical and sexual abuse can be analogous to repeated terrorist attacks. In a study of children who suffered repeated abuse and torture in a day care center, Burgess, et al., (1995) found that childhood trauma affected various levels of biological memory systems for as long as 5 or 10 years after the experience. Memories were expressed as somatic symptoms, behaviorally and verbally. There were a variety of unusual complaints, disorganized and abnormal behaviors, and verbal descriptions of feeling that revealed depression, anxiety disorders, chronic PTSD, and developmental delays.

Research in Canada with refugee children and children who had witnessed their mother being physically abused (children had not been directly abused) revealed parallel and common themes of emotional pain, suffering,

---

BOX 4–4   Strategies for Grief Therapy

The following strategies can be useful in grief therapy (Clark, 1997; Hoff, 2001; Kavanagh, 1990).

- Use of photographs, possessions, and other symbols of the deceased to promote both acknowledgment of the loss and development of an internal relationship
- Encouragement for creative expression by writing or drawing, which can capture feelings that may be difficult to verbalize

- Creating rituals, dioramas, or a memorial box, which can be a means of remembering or commemorating the dead person or lost object
- Promotion of cognitive restructuring, which involves confronting and testing distorted beliefs that may maintain a pathological response
- Review of positive and negative aspects of the relationship to assist with the grieving

feelings of betrayal, uncertainty about the enemy, and lack of a sense of peace (Berman, 1999).

Because childhood physical and sexual abuse is repetitive, or even patterned or ritualized (Valente, 2000), the child is actually experiencing a series of unresolved disasters. It is possible that the consequences of such abuse that have been reported, both in childhood (Ardta, 1999; Clark, 1997; Hoff, 2001) and later consequences in adulthood (Bremmer et al., 1999; Clark, 1997; Clod, 1993; Glaister & Abel, 2001; Heim et al., 2000), may also be found in children who live through repeated terrorist attacks or bombings or who are made to participate in events that inflict violence on others. Hall (1999) found that the multiple maltreatment of sexual abuse and repeated interpersonal trauma contributed to symptoms of disorders of extreme distress. Ardta (1999) found that repeated victimization involving sexual abuse in childhood contributed to a lifetime history of PTSD in adulthood.

Dysfunctional brain changes have been found through PET scans in adult women with PTSD who suffered childhood sexual abuse. These changes were apparent in the prefrontal cortex, hippocampus, motor and visual centers of the brain, and areas of the midbrain associated with memory (Bremmer et al., 1999).

In counseling the child with PTSD, use drawings, toys, and games to allow an outlet for aggression in a structured setting. Ask the child what the drawing, words, or play behavior means but avoid interpretation to the child. Explore with the child ways to avoid repeating of future disasters. Teaching problem solving can help the child feel stronger because he or she survived a trauma and can use what was learned throughout life. A clue that the child has resolved the trauma feelings is when drawings, letters, or words suggest a sense of altruism. If closely observed and listened to, survivors even as young as 18 months can tell through play acting, "art," and words what happened as well as their movement toward resolution (Clark, 1997).

It is essential for adults to control their own anxiety, and convey a sense of calm, stability, and consistency, and to help the child work through anxiety and consequent feelings of frustration and aggressive behavior. The child should be taught that fears and conflicts can be resolved through communication rather than displaced on others, no matter the religion or ethnicity, as well as to be responsible for personal behavior. Through such an approach, we avoid planting the seeds for violence in later generations (Weinstein, 2003). See Chapter 10 for more information on the effects of disaster on children.

Older Adults
Older adults have also been found to be a high-risk population for disaster reactions and at need for interventions. The impact of disaster-related losses has shown that a higher incidence of personal loss, injury, and death are experienced by older adults (Norris, Phifer, & Kaniasty, 1994). The elderly may feel like they cannot start over again when loved ones,

home, and prized possessions are lost. They feel devastated and robbed of what they worked for. If the anger and grief are not resolved, chronic PTSD may occur. Adverse reactions are more intense if the survivors view the disaster as preventable. Some elders never return to the predisaster level of functioning (Hoff, 2001). The more frail the person, the more likely the person is to have difficulty coping emotionally with disaster impact or its consequences. Research has shown that older adults are less likely to evacuate, less likely to heed warnings, less likely to acknowledge hazards and dangerous situations, and are much slower to respond to the full impact of losses (Norris, et al., 1994). The following normal changes in the elderly may interfere with coping with a crisis or disaster and may contribute to physical injury and to adverse mental health outcomes (Murray & Zentner, 2001).

- Existing problems with vision, hearing, balance, mobility, temperature control, and physical disorders
- Memory changes, especially of recent events, health routines, or supportive persons
- Slower reaction time and encoding or getting information into the memory, especially when confronting change, which may contribute to the appearance of confusion or cognitive incompetence
- Changes in motivation level; less initiative or willingness to engage in screening or intervention strategies. The person may say, "Go take care of the young people."
- Greater use of adaptive and defensive mechanisms, such as emotional isolation, repression of feelings but maintaining the ideas, rationalization and denial, or compartmentalization with a narrowing of awareness and focus that causes the elder to seem rigid, repetitive, and resistive
- Being more dependent, demanding, egocentric, and preoccupied with the physical self, as well as with routines that cannot be followed during the impact or early postimpact phases of a disaster
- A prior sense of shame, worthlessness, inadequacy, powerlessness, and loneliness, or depression with or without suicidal thoughts

Yet, elders also have a resilience, sense of coherence, self-reliance, and perseverance that can be tapped and strengthened through the counseling process, even if brief, to promote resolution and adaptation. Reminiscence and soliciting their insights can strengthen self-esteem and resolve to overcome the vicissitudes of the situation.

Refugee and Migrant Populations
The few studies conducted in this area seem to suggest that a disaster may have more negative effect on the mental health of refugees and migrant populations (Bremmer et al., 1999; Hoff, 2001; Sack, 1998; Spector, 2002). Some of the factors that may exacerbate this negative effect include limited social support, limited English language skills, inadequate information about disaster response, anxiety about loss of treasured mementos from the prior country of residence, and

anxiety about loss of documentation about their citizen status. Indigenous people may be adversely affected by disasters because their communities are often suffering from marginal status, poor physical health and housing, problems of cultural loss, and ongoing trauma and grief.

People of Diverse Cultural Backgrounds

Cultural factors may also be powerful in determining the reaction of the affected person and the response of others. There may be cultural rituals and social traditions that help deal with grief, the aftermath of disaster, and healing. They need to be understood and supported. Mourning rituals are culture specific. It is essential that cultural issues be taken into account in understanding responses to disaster in different communities, and that appropriate postdisaster mental health services that are culturally sensitive are provided. Several references give in-depth information about cultural values, responses to crisis, and specific appropriate interventions (Antai-Otong, 2002; Berman, 1999; Lowe, 2002; Sack, 1998; Spector, 2002; Weaver, 1995). Another kind of cultural group is military personnel and their families. Fillion et al. (2002) describe reactions of soldiers in combat (combat stress reaction), manifestations, and ASD and PTSD interventions.

People in Poverty

Consequences of a disaster are especially difficult for people who are in poverty, including (a) those who are in acute poverty with limited economic means because of current circumstances; (b) those who are in chronic poverty, with a long history of inadequate economic means for a variety of reasons; (c) those who are homeless and therefore often have no ready support system or economic means, and now must share shelter space with those who lost housing in a disaster; (d) migrant workers and their families who may lack housing and transportation to move to another area, and are displaced from their marginal employment by a disaster; and (e) refugees seeking homes in a strange land, who fled their home because of persecution and who are only to be again displaced by the disaster without the economic resources or social support systems to provide safety and security. Various agencies that work with refugees may not have a disaster plan or no way to track the people with whom they are working. These individuals may already be suffering from PTSD, depression, or anxiety because of the previous traumatic experience. Often the adult generations of migrants, refugees, and immigrant populations have to rely on their children for the information given and interpretation of announcements, or for explanations related to personal or family status or needs. The sense of powerlessness adds to the trauma effects and may be difficult to resolve.

People of Various Faith Beliefs

Consequences of a disaster may be responded with greater emotional equanimity by some groups of people, including those with a high sense of coherence (Antonovsky, 1979,

1987) or those who belong to faith communities or religious denominations that emphasize reliance on faith beliefs. Depending on the spiritual cultural backgrounds, you may hear individuals calling on God, the Lord Jesus, or Allah. They may be praying loudly for protection; to cast off evil forces, demons of destruction, or disease in the name of Jesus; and laying on hand of healing on those who are injured. The beliefs, practices, and rituals may be different than those of rescue workers and professionals; however, they should not be interfered. The spiritual forces within a person, family, or group are powerful and may bring surprising results.

Physically and Mentally Disabled

Physical, developmental, or emotional limitations or disorders may prevent the person from protecting self in violent situations. Lack of access to public transportation and buildings affects both mobility and obtaining shelter, for emergency or follow-up care. These factors may contribute to feelings of negative self-image, alienation, powerlessness, and grief following losses incurred in disasters and grief reactions may go unnoticed (Hoff, 2001). Previous or current psychiatric illness, inability to understand what is occurring, and presence of hallucinations or delusions may be difficult to determine. Careful observation and listening, a consistent calm approach, interacting with the person from a perspective of apparent strengths rather than focusing on pathology are measures to promote coping and may avert a severe adverse reaction.

PSYCHOLOGICAL INTERVENTIONS

The aim of psychological intervention should be providing supportive care for survivors with the goal of promoting mental health and preventing adverse outcomes, such as PTSD, depression, substance abuse, or relationship difficulties. Recognize individuals' strengths and acknowledge and convey to them their capacity to cope with the experience (Aguilera, 1998; Hoff, 2001).

Some interventions have been interwoven throughout the chapter in relation to responses to assessment. This section summarizes psychosocial interventions for individuals, family units, and small groups that meet the goals to provide supportive counseling, promote mental health, and prevent adverse long-term disorders.

General Guidelines

Box 4–5 presents guidelines applicable to working with a person or family in any crisis or disaster during the impact, postimpact, and recovery phases (Aguilera, 1998; Hoff, 2001; Murray & Zentner, 2001; NWS Health, 2000). Following a disaster, people are generally amenable to a variety of interventions. However, any intervention must always be tailored to the specific person(s) and situation, for example,

BOX 4–5   Crisis Intervention Guidelines

1. **Begin with comfort measures, conveying care and consolation** while attending to physical status as necessary. Recognize the person may be associating this event with other violent situations, which can account for unusual reactions. Listen and observe for such.

2. **Acknowledge and validate, or encourage and facilitate expression of feelings** while assisting with physical care or self-help measures and gathering information. Give time to express feelings in a way that is comfortable. Ask: "What are you thinking?" or "What are you feeling?"

3. **Acknowledge strengths and coping abilities.** State: "Your reactions are normal. This is very overwhelming. You're doing as well as you can." If the person does not express emotions, let the conversation move in the direction comfortable to the person.

4. **Clarify perception of the event, the losses involved, the realities of the situation** to help gain a more realistic view and possible implications or consequences. If the person is reluctant to talk, you might say, "As a child, you may have been told never to talk, but here it is safe to share as much as you want."

5. **Accept statements that reflect denial or distortion. Do not argue.** State: "This was random bad luck that led to trauma. It didn't happen because of you."

6. **Avoid false reassurance.** Don't say, "This won't happen again" or "It's all going to be alright/fine."

7. **Through repetitive, gentle explanations, relay information, convey hope and the importance of working together, and promote problem-solving abilities.** Say: "It takes courage to share what you just said. I see ways in which we can work to get through this."

8. **Encourage ability to manage; explore prior coping strategies and examine alternative ways of coping.** Review realistic plans to help gain a sense of control over future events. Role-playing how to handle situations can be useful.

9. **Involve in activity with specific tasks,** especially related to personal needs, but also in relation to helping others. Set limits and give instructions as needed. Activity can decrease anxiety, and self-help and altruism contribute toward problem solving, increased self-esteem, and a sense of hope and manageability.

10. **Accept suggestions that are useful and relevant** for getting the task at hand done. Collaboration is necessary for completing work but also enhances a sense of normality and positive self-concept and self-confidence, which can strengthen the sense of resilience and coherence.

11. **Foster social relationships and effective use of social support systems or referral agencies.** Encourage seeking and accepting help, as necessary, for current or future needs that are likely to arise. Encourage spiritual expressions and participation in group activities, if appropriate.

12. **Clarify continuing decisions and actions while being supportive.** Recognize that outcomes for initial crisis interaction may not become known but that initial crisis intervention is likely to prevent adverse mental health outcomes.

13. **Do not retaliate to angry, derogatory, accusatory, or bitter statements; this is a way to cope with feelings.** Do not take the statement personally, but consider if there is any accuracy to the statements. If so, correct actions, procedures, or policies, if possible, or do what is possible to convey caring and genuine concern.

14. **Accept lack of responsiveness to directions given, information shared, comforting expressions, and a caring attitude.** These interventions may be remembered and used later.

---

words used, timing, nonverbal behavior, and the emotional, social, and cultural considerations previously described.

Anxiety Management

The following techniques, with rationales, can be used with individuals or a small group to reduce or cope with anxiety (Clark, 1997; Hoff, 2001; Murray & Zentner, 2001, Appendix III).

1. **Deep breathing training.** Teach abdominal breathing to bring about the relaxation response or avoid hyperventilation.

2. **Relaxation training.** Teach systematic relaxation of the major muscle groups to counteract tension associated with anxiety. Avoid beverages, candy, and foods that contain caffeine or other stimulants that interfere with rest and sleep.

3. **Positive self-talk.** Replace negative automatic thoughts with positive thoughts to cope with feelings; enhance self-esteem and coping.

4. **Journals, logs, art, music.** Express feelings, substitute positive expressions that promote self-esteem.

5. **Thought stopping.** Teach distraction techniques such as inwardly saying "Stop," to overcome distressing thoughts.
6. **Meditation, visualization, or imagery exercises.** Focus thoughts on a neutral or pleasant object or situation to reduce anxiety, clarify decisions, and enhance self-esteem and hope.
7. **Assertiveness training.** Teach the person how to express wishes, opinions, and emotions without infringing on the rights of others.
8. **Anticipatory guidance.** Discuss potentially anxiety-provoking situations and how they can be handled. The person may also benefit from a short-term anxiolytic medication.

Cognitive Therapy

Cognitive therapy focuses on helping the person to (a) identify trauma-related negative or distorted thoughts (e.g., unrealistic guilt, distrust of others, catastrophizing every situation) and (b) modify or remove unrealistic assumptions, beliefs, and automatic thoughts that cause disturbed feelings and impaired functioning. The goals are to teach survivors to identify dysfunctional or automatic thoughts, and weight evidence for or against them, and adopt a more realistic thought that will generate more balanced emotions. Cognitive therapy may involve many techniques, including (a) reframing or redescribing a situation, (b) visualizing trigger situations and coping methods, (c) using imagery exercises to reduce anxiety and enhance coping, (d) writing a journal or diary, poem, or song, or writing (but not sending) a letter to an abuser to express feelings or to overcome re-experiencing PTSD flashbacks, (e) visualizing the word STOP or using a rubber band around the wrist to snap, in order to interrupt intrusive thoughts of PTSD, and (f) giving various homework assignments to learn new thought and behavior patterns. The numbing, dissociation, and self-mutilation that are a part of PTSD are miserable for the survivor and difficult for the family to live with. Referral to a skilled therapist is essential for postdisaster recovery to occur.

An example of use of several cognitive techniques after a disaster is described by Dewar (2003) as the strategy of "boosting" to enhance self-esteem and adjust to the emotional, social, and physical effects of disability or disease. Research participants used emotional and spiritual boosting strategies that included (a) comparing self and condition favorably to that observed in other sufferers, (b) focusing on the positive aspects of circumstances, (c) building courage to cope with difficult times and to prepare for even more difficult times, (d) visualizing improvement through self-comforting talk, and (e) doing "emotional weight-lifting," visualizing problems as a series of weights on the floor and then imagining self lifting each one and putting it aside.

Cognitive-behavioral therapy involves some combination of previously described cognitive methods and emphasis on behavior management, including healthy coping with anger, assertive communication, and developing social skills. These methods, combined with education about symptoms and management of the problem, and development of a therapeutic counseling relationship, can be effective in treating adverse mental health disorders.

Research suggests that relatively brief but specialized interventions may effectively prevent PTSD in some subgroups of trauma patients. Several controlled trials have suggested that brief (e.g., four to five sessions) cognitive-behavioral treatment comprised of education, breathing training and relaxation, imagery and real-life exposure, and cognitive restructuring, delivered within weeks of the traumatic event, can prevent PTSD in survivors of sexual and nonsexual assault (Foa, Hearst-Ikeda, & Perry, 1995) and after motor vehicle and industrial accidents (Bryant, et al., 1998; Bryant, Sackville, Dang, Moulds, & Guthrie, 1999).

Expressive therapy principles can be used with adults as well as children. It involves use of games, art, music, books, puppets, and toys to introduce topics that cannot be effectively addressed more directly and to facilitate exposure to and reprocessing of traumatic memories. Expressive therapy can tap into emotions that are often difficult to verbalize and promote behavior change.

MENTAL HEALTH VULNERABILITY OF THE NURSE AS DISASTER WORKER

Working with disaster survivors is stressful and crisis-provoking; often the nurse is simultaneously suffering a disaster while caring for survivors and working amidst disaster impact. The nurse may feel as overwhelmed and traumatized as the population for whom she or he is caring. The nurse, as a member of the rescue and caretaking team, must recognize that mental health workers are also vulnerable to and may experience any of the reactions to crisis and disaster that have been described earlier. Observe the signs and symptoms and seek help from others. Periodically leave the immediate disaster scene and follow the rules established for workers, such as taking time to eat and sleep. Avoid taking on the "martyr role" or engaging in "rescue fantasy." No person can be the only or primary one to assume responsibility or engage in all facets of disaster intervention. A team approach is mandatory; each worker contributes toward the whole recovery effort—physically and emotionally.

Workers assigned to recover human remains from wreckage or bombing sites can tolerate only a few hours at a time of confronting the horror. They need time away from the work and an opportunity to process what they witnessed (Hoff, 2001; Taylor & Frazer, 1981).

Following a disaster, whether natural or of human origin, an area-wide memorial service can be important for survivors. People are supported by each other. Perhaps all will want to cry and release pent-up emotions. The message to sing and pray, overcome grief, and rejoice in what remains will help survivors and the community, to carry on with life, while remembering and honoring those who lost life (Hoff, 2001).

Risks for Nurses Working with Trauma Survivors

Nurses who work with survivors of disasters may be at risk for vicarious traumatization. Vicarious traumatization occurs in response to listening to survivors' stories of the traumatic event. These accounts elicit strong feelings. Emotional reactions that overwhelm the nurse may interfere with the ability to function. Nurses who experience vicarious traumatization may experience psychological responses that can be disruptive and painful, and persist after working with trauma victims (Blair & Ramones, 1996; McCann & Peralman, 1990; Rand, 2002).

Protection against vicarious victimization involves recognition of the impact of the material on personal beliefs and identity, developing a support network, and ventilation of feelings in a supportive environment with coworkers and other professionals. Prevention and management involve constructing mental and, if possible, physical boundaries between personal and professional activities and having variety in each component. Additionally, trauma therapists might want to carefully monitor their time with disaster victims to defuse some of the traumatic impact.

Self-Care

Disaster work should not be done in isolation. Be aware of the fatigue from the physical work and the emotional drain from seeing wreckage and repeatedly listening to trauma stories. Nurses cannot be totally immune to the effects of helping survivors work through their trauma. However, they can take some steps to provide some degree of protection and relief from becoming totally overwhelmed and ineffective in their care. It is essential to take time to eat, sleep, and do exercises unrelated to disaster work.

Hutchinson (1987) discussed the strategies of (a) acting assertively, (b) encouraging goodwill, (c) discharging pent-up emotions, (d) taking mental health breaks by creating a distance between or withdrawing of self, even if temporarily, and (e) using of humor and meditation. These strategies can be taught to individuals, families, and groups, as well as applied to self and rescue workers. The methods to cope with crises and interventions discussed in

the previous sections can be applied by the nurse to self as well as taught to survivors.

SUMMARY

Disasters, whether of natural or human origin, evoke predictable emotional and cognitive responses in survivors. These responses are described in terms of levels of victims, phases of disasters, stress responses, and phases of and reactions to crises, which are inherent in disaster. These reactions are emotional, cognitive, and behavioral in nature. Several factors influence perception and outcome of the crisis or disaster. Most people return to the level of function that was evidenced prior to the disaster or crisis. Antonovsky's Salutogenic Model explains why some people endure situations. However, crisis intervention methods and specific cognitive therapy and cognitive-behavioral therapy methods can maintain function and prevent reactions such as acute stress disorder, as well as treat adverse mental health outcomes, such as complicated grief and bereavement reactions and post-traumatic stress disorder. The therapeutic approaches used by nurses during disasters address the needs of the individual, family, and/or group. Nurses must also recognize needs of caregivers, including themselves, and utilize measures to promote self-care and avoid secondary traumatization.

CASE STUDY

PTSD Patient in the ICU

A.P. was a 23-year-old Israeli army medic who was severely injured while at home on leave when a suicide bomber detonated a bomb. A.P. was admitted to Hadassah Hospital and underwent emergency surgery on both arms and one leg. He was admitted intubated to the ICU after 19 hours of surgery. After 24 hours, he was extubated and immediately calmed his family by stating that he was fine. A.P. was very cooperative, helping the nursing staff in moving and washing, even when undergoing painful procedures, such as getting out of bed to sit in a chair. After 3 days in the ICU, A.P. began complaining of constant pain that was unrelieved by pain medication. Until his third hospital day, he had refused pain medication, stating that he didn't need anything, and he was coping easily. The nursing staff felt that this behavior was unusual and decided to investigate. In-depth discussion with A.P. revealed that he had heard the housekeeper in the department talking in Arabic and this triggered a sharp stress and anxiety reaction. A psychiatric consultant was called, and an antistress medication was prescribed. A.P. was eventually discharged. For the first few months, A.P. was never left alone. Whenever his parents left the house, even briefly to visit neighbors, A.P. called them, asking them to return within a few minutes. With counseling, he recovered from his PTSD. After 5 months, he could be left alone at home and resumed driving to see his friends and maintaining his social life.

The sooner PTSD is diagnosed and treated, the faster the recovery. The symptoms of PTSD are varied and can be any signs of behavior changes related to stress. For example, a bomb victim who was admitted to ICU spent several days intubated and sedated. After being extubated, she could not speak. CT scans were ordered; the director of ear, nose, and throat examined her; and finally a neurologist was consulted. No obvious injury was seen. After a period of time, the nurses suspected that she was suffering from PTSD and a psychiatrist was consulted.

1. Responses of survivors following disasters are frequently complex. How is that concept expressed in this case?
2. What nursing interventions should be implemented?

TEST YOUR KNOWLEDGE

1. During the honeymoon phase in a disaster, people
   A. Do everything possible to prevent loss of life and property
   B. Complain about the lack of government response but are hopeful for aid
   C. Are busy solving their own problems
   D. Are in an optimistic mood and persist in doing what is absolutely necessary in daily routines

2. The person in the Alarm Stage of the General Adaptation Syndrome and the impact phase of a disaster have similar reactions, except
   A. Increased neuromuscular response
   B. Sense of anxiety and helplessness
   C. Sense of high self-esteem
   D. Disorganized thinking

3. The intervention that is not considered psychological first-aid is
   A. Providing for physical needs and shelter
   B. Implementing cognitive behavioral therapy sessions
   C. Connecting survivors with family members
   D. Allowing spontaneous sharing of feelings and experiences

4. An important attribute of the nurse when interviewing a survivor is
   A. Always be in a position of authority
   B. Keep emotional distance from the survivor
   C. Be a good listener
   D. Maintain control by making all decisions

5. Which of the following statements about assessing for suicide is false?
   A. Directly ask if the client has thoughts of harming self
   B. Be supportive
   C. Only ask about suicide if the survivor brings it up
   D. Ask specific questions about a suicide plan

6. Which of the following is not a high risk factor for difficulty with postdisaster recovery?
   A. Exposure to gruesome or massive death
   B. History of mental illness
   C. Use of dissociation during the traumatic event
   D. Mastery of previous traumatic events

7. Unresolved grief following a disaster is characterized by all of the following except
   A. Continued social isolation
   B. Maintenance of illusion that a person is not dead
   C. Reorganization of behavior directed toward new persons/objects
   D. Development of symptoms similar to those of the deceased

8. Principles of crisis intervention include all except
   A. Assessing accurately the crisis event
   B. Clarifying psychodynamics of person's behavior
   C. Exploring coping mechanisms and realistic problem solving by the client
   D. Collaborating with the client in forming a short-term realistic plan

9. All of the following symptoms are reflective of the diagnosis of post-traumatic stress disorder (PTSD) except
   A. Reexperiencing distressing thoughts, dreams, or flashbacks
   B. Feeling numb
   C. Being jumpy or easily startled
   D. Fantasy orientation toward the future

10. Julie has recently survived an explosion at her place of employment. Many people died; however, she has no physical injuries. She appears distraught but insists that she is fine. Which of these interventions would be inappropriate?
   A. Provide her the opportunity to talk about the experience
   B. Help her connect with family and significant others
   C. Mandate that she attend a formal debriefing within 48 to 72 hours
   D. Provide information about support systems she can access later

See Test Your Knowledge answers in Appendix B.

EXPLORE 🌐 MEDIALINK

Interactive resources and an audio glossary for this chapter can be found on the Companion Website at http://www.prenhall.com/langan. Click on Chapter 4 to select the activities for this chapter.

REFERENCES

Aguilera, D. C. (1998). *Crises intervention: Theory and methodology* (8th ed.) (pp. 32–71). St. Louis: Mosby.

American Psychiatric Association. (2000). *Diagnostic and statistical manual of mental disorders* (4th ed.). Text Revision. Washington, DC: Author.

Antai-Otong, D. (2002). Culture and traumatic events. *Journal of American Psychiatric Nurses Association, 8,* 203–208.

Antonovsky, A. (1979). *Health, stress, and coping: Perspectives in mental and physical well-being.* San Francisco: Jossey-Bass.

Antonovsky, A. (1987). *Unraveling the mystery of health: How people manage stress and stay well.* San Francisco: Jossey-Bass.

Ardta, A. (1999). Repeated sexual victimization and mental disorders in women. *Journal of Child Sexual Abuse, 7*(3), 1–17.

Asaro, M. R. (2001a). Working with homicide survivors, Part 1: Impact and sequela of murder. *Perspectives in Psychiatric Care, 37*(3), 95–101.

Asaro, M. R. (2001b). Working with adult homicide survivors, Part II: Helping family members cope with murder. *Perspectives in Psychiatric Care, 37*(4), 115–124.

Bengtsson-Tops, A., & Hansson, L. (2001). The validity of Antonovsky's sense of coherence measure in a sample of schizophrenic patients living in the community. *Journal of Advanced Nursing, 33*(4), 432–438.

Berman, H. (1999). Stories of growing up amid violence by refugee children of war and children of battered women living in Canada. *Image: Journal of Nursing Scholarship, 31*(1), 57–63.

Bisson, J. I., McFarlane, A., Rose, S. (2000). Effective treatment for PTSD: Practice guidelines from the International Society for Traumatic Stress Studies. In E. B. Foa, T. M. Keane, & M. J. Friedman (Eds.). *Psychological Debriefing* (pp. 39–59). New York: Guilford Press.

Blair, D., & Ramones, V. (1996). Understanding vicarious traumatization. *Journal of Psychosocial Nursing, 34*(11), 24–30.

Boyle, J. (2002). Emergency and disaster preparedness: Where is transcultural nursing? *Journal of Transcultural Nursing, 13*(4), 273.

Bremmer, J. et al. (1999). Neural correlates of memories of childhood sexual abuse in women with and without post-traumatic stress disorder. *American Journal of Psychiatry, 156*(11), 1787–1795.

Bryant, R. A., & Harvey, A. G. (2000). *Acute stress disorder: A handbook of theory, assessment and treatment.* Washington, DC: American Psychological Association.

Bryant, R. A., Harvey, A. G., Dang, S., Sackville, T., & Basten, C. (1998). Treatment of acute stress disorder: A comparison of cognitive-behavioral therapy and supportive counseling. *Journal of Consulting and Clinical Psychology, 66,* 862–866.

Bryant, R. A., Sackville, T., Dang, S., Moulds, M., & Guthrie, R. (1999). Treating acute stress disorder: An evaluation of cognitive behavior therapy and counseling techniques. *American Journal of Psychiatry, 156,* 1780–1786.

Burgess, A. W., Hartman, C. R., & Baker, T. (1995). Memory presentations of childhood sexual abuse. *Journal of Psychosocial Nursing and Mental Health Services, 33*(9), 9–16.

Burkle, F. M. (1996). Acute-phase mental health consequences of disasters: Implications for triage and emergency medical services. *Annals of Emergency Medicine, 28,* 119–128.

Caplan, G. (1964). *Principles of preventive psychiatry.* New York: Basic Books.

Carlson, E. B., & Dalenberg, C. J. (2000). A conceptual framework for the impact of traumatic experiences. *Trauma, Violence, and Abuse, 1,* 4–28.

Carr, V. J., Lewin, T. J., Webster, R. A., Kenardy, J. A. (1997). A synthesis of the findings from the Quake Impact Study: A two-year investigation of the psychosocial sequelae of the 1989 Newcastle earthquake. *Social Psychiatry and Psychiatric Epidemiology, 32,* 123–136.

Clark, C. (1997). Post-traumatic stress disorder: How to support healing. *American Journal of Nursing, 97*(8), 27–32.

Clod, C. (1993). Long-term consequences of childhood physical and sexual abuse. *Archives of Psychiatric Nursing, 7*(3), 163–173.

Davidhizar, R., & Shearer, R. (2002). Helping children cope with public disaster: Support given immediately after a traumatic event can counteract or even negate long-term adverse effects. *American Journal of Nursing, 102*(3), 26–33.

De Bellis, K. M. et al. (1999). Developmental traumatology: Brain development. *Biological Psychiatry, 45*(10), 1271–1284.

Dewar, A. (2003). Boosting strategies: Enhancing the self-esteem of individuals with catastrophic illnesses and injuries. *Journal of Psychosocial Nursing, 41*(3), 24–32.

Drell, M. J., Siegel, C. H., & Gaensbauer, T. J. (1993). Posttraumatic stress disorder. In C. H. Zeanah (Ed.), *Handbook of Infant Mental Health.* New York: Guilford.

Figley, C., Giel, R., Borgo, S., Briggs, S., & Harotis-Fatouros, M. (1995). Prevention and treatment of community stress: How to be a mental health expert at the time of disaster. In S. E. Hobfoll & M. W. de Vries (Eds.), *Extreme stress and communities: Impact and intervention.* London: Kluwer Academic Publishers.

Fillion, J., Clements, P., Averill, J., & Vigil, G. (2002). Talking as a primary method of peer defusing in military personnel exposed to combat trauma. *Journal of Psychosocial Nursing, 40*(8), 41–49.

Fink, S. (1967). Crisis and motivation: A theoretical model. *Archives of Physical Medicine and Rehabilitation, 48*(11), 592–597.

Fischhoff, B., Crowell, N. A., & Kipke, M. (Eds.). (1999). *Adolescent decision making: Implications for prevention programs.* Washington, DC: National Academy Press.

Flick, L., & Homan, S. (1994). Sense of coherence as a predictor of family functioning and child problems. In H. McCubbin (Ed.), *Sense of coherence and resiliency* (pp. 7–124). Madison, WI: University of Wisconsin.

Foa, E. B., Davidson, J. R. T., & Frances, A. (1999). Expert consensus guidelines series: Treatment of posttraumatic stress disorder. *Journal of Clinical Psychiatry, 60* (Suppl. 16), 4–76.

Foa, E. B., Hearst-Ikeda, D., & Perry, K. J. (1995). Evaluation of a brief cognitive-behavioral program for the prevention of chronic PTSD in recent assault victims. *Journal of Consulting and Clinical Psychology, 63,* 948–955.

Freedy, J. R., & Kilpatrick, D. G. (1994). Everything you ever wanted to know about natural disasters and mental health. *National Center for PTSD Quarterly, 4,* 6–8.

Freedy, J. R., Saladin, M. E., Kilpatrick, D. G., Resnick, H. S., & Saunders, B. E. (1994). Understanding acute psychological distress following natural disaster. *Journal of Traumatic Stress, 7,* 257–274.

Ganong, W. (1999). *Review of medical physiology* (19th ed.). Stamford, CT: Appleton and Lange.

Glaister, J., & Abel, E. (2001). Experiences of women healing from childhood sexual abuse. *Archives of Psychiatric Nursing, 15*(4), 188–194.

Green, B. L. (1993). Identifying survivors at risk: Trauma and stressors across events. In J. P. Wilson & B. Raphael (Eds.), *International handbook of traumatic stress syndromes.* New York: Plenum Press.

Green, B. L., & Lindy, J. D. (1994). Posttraumatic stress disorder in victims of disasters. *Psychiatric Clinics of North America, 17,* 301–309.

Hall, D. K. (1999). Complex PTSD/ Disorders of extreme stress in sexually abused children. *Journal of Child Sexual Abuse, 8*(4), 51–71.

Heim, C., Newport, D. J., Heit, S., Graham, Y. P., Wilcox, M., Bonsall, R. et al. (2000). Pituitary-adrenal and autonomic responses to stress in women after sexual and physical abuse in childhood. *Journal of American Medical Association, 284*(5), 592–597.

Hoff, L. (2001). *People in crisis: Clinical and public health perspectives* (5th ed.) (pp. 292–345). San Francisco: Jossey-Bass.

Hutchinson, S. (1987). Self-care and job stress. *Image: Journal of Nursing Scholarship, 19*(4), 192–196.

Ignacio, L. L., & Perlas, A. P. (1994). *From victims to survivors. Psychosocial intervention in disaster management.* Manila: UP Manila Information, Publication and Public Affairs Office (IPPAQ).

James, R. K., & Gilliland, B. E. (2001). *Crisis intervention strategies* (4th ed.). Belmont, CA: Wadsworth/Thomson Learning.

Janoff-Bulman, R. (1992). *Shattered assumptions: Toward a new psychology of trauma.* New York: Free Press.

Kavanagh, D. G. (1990). Towards a cognitive-behavioral intervention for adult grief reactions. *British Journal of Psychiatry, 157,* 373–383.

Koopman, C., Classen, C., Cardena, E., & Spiegel, D. (1995). When disaster strikes, acute stress may follow. *Journal of Traumatic Stress, 8,* 29–46.

Koren, D., Arnon, I., & Klein, E. (1999). Acute stress response and posttraumatic stress disorder in traffic accident victims: A one-year prospective, follow-up study. *American Journal of Psychiatry, 151,* 888–894.

Landsverk, S. S., & Kane, C. F. (1998). Antonovsky's sense of coherence: Theoretical basis of psychoeducation in schizophrenia. *Issues in Mental Health Nursing, 19*(5), 419–431.

Lowe, J. (2002). Cherokee self-reliance. *Journal of Transcultural Nursing, 13*(4), 287–295.

Ludin, T. (1994). The treatment of acute trauma: Posttraumatic stress disorder prevention. *Psychiatric Clinics of North America, 17,* 385–391.

Maslow, A. (1968). *Toward a psychology of being* (2nd ed.). New York: D. Van Nostrand.

Maslow, A. (1971). *The further reaches of human nature.* New York: Viking Press.

McCann, L., & Peralman, L. (1990). Vicarious traumatization: A framework for understanding the psychological effect of working with victims. *Journal of Traumatic Stress, 3,* 131–149.

McFarlane, A. C. (1987). Posttraumatic phenomena in a longitudinal study of children following natural disaster. *Journal of the American Academy of Child Adolescent Psychiatry, 26,* 764–769.

McFarlane, A. C. (1995). Stress and disaster. In S. E. Hobfoll, & M. W. de Vries (Eds.), *Extreme stress and communities: Impact and intervention.* London: Kluwer Academic Publishers.

Mitchell, J. T., & Everly, G. S. (2000). Critical incident stress management and critical incident stress debriefing: Evolutions, effects and outcomes. In B. Raphael & J. P. Wilson (Eds.). *Psychological debriefing: Theory, practice, and evidence.* Cambridge, UK: Cambridge University Press.

Motzer, S., & Stewart, B. (1996). Sense of coherence as a predictor of quality of life in persons with coronary heart disease surviving cardiac arrest. *Research in Nursing and Health, 19,* 287–298.

Murray R. B., & Zentner, J. (2001). *Health promotion strategies through the life span* (7th ed.). Upper Saddle River, NJ: Prentice Hall.

Nagata, D., & Takeshita, Y. (1998). Coping and resilience across generations. Japanese-Americans and the World War II internment. *Psychoanalytic Review, 85,* 587–613.

National Institute of Mental Health. (2002). *Mental health and mass violence: Evidence-based early psychological interventions for victims/survivors of mass violence. A workshop to reach consensus on best practices* (NIH publication no. 02-5138). Washington, DC: U.S. Government Printing Office.

Norris, F. H., Phifer, J. F., & Kaniasty, K, (1994). Individual and community reaction to the Kentucky floods; Findings from a longitudinal study of older adults. In R. J. Ursano, B. G. McCaughey & C. S. Fullerton (Eds.), *Individual and community responses to trauma and disaster: The structure of human chaos.* New York: Cambridge University Press.

North, C. S., Smith, E. M., & Spitznagel, E. L. (1997). One-year follow-up of survivors of a mass shooting. *American Journal of Psychiatry, 154,* 1696–1702.

NSW Health. (2000). *Disaster mental health response handbook: An educational resource for mental health professionals involved in disaster management.* (State Health Publication No. [CMH] 00145). Retrieved June 26, 2003 http://www.nswiop.nsw.edu.au/Resources/Disaster_Handbook.pdf

Parkes, C. M., & Weiss, R. S. (1983). *Recovery from bereavement.* New York: Basic Books.

Pennebaker, J.W. (1997). *Opening up: The healing power of expressing emotions.* New York: The Guilford Press.

Rand, M. (2002). What is somatic attunement? *Annals of American Psychotherapy Association, 5*(6), 30.

Rando, T. A. (1984). *Grief, dying, and death: Clinical interventions for caregivers.* Champaign: Illinois Research Press.

Raphael, B. (1986). *When disaster strikes.* New York: Basic Books.

Raphael, B. (1993). *Disaster management. National Health and Medical Research Council publication.* Canberra: Australian Government Publishing Service.

Raphael, B. (1996). Social re-integration and political action. In E. L. Giller & L. Weisaeth (Eds.) *Post-traumatic stress disorder.* London: Bailliere Tindall.

Raphael, B., & Martinek, N. (1997). Assessing traumatic bereavement and posttraumatic stress disorder. In J. P. Wilson & T. M. Keane (Eds.), *Assessing trauma and PTSD.* New York: The Guilford Press.

Raphael, B., & Minkov, C. (1999). Abnormal grief. *Current Opinion in Psychiatry, 12,* 99–102.

Raphael, B., & Wilson, J. P. (2000). *Psychological debriefing: Theory, practice, and evidence.* Cambridge, UK: Cambridge University Press.

Riggs, D. S., Rothbaum, B. O., & Foa, E. B. (1995). A prospective examination of symptoms of posttraumatic stress disorder in victims of nonsexual assault. *Journal of Interpersonal Violence, 10,* 201–213.

Rose, S., & Bisson, J. (1998). Brief early psychological interventions following trauma: A systematic review of the literature. *Journal of Traumatic Stress, 11,* 697–710.

Roth, S., Newman, E., Pelcovitz, D., van der Kolk, B., & Mandel, F. S. (1997). Complex PTSD in victims exposed to sexual and physical abuse: Results from the DSM-IV field trial for posttraumatic stress disorder. *Journal of Traumatic Stress, 10,* 539–555.

Sack, W. H. (1998). Multiple forms of stress in refugee and immigrant children. *Child and Adolescent Psychiatric Clinics of North America, 2,* 153–167.

Schiraldi, G. R. (2000). *The post-traumatic stress disorder source book: A guide to healing, recovery, and growth.* Los Angeles: Lowell House.

Selye, H. (1965). Stress syndrome. *American Journal of Nursing, 65*(3), 97–99.

Selye, H. (1980). The stress concept today. In I. C. Kutash and L. B. Schlesinger (Eds.), *Handbook on stress and anxiety* (pp. 127–144). New York: Jossey Bass.

Singh, B.S., & Raphael, B. (1981). Postdisaster morbidity of the bereaved: A possible role for preventive psychiatry. *Journal of Nervous and Mental Disease, 169,* 203–212.

Solomon, S. D. (1999). Interventions for acute trauma response. *Current Opinion in Psychiatry, 12,* 175–180.

Solomon, Z., & Benbenishty, R. (1986). The role of proximity, immediacy, and expectancy in frontline treatment of combat stress reaction among Israelis in the Lebanon War. *American Journal of Psychiatry, 143,* 613–617.

Spector, R. (2002). *Cultural diversity in health and illness* (5th ed.). Upper Saddle River, NJ: Prentice Hall.

Taylor, S. J. W., & Frazer, A. G. (1981). The stress of post-disaster body handling and victim identification. *Journal of Human Stress, 8,* 4–12.

Ursano, R. J., Fullerton, C. S., Vance, K., & Wang, L. (2000). Debriefing: Its role in the spectrum of prevention and acute management of psychological trauma. In B. Raphael & J. P. Wilson (Eds.), *Psychological debriefing: Theory, practice, evidence.* Cambridge, UK: Cambridge University Press.

Ursano, R. J., Grieger, T. A., & McCarroll, J. E. (1996). Prevention of posttraumatic stress: Consultation, training, and early treatment. In B. van der Kolk, A. McFarlane, & L. Weisaeth (Eds.), *Traumatic stress: The effects of overwhelming experience on mind, body, and society* (pp.441–462). New York: Guilford.

Valente, S. (2000). Controversies and challenges of ritual abuse. *Journal of Psychosocial Nursing, 18*(11), 8–17.

Weaver, J. D. (1995). *Disasters: Mental health interventions.* Sarasota, FL: Professional Resource Exchange.

Weinstein, M. (2003, Spring). Terrorism and our children. *Annals of American Psychological Association,* p. 38.

Weisaeth, L. (1994). Technological disasters: Psychological and psychiatric effects. In R. Ursano, B. McCaughey, & C. Fullerton, (Eds.), *Individual and community responses to trauma and disaster: The structure of human chaos.* London: Cambridge University Press.

Zook, R. (1998). Learning how to use positive defense mechanisms. *American Journal of Nursing, 98*(3), 16B–16H.

CHAPTER 5

Preparing Nursing Administrators, Faculty, and Students for Disasters

Joanne C. Langan, Vered Kater, and Ayala Aharoni

LEARNING OBJECTIVES

1. Discuss the necessity of nursing administrator, faculty, and student involvement in nursing's disaster preparation and response.
2. Identify the roles of nursing education and service administrators, faculty, and students before, during, and after emergency and disaster events.
3. Create a checklist of activities or questions to determine the organization's readiness for disaster response.
4. Apply evaluation criteria, specific to the organization's goals and objectives, to emergency and disaster response plans, policies, and procedures.

MEDIALINK www.prenhall.com/langan

Resources for this chapter can be found on the Companion Website at http://www.prenhall.com/langan. Click on Chapter 5 to select the activities for this chapter.

CHAPTER OUTLINE

Know Your Terms
Audio Glossary
Web Links
    Evacuation Resources
    School Resources
MediaLink Applications

GLOSSARY

American Hospital Association (AHA). The AHA leads, represents, and serves hospitals, health systems, and other related organizations that are accountable to the community and committed to health improvement. Their mission is to advance the health of individuals and communities

American Organization of Nurse Executives (AONE). Founded in 1967, the AONE is a subsidiary of the American Hospital Association. It is a national organization of nearly 4,000 nurses who design, facilitate, and manage care. Its mission is to represent nurse leaders who improve health care

Bioterrorism/disaster preparedness policy. A statement or description of actions, roles, and expectations of administrators, faculty, staff, students, and volunteers related to bioterrorism or disaster events

Hospital emergency mutual aid memorandum of understanding. Procedure describing how hospitals will share workers during a disaster, in the event that some workers may be unable to reach their primary place of employment

International Nursing Coalition for Mass Casualty Education (INCMCE). The purpose is to facilitate the systematic development of policies related to mass casualty events as they influence the public health infrastructure and impact on nursing practice, education, research, and regulation. It is coordinated by Vanderbilt University School of Nursing. It was founded in response to recognition of the need for nurses to be more adequately prepared to respond to mass casualty events

Joint Commission on the Accreditation of Healthcare Organizations (JCAHO). Evaluates and accredits more than 16,000 health care organizations and programs in the United States. An independent, not-for-profit organization, JCAHO is the nation's predominant standards-setting and accrediting body in health care

MedComm. The St. Louis Region Metropolitan Medical Response System's medical emergency operations center, a central point of information and control in a disaster

Memorandum of Understanding (MOU)/ Memorandum of Agreement (MOA). A type of contract, a voluntary agreement between two or more agencies

St. Louis Region Metropolitan Medical Response System (SLMMRS). One of the Metropolitan Medical Response Systems created for the greater St. Louis region so that in the event of a significant incident such as a terrorist act, natural disaster, public health crisis, or mass casualty, there is no hesitation in providing an integrated, coordinated response of local law enforcement, fire, rescue, HAZMAT, EMS, hospital, public health, dispatch, media, and other health and response entities that provide critical first response capabilities

INTRODUCTION

While health care agency administrators are greatly concerned about their ability to provide timely access to non-emergency as well as emergency services on a "normal," daily basis, they are gravely concerned about their ability to provide essential services during a response to mass casualty events. Some of the solutions offered to alleviate the impact of the nursing shortage in times of disaster include the recruitment of inactive licensed nurses, nurse administrators, educators, and nursing students. These nurses and students could prove to be valuable and effective in getting mass numbers of citizens immunized or to assist in disaster response efforts such as in the decontamination area, in the event of a mass casualty disaster.

Specific competencies for emergency and disaster preparedness for nurses were outlined in Chapter 1. Additional core competencies specific to nurses who have formal managerial or formal leadership responsibilities will be discussed in this chapter, as well as assessment strategies and suggestions for policy to assist education and service administrators as well as faculty and students to be better prepared for disasters.

Representatives of the American Hospital Association (AHA) and the American Organization of Nurse Executives (AONE) wrote a letter dated June 10, 2003, to the Honorable Michael Capuano of the U.S. House of Representatives. The letter focused on the impact of the escalating nursing shortage. The following is an excerpt of the letter.

Hospitals and health care facilities across America are experiencing a critical shortage of nurses. Over the past five years, enrollments in nursing programs have declined and this trend is expected to continue for the foreseeable future. The average age of a working registered nurse is 43 years old, and is expected to continue to increase before peaking at age 45.5 in 2010, when many RNs will begin to retire. The need for nurses will be further compounded by the potential health care demands of the looming 78 million aging "baby boomers" who also will begin to retire in 2010.

The current nursing shortage is creating an environment with the potential to jeopardize hospitals' ability to provide timely access to non-emergency as well as emergency services. An inadequate number and mix of personnel has forced some facilities to close beds, put emergency rooms on "divert" status, delay elective surgeries, and curtail hospital services. (Pollack & Thompson, 2003)

This situation places hospitals and other agencies in a precarious position. If a facility cannot maintain nonemergency capabilities, how will it fare in times of crisis? Nurse administrators, faculty, and students are in an ideal position to make a contribution during a mass casualty event. However, these nurses and students need to know what is expected of them and be educated in specific skills required to assist appropriately.

ADMINISTRATORS

Emergency and disaster preparedness core competencies for nurses were identified in Chapter 1. Additional core competencies exist that should be of special interest to those who have formal managerial or leadership responsibilities (Gebbie & Qureshi, 2002). The core competencies for administrators are as follows:

1. Ensure that there is a written plan for major categories of emergencies.
2. Ensure that all parts of the emergency plan are practiced regularly.
3. Ensure that identified gaps in knowledge or skills are filled. (p. 51)

It is the responsibility of the nurse administrator to be sure that each unit for which he or she is responsible has a written emergency and disaster plan. The plan will have specific duties for each level of the organization. For example, the nurse representative on the agency's emergency preparedness committee needs to communicate whether the plan is feasible for individual units, departments, or the overall organization. Organizational structures such as flat, centralized, and decentralized will have great bearing on how the plan looks and is implemented. The plan must also be compatible with the plan in the community where the agency is located.

Disaster plans are most effective when they are practiced on a regular basis, critiqued, modified, and practiced again. As previously cited, approximately 20 drills are held in hospitals each year in Israel. In the United States, the Joint Commission on the Accreditation of Healthcare Organizations (JCAHO) requires annual emergency management drills. This requirement provides an impetus to review the disaster plan and conduct the exercises regularly, yet one drill per year is not enough. When a disaster occurs, the responders must react automatically. Response activities should be swift and accurate, and repeated drills are necessary to achieve optimum implementation.

Debriefing following a drill or emergency response is important to achieve an effective disaster response plan. Though plans and procedures may look acceptable in a written disaster plan, they may not execute well. If the procedures did not execute well in a drill, they may be more harmful than beneficial during an actual disaster.

Assessment of Needs

Assessment, the first step in the nursing process, begins with gathering information about clients. The needs of institutions regarding disaster preparedness should be assessed regularly. Begin by asking key questions.

1. Does your agency have a disaster preparedness team or task force?
2. Is there a disaster preparedness policy?
3. Where is the policy located?
4. Do all persons to whom the policy refers have access to the policy?
5. What is the schedule of review and update of policy?
6. Does the policy call for mock disaster exercises?
7. Who creates the exercises?
8. How often are the exercises practiced?
9. Who reviews the exercises after they have been conducted?
10. To whom are modifications recommended?
11. Is there a budget component? Does the agency's financial officer have monies earmarked for disaster preparedness?
12. What kind of budget do you need?
13. What supplies and equipment are required to be prepared?
14. What other agencies are partners in your disaster policy? For example, if you are a school of nursing, do you have a fire department, security/police station or hospital in close proximity to your school?
15. What is your communication system?
16. Who calls whom in the event of a disaster?
17. Where do you report in the event of a natural or terror related disaster?
18. Is there a specified meeting place outside of the building where you work where you are to meet (such as in the event of a fire)? See Figure 5–1.
19. How do you account for numbers of persons outside of the building if you do not know how many entered the building?
20. Is there a disaster "go" box containing the building occupants' emergency information?
21. Who is designated to update the information in the "go" box and to carry it out of the building?
22. Who has the power to make decisions? Is decision-making authority transferable during times of disaster? To whom may this authority be transferred?

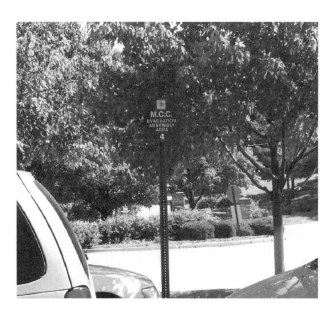

Figure 5–1. Sign designating meeting place in case of evacuation.

If the leadership within an organization is unable to answer these questions, a disaster planning committee may be charged with creating a disaster plan and policies. As the above questions are answered, additional issues may arise. Do not hesitate to involve experts from the community. There are many tools available to assist organizations with assessment, planning, exercises, and evaluation. Some of these tools are discussed in Chapter 2.

Langan (2003) found that clinical agencies often assume that schools of nursing have policies in place regarding both clinical faculty and nursing student behaviors and activities covering most instances. Schools of nursing assume that the clinical agencies have distinct policies regarding clinical faculty and nursing students. The research study suggests that both agencies and schools of nursing are partially correct. Communication among schools and agencies is often inconsistent. Expectations among administrators, faculty and students may be unknown or ambiguous. Lack of clear communication and delineation of expectations were cited as major factors in perceived role problems. This ambiguity of expectations would wreak havoc in an emergency or disaster situation where clinical agencies, faculty, and students must work together effectively and efficiently in a rapid response.

SCHOOLS OF NURSING: ADMINISTRATION, FACULTY, STAFF AND STUDENTS

On September 11, 2001, it became apparent that schools of nursing needed disaster preparedness plans or at least some type of policy. It may be unclear in schools of nursing what the roles of clinical nursing faculty, nursing students, or faculty in general would be in the clinical agencies or in the community in the event of a mass casualty event. Preliminary informal surveys with hospitals found that most hospitals would expect the faculty members and students to remain in the facility and assist in the care of disaster victims. The author sent an informal e-mail survey to 47 schools of nursing within the United States and posed the question, "Do you have a disaster policy in place that addresses what is to be done if a disaster occurs in the community where students and faculty members are in clinical agencies?" Additionally, schools were asked to share the policy if one existed. Of the 47 schools questioned, 14 responded. Eight schools responded that they had no policy. Some schools of nursing were working toward a written policy, but had only verbal instructions at the time of the query.

One respondent stated that the faculty and students would defer to the agency disaster plans in which the faculty and students were working. It is unknown whether those agencies mention faculty and students in their plans. Faculty and students are instructed to "Do what the employees do." Another stated that staying in the agency and providing assistance would be acceptable, but there was no written policy. However, there was a disaster planning committee in the

school. A third stated that there was no policy regarding students, but as faculty and employees teaching in a program associated with a health care system, the faculty members are instructed to report to the nearest health care facility and to stay and assist as directed. An interesting reply came from a fourth school of nursing; the school responder admitted there was no official written policy on the subject, however, when their nursing students are in clinical practicum experiences out of the country, they are instructed to carry their passports with them and to meet at the American embassy in the event of a disaster or emergency. Following a conversation with its legal department, another school stated that it had a disaster plan for students, faculty, and staff for on-campus and external disasters. External disasters were described as natural disasters such as tornadoes. When students are in the community engaging in clinical experiences, they are to defer to the agency's disaster plan. There was some confusion about what the students would do if they were out of state or out of the country for additional school-related experiences. The final school reported having no policy for disaster preparedness for faculty and students, but faculty and students would follow the hospital policy if a disaster should occur while the students are in clinical. This school had developed some internal policies regarding document preservation and storage offsite, in the case of a disaster, so that records would be preserved. Additionally, the school has a policy to copy each form or document on backup tapes or discs offsite in the case of a disaster.

These communications suggest that the schools are interested in language development for a policy regarding expectations of clinical faculty and nursing students in clinical agencies during disaster events. Most appreciated the discussions that were generated as a result of the query. It was surprising to find that documents were being preserved in the event of a catastrophe through policy, but human lives and actions were not addressed. Hopefully, ongoing discussions will be prompted among nursing service and education facilities.

Review of Contracts Between Agencies (Memoranda of Agreement)

It is recommended that both the clinical agency and the school of nursing review the memoranda of agreement or contracts shared between the entities. When reviewing the contracts, seek answers for the following questions:

1. Is there any language in the contracts that indicates behaviors that are expected of either the clinical nursing faculty or students?
2. What are the expectations of agency employees?
3. Is there a difference in expectations among professional and nonprofessional staff?
4. What policy is to be followed if the clinical faculty member is both an employee of the clinical agency and an employee of the school of nursing?

5. Are the expectations of both agencies compatible?
6. Must the clinical nursing faculty member choose between the school and agency when deciding which action to take?
7. What policy is to be followed if the nursing student is an employee of the clinical agency but is at the agency in a student role at the time of a disaster?
8. Does the school of nursing have different expectations for different categories of employees? For example, are clinical faculty expected to react to a disaster event differently than nonclinical faculty?
9. What are the staff persons to do in the event of a disaster?
10. What are the students, faculty members, and administrators expected to do if a disaster occurs in the school's community? Are they to stay in the building, evacuate to a specified location, or report to the nearest hospital to assist, or go home if feasible?
11. Who is to communicate directions in the event of a disaster and how will communications be achieved?

Request the assistance of the institution's or academic counsel to amend the contracts, if necessary, to include language that addresses the issue of emergency and disaster preparedness. Policies created regarding disaster preparedness should address the best interest and safety of all involved. The contracts among agencies are a start; the policies and procedures developed by the agencies will address specific issues and actions.

Development, Implementation, and Evaluation of Policies and Procedures

If there is no specific language in the memoranda of agreement or contracts between the school of nursing and the clinical agencies regarding disaster preparedness, then the schools must develop policies and procedures and share them with the agencies. Or, the agencies should develop the policies and share them with the schools prior to each semester. All parties must be clear about expectations prior to the commencement of each semester. This is essential as there is no time for debate or discussion once a disaster hits.

Schools of nursing must decide among several scenarios in choosing a disaster policy regarding clinical faculty and nursing students in various clinical agencies.

1. The school of nursing may choose to have all clinical faculty and students leave the clinical agencies and return to the school campus's designated area.
2. If the agency wishes the faculty and students to stay in the facility to assist with disaster victims, appropriate training must be provided during orientation.
3. If the agency wishes the faculty and students to leave, the faculty and students will receive evacuation details during orientation.
4. If the disaster directly affects the clinical agency and faculty members or students are injured, it must be determined whether the agency will be responsible for emergency medical attention and subsequent care, if necessary.
5. Determine whether the faculty and students, as individuals, have the right to refuse to assist in disaster relief at the assigned clinical agency.
6. Determine the method of informing students' parents, spouses, etc. of the policy and how they may obtain information regarding students' activities and status.
7. Determine the students' obligations to the agency should they be employees of the agency.
8. Determine faculty members' obligations to the agency should they be part-time employees of the agency.

See Box 5–1 for a sample bioterrorism/disaster preparedness policy. This language may be used as a template or the language may be modified to best suit the needs of specific schools and/or agencies.

BOX 5–1   Bioterrorism/Disaster Preparedness Policy

This memorandum addresses the appropriate steps "School of Nursing" faculty and students should take in the event that they are engaged in clinical activities at an external health care facility or agency during a natural or terror-related disaster. More precisely, this memorandum addresses whether such faculty and students should remain at the facility or agency in order to assist in responding to the disaster or should leave the facility.

As a general principle, the affiliation agreement between "Your School" and the facility or agency will require that faculty and students follow the policies of the facility or agency that address the appropriate response to such disasters. In such cases, faculty and students should follow the facility or agency policies. Confusion arises, however, when the disaster response policy of the facility or agency does not specifically address the actions that are required of faculty and students. In order to avoid such confusion, this [legal] office recommends proactively addressing this issue with each facility or agency affiliated with "School of Nursing." Such proactive steps will help to mitigate the scope of the confusion that will undoubtedly occur in the event of such a disaster.

Expectations of Clinical Agencies During Disasters:
For Staff Nurses:

For Clinical Faculty:

For Students:

For Professional and Non-Professional Staff:

Expectations of Schools of Nursing During Disasters:
For Clinical Faculty:

For Non-Clinical Faculty:

For Students:

For Staff:

Figure 5–2. Clinical agency and school of nursing exercise.

The expectations of the clinical faculty, nonclinical faculty, staff, and students must be communicated to the students, staff, faculty, and clinical agencies. Additionally, significant others, parents, and family members need the information so that they will understand what is taking place in the event of a disaster in the school's community.

Figure 5–2 shows an exercise that clinical agencies and schools of nursing may discuss in communicating expectations among agency and school personnel and students.

Following the determination of expectations and roles in disaster relief activities in both clinical agencies and schools of nursing, the use of Figure 5–3 is suggested. The school of nursing may use this form as a means of proac-

SAINT LOUIS UNIVERSITY
SCHOOL OF NURSING
BIOTERRORISM/DISASTER PREPAREDNESS PROCEDURE

SEMESTER: _____   DATE: _____

FACULTY: _____

COURSE #/NAME: _____

CLINICAL AGENCY: _____

NAME(S) OF STUDENT(S) PLACED IN AGENCY:

_____   _____

_____   _____

_____   _____

_____   _____

TECHNOLOGIES/SKILLS:

In the event that you are engaged in clinical activities at an external health care facility or agency during a natural or terror related disaster, the health care facility expects the clinical faculty member and students to:

_____

_____

_____

_____

Figure 5–3. Bioterrorism/disaster preparedness procedure.

tively determining what actions should be taken by both clinical faculty and students during and following a natural or terror related disaster. The procedure must also consider actions to be taken by faculty and students working in community settings, including rural areas.

A review of the current policies and procedures must be scheduled on a regular basis. The disaster preparedness committee must schedule meetings with a review of the policies and procedures on the agenda. Outdated or obsolete directives are distracting at a minimum and can have devastating results in a true disaster.

Disaster Nursing Curriculum

Disaster nursing should be a required content for all nursing students at both undergraduate and graduate levels. The International Nursing Coalition for Mass Casualty Education (INCMCE) distributed an electronic survey to schools of nursing to determine the types of content and instruction that have been offered since 2000 specific to disaster preparedness. Efforts such as this will assist schools in pooling resources and increasing awareness for additional curriculum and instruction efforts in disaster preparedness.

NURSING VIGNETTE 5–1   Israeli Faculty and Student Activity in Disaster Response

Vered Kater, RN

A wedding hall collapsed in Jerusalem, and about 600 persons were injured. I was in Tel Aviv at the time. It was 11:00 P.M., but I went right to the emergency room of the hospital. I am not an ER nurse, but I went to help anyway as most of the nurses do. Several students walked in; they might have been working elsewhere in the hospital. They asked, "What can we do?" I told one to prepare IV solutions, and another to draw up medicines. My directions were very concrete. I gave them very limited, specific directions until they calmed down. That helped them cope and perform better.

Usually, a single nurse is assigned to a sick bay. A nursing student may be assigned to work with that nurse and take vital signs every 15 minutes, or start an IV, if qualified to do so. The students may not give medicines without their faculty member present. The faculty maintain responsibility for the students. They must follow the protocols, A-B-C, A-B-C, as if on automatic pilot. Everyone is important in the disaster response. Even the kitchen staff pitch in and bring trolleys of water, coffee, tea, and sandwiches.

Afterwards, we talked. The students appreciated the short, clear, concrete directions. I gave them a lot of positive stroking. That always helps.

At the George Mason University College of Nursing and Health Science, Dr. Charlene Douglas incorporates an in-class disaster management exercise as part of her community health and epidemiology class. The earthquake in Kobe, Japan, is used to determine immediate priorities, and priorities 8, 24, and 72 hours after impact. Students complete a community assessment tool from their clinical section of the course using information reported on the earthquake (Douglas, 2002). This type of exercise strengthens students' abilities to be effective volunteers in disaster response efforts.

See Box 5–2 for a disaster nursing curriculum outline from the Henrietta Szold Hadassah-Hebrew University School Of Nursing.

STUDENT NURSE VOLUNTEERS IN THE AMERICAN RED CROSS

The American Red Cross has a formal program in place to prepare nursing students as volunteers, before they receive their nursing license. Schools of nursing may wish to review what the ARC proposes in its program to augment public health nursing curriculum. The ARC suggests that during a disaster, whether natural or man made, nursing students can be valuable to the recovery of a stricken community. See Nursing Vignette 5–1. Areas in which nursing students can assist are as follows:

1. Blood, organ, and tissue collection
2. In health and safety services as leaders or project managers
3. As direct providers of services in health and safety educational courses: first aid; CPR; HIV/AIDS education; nurse assistant training; Healthy Pregnancy, Healthy Baby; basic aid

training (BAT); First Aid for Children Today (FACT); and water safety.

4. In health promotion and disease prevention, to help coordinate or administer immunization programs, blood pressure screening, health monitoring programs, and first aid teams
5. As participants in chapter health project planning committees to provide counseling and referrals (American Red Cross, 1995)

To accomplish these tasks, the ARC provides disaster nursing information and educational opportunities. While this education would be a necessity for students participating in the volunteer program, it would also be helpful for nursing faculty to be aware of appropriate actions to take in a disaster. One ARC program available to nursing faculty is called, "Preparing for the Unexpected." It deals with planning for disasters, family disaster kits, escape routes, and necessary items to have on hand in any emergency (S. Shorkley, personal communication, April 8, 2003).

If a disaster of sufficient magnitude occurred in the community and there was a need for additional Disaster Health Services support, the local ARC chapter would notify the school of nursing. The school of nursing would then notify the nursing students who have completed the preparation courses of the volunteer opportunities available with the Disaster Health Services and advise them how to access their local chapter of the ARC. A "letter of cooperation" would outline the expectations of the school of nursing and the local chapter of the ARC (D. Wallace, personal communication, April 8, 2003).

This valuable experience and opportunity could be rewarded with clinical hours granted to the students. The content covered in the educational offerings is a definite fit in the public health nursing curriculum and would assist in

BOX 5–2   Disaster Nursing: An Outline of a Curriculum and Considerations in Training Nurses in Hadassah

Ayala Aharoni RN, BA. MPH., ICU
Coordinator of Emergency Nursing Training
Henrietta Szold Hadassah
Hebrew University School Of Nursing

In recent years Israeli hospitals have been treating a large number of victims of terrorism. We have been exposed to a variety of traumas and injuries including many of the multi-trauma types such as blast injuries. We have also received numerous patients with shock traumas but no physical injuries. Such traumas change the lives of the victims, their families, and society. The exposure to these traumas also leaves scars on the professional and personal lives of the nurses.

The training needs of a "regular" nurse are different than those of a trauma nurse. However, too often "regular nurses" have to face and handle cases of trauma. This is why we include units about trauma in the education of all nurses.

Every nursing student takes a trauma course in the last year of study. We are also designing an advanced trauma course to be offered in the future. What should be included in the preparation of a nurse to handle traumas? In addition to expanding the knowledge of injuries and physical damage, we prepare the nurse for unique Israeli difficulties. In the following, I present some of the major training needs of nurses to handle trauma more effectively, and the curriculum outline for satisfying these needs.

Training needs for better handling of major traumas after a terror attack include

1. The need to increase the nurse's ability to function while under heightened tension, both internal and external, due to possible increased friction among colleagues.
2. The need to instill ethical rules for nurses, despite their ambivalence, to treat all patients of a terror attack regardless of their national identity, e.g. when:
   A. The nurse is Jewish and the injured is Arab, and the suicide bomber was also an Arab;
   B. The nurse is Jewish and has to prioritize treatment of two patients, one Arab and one Jewish;
   C. The nurse is Arab, surrounded by Jewish victims of an Arab bomber;
   D. The nurse must care for a patient who might actually have been the terrorist.
3. The need to handle the nurse's personal fears, often, in cases of a terrorist attack, the nurse is expected to function while worrying about her family members who might have been on the scene of the attack.

Rationale and considerations

1. **Stress and capacity to handle it.** In training nurses for "normal" situations, we emphasize order, procedures, and caring for details. However, terror attacks create havoc. Communications with colleagues and patients are complex, often unclear, and thus put the student nurse in very stressful situations. We have to prepare the students for functioning in situations of uncertainty, when there is no one to comfort them. Instead, the student nurses have to comfort others while not knowing the full extent of the event.
2. **Treating with disregard to the national identity of the patient.** The major ingredient in the current conflict in the Middle East is the definition of national identity. Too often the feelings of each side of the conflict are "We" against "Them." It is so common, unfortunately, to generalize. Each side tends to hate all who belong to the "other" side. Against this background, the student nurses have to treat people who belong to the "Them." We try to instill in our students the values and codes of nursing—placing these values above and before any definition of national identity of the patient.

   At the same time, we work hard on advocating mutual respect among the student nurses; Jewish, Christian, and Arab students study together and work together even in cases of terror attacks to help the victim. Our clear message to all of the students is that the national identity of the patient is completely irrelevant; we help all regardless of who they are.
3. **Relatives of the student nurses might be among the victims.** This is often the fear of the nurses and a major cause for stress. We cannot do much about it, but try to improve information channels. We allow them to open cellular phones, and try to bolster their sense of responsibility to give the proper attention to those they treat, even when they themselves are engulfed by fear of the situation.

From concepts to a curriculum

A. Educational considerations
   The following are some of the questions we asked ourselves during the curriculum design:
   1. What are the skills the nurse has to acquire in order to handle various traumas?
   2. How do we prepare the nurses for the mental challenges in handling traumas? (e.g. how to deal

(continued)

BOX 5–2   (continued)

with stress, how to be able to 'detach' from the horror in order to function?)

3. How do we prepare nurses to function on the scene without consideration of the national identity of the victim?

4. What is the role of the teacher supervising nursing students while a traumatic event takes place?

5. How do the teachers evaluate the performance of their students in a real traumatic event?

6. What is the psychological/social help student nurses need before and after handling cases of trauma?

B. Content

The basic trauma curriculum of the last year of school studies included, among others, the following:

Handling of various injuries, treating patients with head, chest and other injuries who are in shock, victims of non-conventional injuries (gases, etc.), and catering to the mental needs of trauma patients. We utilized exercise and role-playing and emphasized the importance of the nurses' functioning in such traumatic events.

We have started to prepare the students for emergency situations, when regular functioning structures and routines are disturbed or gone. They learn how to discharge patients from the emergency room in order to make room for the incoming trauma victims. They learn the importance of documenting and reporting all available data. If we do not keep accurate records of emergency cases while lines of communications are disrupted, the results can be grave.

In the advanced trauma course, we plan to expand the psychological preparation of the nurses. A special emphasis is placed on communications skills. In my MA thesis I researched the quality of the communications the student nurses experience in their daily work. The findings indicate many stressful situations whereby the student nurse feels that she/he is abused and communications go sour. If this is the situation in "normal" settings, it is far worse in cases of emergency when many students experienced panic. In our advanced course, students will attend special workshops and perform simulations of positive communication skills in situations of panic and uncertainty.

We further encourage our students to be tuned in to and to respect their emotional needs, to express these needs, and not to feel that a need for help is a sign of weakness.

We are currently developing procedures, with the nursing students, for analyzing the traumatic situations they have handled or experienced. In the training, we include the sharing of emotional experiences, expression and legitimization of fear, and increasing the ability of the students to evaluate themselves without fear. We encourage peer analysis and support.

A challenge for the teachers

It is difficult for us as the teachers to assess objectively the performance of the students in real traumatic events. Hence, we constantly remind ourselves to act as role models both in the way we function in traumatic situations, and later, when we evaluate the performance of the nursing students. We have found that openness and a willingness not only to teach the students but also to learn from them make us all more open and allow all of us to grow.

Summary

The test of any educational program, including educating nurses, lies in the real world when the graduate has to handle real challenges. One can never fully prepare a nursing student for a real life major catastrophe. The reality is often more complicated than the simulation. However, based on the all too frequent traumas our nurses have endured, we sense that they have succeeded in internalizing high levels of commitment. Additionally, most of them seem to have managed to put nursing moral codes above national tensions, and most have managed to concentrate relatively well on their duties.

In all major emergencies we have experienced, students and nurses rushed to the scene or the hospital to help, even if they were not summoned. Somehow, the unfortunate plethora of terror attacks and catastrophes bolster the commitment and the "nursing fiber" of our students and nurses and make them socialize and mature faster in their chosen profession.

We, their teachers, are proud of them, but somehow wish for peaceful times when such maturity of nurses takes longer, and when there are not so many occasions for nurses to show their professional dedication in handling emergencies and traumas.

St. Louis Metropolitan Medical Response System Disaster Team

Development and Deployment of a Voluntary Health Care Worker Group Available for Inter-Hospital Work During a Disaster

Purpose: During a disaster, whether from natural causes or due to terrorist activity, it is possible for any hospital in the St. Louis region to require additional manpower. St. Louis region hospitals ("Participating Hospital") have entered into a Hospital Emergency Mutual Aid Memorandum of Understanding which describes their willingness to help each other during a disaster. The following procedure describes the process for establishing and using a mobile disaster team of health care workers in conjunction with the St. Louis Region Metropolitan Medical Response System (SLMMRS).

1. Each Participating Hospital's CEO will designate up to 25 people from their hospital who would be willing to volunteer their assistance through SLMMRS to work at another area hospital during a disaster. These would include predominantly physicians and nurses in the areas of emergency and critical care medicine and surgery. Others with special expertise (i.e. toxicology, radiation, smallpox) would also be recruited.

2. These health care professionals would complete a data collection sheet with their identification and credentialing information which would be entered into the SLMMRS database. They would then receive a badge identifying them as an SLMMRS Disaster Team Volunteer.

3. During a disaster, an affected Participating Hospital would call MedComm requesting assistance. MedComm would contact other area Participating Hospitals asking them to contact their disaster team members (or MedComm could assist in this call-up). Willing volunteers who are not needed by their home hospital would be asked to report to the recipient hospital.

4. MedComm would send a list of all possible volunteers and their basic information to the affected hospital via fax or email. The recipient hospital would verify disaster team members' identity by SLMMRS badge and the list.

5. Use, supervision and responsibility for volunteer healthcare personnel would be governed by recipient hospital's policies and procedures.

Figure 5–4. St. Louis Metropolitan Medical Response System Disaster Team MOU. *(From K. Webb, MD, Chief Medical Officer at Saint Louis University Hospital. Reprinted with permission.)*

helping the students to meet the essential disaster and emergency preparedness competencies.

ST. LOUIS REGION METROPOLITAN MEDICAL RESPONSE SYSTEM

The St. Louis Metropolitan Medical Response System (SLMMRS) is formulating plans to develop an area-wide team of health care volunteers to donate time in assisting with disaster response. This group has created a number of forms—fact and explanation sheets—to inform persons interested in this type of activity. Nursing faculty members and nursing students are invited to participate in this volunteer activity. The forms address frequently asked questions as well as legal issues. The first sheet (Figure 5–4) describes the SLMMRS need for volunteers and the Hospital Emergency Mutual Aid Memorandum of Under-standing. The procedure describes how hospitals will share workers during a disaster. This is deemed necessary as some workers may be able to reach a health care facility that is not their primary place of employment. However, they may not be able to reach their primary place of employment due to road closures, health care facility closure, and transportation difficulties (K. Webb, personal communication, June 27, 2003).

Figure 5–5 explains the step-by-step process that would be executed by hospitals in need of disaster volunteers. For example, if a hospital is in a declared state of emergency, the chief executive officer (CEO) would contact the communications center (MedComm) which organizes and dispatches disaster team members. The CEO would indicate that more nurses are needed and ask for help in contacting those volunteers. The verification process includes having an MMRS badge, which is similar to the patient tracking band with a bar code system that may be scanned.

REQUEST AND VERIFICATION
VOLUNTEER SLMMRS
DISASTER TEAM

1. Hospital should be in a declared state of emergency per Emergency Management Plan in order to utilize SLMMRS Disaster Team Volunteers.

2. The Hospital CEO or designated Incident Commander may request SLMMRS Disaster Team Volunteers by contacting MedComm.

3. This request should include the number and type of volunteers.

4. SLMMRS designates five general types of hospital volunteers as part of its Disaster Team: Physicians, Nurses, Pharmacists, other clinical personnel, and other non-clinical personnel. Each type of personnel has a separate color identity badge. Pictures of the different identity badges follow.

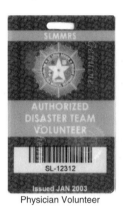 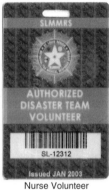  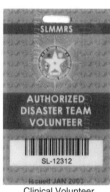 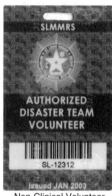

| Physician Volunteer | Nurse Volunteer | Pharmacist Volunteer | Clinical Volunteer | Non-Clinical Volunteer |

5. Disaster team personnel will report to hospital security for identity verification.

6. Disaster team personnel will present their MMRS badge and their primary hospital badge as verification of their profession and identity. If their hospital badge does not contain their picture, security should request identity verification by driver's license.

7. Security will maintain a log similar to that shown. (See Appendix C for Volunteer Log.)

8. If there are questions regarding identity of a volunteer, MedComm maintains a list of mother's maiden name for security clearance.

9. Volunteers will be issued a hospital specific temporary badge, which contains their name and profession.

10. Volunteers will be directed to the personnel pool for assignment per Emergency Management Plan.

11. Volunteers should be paired with a hospital staff member of similar specialty who would be their immediate supervisor for the period. They should not work unsupervised.

12. After the disaster, all volunteers should be credentialed according to JCAHO standards.

Figure 5–5. St. Louis Metropolitan Medical Response System volunteer form. *(From K. Webb, MD, Chief Medical Officer, Saint Louis University Hospital. Reprinted with permission, Sanjay Jain, LaserBand LLC.)*

FREQUENTLY ASKED QUESTIONS AND ANSWERS

1. **What kinds of things would I do as part of the Disaster Team?**

   Whatever you do in your regular job (scope of expertise). Your specific assignment will be determined by the hospital CEO or site commander. Your service would be in the St. Louis region only.

2. **Do I have to come if I'm called up?**

   No, you may already be working or otherwise committed, either professionally or personally. This is voluntary although the system would not be activated unless you were needed. [Family care centers are discussed in Chapter 2.]

3. **How would I be contacted?**

   St. Louis Metropolitan Medical Response System (SLMMRS) would call your primary hospital and they would contact you to see if you were available.

4. **Would I be paid?**

   No, this is a voluntary community service.

5. **How would I be identified as an authorized volunteer?**

   You'll receive a badge identifying you as a member of the SLMMRS disaster team that you could keep in your wallet or on the back of your regular badge. You also need to bring your regular hospital photo ID.

6. **Do I get any training?**

   We anticipate offering in-service training programs for selected groups.

7. **What about professional liability coverage?**

   Under Missouri law, Section 537.118 RSMO, Volunteers of a non-profit organization have limited immunity from personal liability for good faith acts or omissions of the volunteer while performing official functions on behalf of the non-profit which result in damage or injury to persons who receive services from the volunteer. SLMMRS is a non-profit organization. This is not an absolute immunity in that the statutory immunity does not apply to liability for intentional or malicious conduct or negligence.

Figure 5–6. St. Louis Metropolitan Medical Response System FAQ Sheet. *(From K. Webb, MD, Chief Medical Officer, Saint Louis University Hospital. Reprinted with permission.)*

Many questions regarding the disaster volunteer system are anticipated. The following sheet (Figure 5–6) was created to address many of these questions and concerns.

The policies and procedures outlined by the SLMMRS group are the foundation for organizing volunteer disaster responders. The system will need to be tested through drills to determine whether any steps have been missed or may be in need of modification. Other frequently asked questions are, "Can I bring my family?" and "Who will take care of my family?" Hopefully, the disaster plan

has family care provisions that will be clearly communicated with employees and volunteers.

It is only through the assistance of volunteers, specific education, practice, collaboration and a willingness to modify policies and actions that a successful response is implemented. Administrators, students, faculty, and staff are valuable assets in this concerted effort.

The following Nursing Vignette describes a system of volunteers in Israel that is very similar to the SLMMRS volunteer system for nurse faculty members and students.

NURSING VIGNETTE 5–2   Preparedness and Involvement of the Faculty in Times of Disaster at the Henrietta Szold School of Nursing, Jerusalem, Israel

In times of emergency, nursing faculty members become part of the teams that treat the injured. The nursing school is part of the Hadassah Hebrew University Hospital. Some of the faculty have university appointments while the majority are employed by the hospital. Several educators have dual appointments. They work part time on a ward and teach part time. Regardless of the way they are employed, the entire faculty is active in emergency situations. One of the hospital nurse supervisors has the task of finding the units best suited to the abilities of all Hadassah nurses, including the faculty of the school. A computerized list is distributed to all departments and to the school of nursing. This list specifies the location of each nurse in times of emergency. The placements take into consideration the education and experience of the faculty and the needs of the different units/wards.

The unit assignment list is regularly updated and all nurses know where to go and who will be the nurse in charge of their specific unit. Each faculty member receives a list with the names and phone numbers of the emergency team on which he or she will be a member.

During the year, several practice drills are held. These drills are unit specific and are announced to the team members in advance. This is to ensure maximum participation. Two types of drills clarify the way in which these drills operate. The "Family Room" team had an in-service training on the use of computers in June 2003, relevant only for that specific group. On the other hand, there are four additional emergency rooms in times of disasters. The emergency room teams practice several times each year with healthy soldiers who act as victims. These drills are vital, as they enable the nurses to work well together as a team. Coming together for drills builds a sense of cohesiveness as a team, as the team members in disasters do not have the opportunity to work together during "normal" circumstances.

During times of disasters, faculty members do not have responsibility for the students from the school of nursing, because the faculty is recruited for active nursing care and the nursing students are recruited for hospital services.

At the beginning of their nursing studies, the students are asked to volunteer in the hospital during times of disaster. In addition, they are requested to sign a statement that confirms their willingness to work in the hospital during times of need. The majority of nursing students sign this statement. Once they have signed this contract, they are put on an emergency list, similar to the list of faculty members. Each year, the lists are updated. During the first year of nursing school, many students are active in patient transport or the registration of victims. As the students' nursing skills improve, they are more involved in direct patient care. In times of emergency, the Ministry of Health grants temporary permits for these nursing students. In this way, the students are allowed to perform specific nursing actions independently, based on the years of study and their competence.

Written by Vered Kater, RN, MSN, faculty at the school, based on a lecture by and with the permission of Aviva Friedman-Kalmovitcz, RN, MA, Assistant Director at the Hadassah-Hebrew University Henrietta Szold School of Nursing, Jerusalem, Israel.

SUMMARY

Nursing administrators, educators and students are all valuable assets in any health care system. They must all work collaboratively in the disaster response effort to create timely and effective policies and procedures that will enhance the disaster response efforts of their communities. We have an obligation to be prepared for unknown future catastrophic events to enhance the ability of health care providers to save lives.

CASE STUDY

Students and Faculty Respond to Hospital Disaster

A group of 10 nursing students is working on a medical-surgical unit with their clinical faculty member. It is the summer between their junior and senior years in a four-year baccalaureate program. Just as the faculty member was concluding the post-conference session with the students, the patient care director entered the conference room and asked if anyone would be staying on the unit. The hospital received word that a tour bus had overturned on the nearby highway. The hospital expected to receive 62 injured older adults. Three of the 10 students worked as nursing assistants on the weekends at that particular hospital and immediately offered to volunteer. Two additional students stated they would volunteer as well.

1. What should the clinical faculty member do?
2. What should the five students who did not offer to stay and help do?
3. What kinds of technologies might the students be asked to perform?
4. What kinds of technologies would the students not be expected to perform?

5. Would this scenario be any different if the request for help came at 10 A.M. during a 7 A.M. to 3 P.M. clinical shift?

6. What should the nurse administrator and the clinical faculty member have discussed prior to the nursing students' first day on this unit?

TEST YOUR KNOWLEDGE

1. Which of the following statements is *not* a statement of a core competency for administrators?

   A. Ensure that every nursing student receives education to perform decontamination on disaster victims.
   B. Ensure that there is a written plan for major categories of emergencies.
   C. Ensure that all parts of the emergency plan are practiced regularly.
   D. Ensure that identified gaps in knowledge or skills are filled.

2. The needs of an organization regarding disaster preparedness should be assessed regularly.

   A. True
   B. False

3. In which of the following activities may nursing students participate if they have successfully completed the American Red Cross' formal program to prepare students as volunteers?

   A. Starting IVs at their community hospital where they work as a nurse's aide
   B. Giving insulin injections to their neighbor's child
   C. Teaching in the community center about health promotion and disease prevention
   D. Prescribing medicines for minor injuries and complaints

4. Which of the following questions would be appropriate to ask to determine an organization's readiness for disaster response?

   A. Is there a disaster preparedness policy?
   B. Does the policy call for mock disaster exercises?
   C. Who reviews the exercises after they have been conducted?
   D. What is your communication system?
   E. All of the above

5. If your agency does not have a formal written disaster policy, it is probably of no consequence because the risk of disaster in your area is very low.

   A. True
   B. False

6. If a very anxious nurse responded to the Emergency Department to assist with the treatment of victims from a mass casualty event and stated, "I don't know if I can do this, I have never worked in the ICU or the Emergency Department!" how would you respond?

   A. Speak in a reassuring voice
   B. Tell him/her that he/she will be taking vital signs every 15 minutes on a specified number of patients
   C. Assign a simple, repetitive activity initially
   D. Assign more challenging activities when the nurse calms down
   E. All of the above

7. In a mass casualty disaster response, who may be recruited in the disaster relief effort?

   A. Inactive licensed nurses
   B. Nurse administrators
   C. Nurse educators
   D. Nursing students
   E. All of the above

8. One of the goals of the International Coalition for Mass Casualty Education (INCMCE) is to

   A. Assist all registered nurses in becoming trauma specialists
   B. Discourage retired nurses from responding to calls for disaster assistance
   C. Remind registered nurses that they are few in number and cannot make a difference in disaster relief efforts
   D. Make education about mass casualty events and response free and available to all nurses

9. It is the responsibility of the nurse administrator to be sure that each unit for which he or she is responsible has a written emergency and disaster plan.

   A. True
   B. False

10. The agency administrator does *not* need to ensure that the organization's emergency and disaster plan is compatible with the plan in the community where the agency is located.

    A. True
    B. False

See Test Your Knowledge Answers in Appendix B.

EXPLORE MEDIALINK

Interactive resources and an audio glossary for this chapter can be found on the Companion Website at http://www.prenhall.com/langan. Click on Chapter 5 to select the activities for this chapter.

REFERENCES

American Red Cross. (1995). *Student nurse volunteers in the American Red Cross: Nursing as you dreamed it would be.* Washington, DC: Author.

Conway-Welch, C. (2002). Nurses and mass casualty management: Filling an educational gap. *Policy, politics, and Nursing Practice, 3*(4), 289–293.

Douglas, C. Y. (2002). Disaster management in community health. *George Mason University College of Nursing and Health Science Dimensions, 9,* 5.

Gebbie, K. M., & Qureshi, K. (2002). Emergency and disaster preparedness: Core competencies for nurses: What every nurse should but may not know. *American Journal of Nursing, 102,* 46–51.

Institute of Medicine National Research Council. (1998). *Improving civilian medical response to chemical or biological terrorist incidents: Interim report on current capabilities.* Washington, DC: National Academy Press.

Langan, J. C. (2003). Faculty practice and roles of staff nurses and clinical faculty in nursing student learning. *Journal of Professional Nursing, 19*(2), 76–84.

Pollack, R., & Thompson, P. (2003). *Letter to the Honorable Michael Capuano, U.S. House of Representatives, Washington, DC.* Retrieved June 14, 2003 from http://www.hospitalconnect.com/aone/docs/fletcher_capuano.doc

CHAPTER 6

Preparing Staff and Inactive Registered Nurses to Manage Casualties

Dotti C. James, Joanne C. Langan, Helen Sandkuhl, and Julie Benbenishty

LEARNING OBJECTIVES

1. Discuss the responsibilities of the organizations charged with preparing the United States for mass casualty events.
2. Differentiate between traditional triage and triage following a mass casualty event.
3. Identify the core competencies necessary for effective and efficient management of large numbers of casualties.
4. Discuss ways of minimizing obstacles to assessing and treating efficiently.
5. Explore methods for determining the number and types of casualties to be expected following a disaster.
6. Analyze the logistics of decontaminating mass numbers of disaster victims, ambulatory and non-ambulatory.
7. Discuss the most common types of injuries following terrorist bombings and key assessment parameters for each.
8. Explore ways of identifying and tracking victims after they enter the health care system.
9. Discuss methods of recruiting and caring for agency and inactive registered nurses needed during a disaster response effort.

MEDIALINK www.prenhall.com/langan

Resources for this chapter can be found on the Companion Website at http://www.prenhall.com/langan. Click on Chapter 6 to select the activities for this chapter.

CHAPTER OUTLINE

Know Your Terms
Audio Glossary
Web Link
    Emergency Preparedness and Response Resources
MediaLink Applications
    Role Play: Receiving MCE Victims at Your Hospital

GLOSSARY

Core competencies. The basic skills for effectively handling a disaster

Decontamination. The process of removing pathogenic organisms, chemical agents, or radioactive substances from persons or objects

95

Primary blast injury. Injury sustained from a high-order explosive affecting primarily gas-filled structures such as lungs, GI tract, and tympanic membrane

Quaternary blast injury. Injuries not encompassed by other blast injury categories, such as burns, respiratory, and cardiac complications

Secondary blast injury. Injury resulting from flying debris and bomb fragments

Shock. Lowered blood pressure due to peripheral vasoconstriction as the body attempts to compensate for circulatory fluid loss. May result from loss of blood, disruption of autonomic nervous system control over vasoconstriction, inadequate cardiac function, or exposure to a substance to which the victim is sensitive

Tertiary blast injury. Injury resulting from individuals being thrown by the blast wind

Triage. A continuous process of sorting or assigning and reassigning treatment priorities for victims

INTRODUCTION

Prior to September 11, 2001 widespread disasters in the United States were limited to natural disasters, with the exception of the Oklahoma City bombing. Following 9-11, the United States embarked on a serious reorganization of emergency services coordination and preparation.

In the last twenty years, the United States has seen dangers escalate. Industrial disasters are increasing due to the increased scale and lethal potential of industry. Deliberate disasters are escalating because of unrest worldwide, the presence of terrorist cells in the United States, and the availability and lethality of chemical, biological, and nuclear weapons. Even though these threats have been in existence for decades, the overall threat to our nation is growing. The question is, will nurses know how to care for survivors? If chemical agents, biological agents, or a radiation event occur, will receiving hospitals have the capacity to safely respond? Emergency departments will become the front line for emergency care and disaster response. Nurses, as the largest body of health care providers, must take an active role in preparation activities for mass disasters. To be effective in that role, nurses must understand the current state of ED, hospital, and agency functioning in order to develop a realistic and effective plan for disasters.

The emergency department (ED) is unique from other hospital departments in that it is open 24 hours a day, provides unplanned and unscheduled care, and has an uncontrolled environment in which the doors cannot be closed when beds are full and patients continue to arrive. The emergency department accessibility also leads to vulnerability of the hospital and the ED itself. For example, patients and staff can be potential hostages because narcotics are widely available within the department. This potential can be magnified during civil disturbances. In addition, the surge capacity of the hospital and the ED can rapidly be exceeded during and following mass casualty events. Therefore, planning is necessary to determine how resources and personnel will be used in the event of a disaster.

The goal is to develop a flexible system that can be tested for response ability, is adaptable to meet the needs of a variety of disasters, and provides a system that is not too complex so that the training of staff to perform specific roles can be realistically accomplished. This should be built into the hospital's response plan for disasters.

During everyday operations, emergency departments should be constantly alert for cues suggestive of an impending situation, and proactive in developing processes to meet the needs of everyone who enters the hospital doors. The emphasis on preparedness activities should be incorporated into the department's orientation program and into daily routines. An example, on a smaller scale to mass casualty incidents, is the extensive problem of ED overcrowding nationwide. Many EDs have developed processes to avoid diversion of emergency patients through a bed capacity management program. ED overcrowding is not just an ED problem, but a hospital-wide problem that needs to be addressed with a multidisciplinary team (Giorgianni, Grana, & Scipioni, 2002). The question remains, if we cannot manage daily ED overcrowding, how will we be able to manage the influx of patients from mass casualty events?

In January 2001, the Joint Commission on Accreditation of Healthcare Organizations (JCAHO, 2001a, 2001b) introduced standards that defined institutional responsibilities for emergency management of casualties and community involvement in this process. These standards suggest that the current state of health care readiness varies from highly sophisticated to nonexistent, and that preparedness should take an "all-hazards" approach, analyzing all hazards that are credible threats to a community. These standards emphasize the importance of emergency management and challenge health care organizations to look at the relationships and collaborative efforts between medical care systems and public health systems, and to become better prepared to meet incidents of terrorism. After 9/11, JCAHO required health care organizations to communicate and coordinate efforts with each other. Health care organizations must develop effective plans for the following four phases of disaster management.

- **Mitigation:**   to lessen the impact of potential emergencies, supporting vulnerable areas within the organization
- **Preparedness:**   to build capacity to manage the after-effects of disasters
- **Response:**   to develop a control plan for anticipated negative effects
- **Recovery:**   to restore essential services and operations

GOVERNMENTAL INFLUENCE AND RESPONSIBILITY

Health care agencies do not have to plan alone. Certain governmental efforts focus on preparing for the management of large numbers of casualties and avoidance of unnecessary duplication of efforts. In March 2003, the Department of Homeland Security assumed the primary responsibility for ensuring that emergency response professionals are adequately prepared. Its responsibilities are identified in Box 6–1.

The National Disaster Medical System (NDMS) is responsible for managing and coordinating the federal health, medical, and related social services and recovery for any major emergencies and federally declared disasters. These include natural disasters, technological disasters, major transportation accidents, and terrorism (NDMS, 2004). This broad mandate challenges health care providers who will be responsible for managing large numbers of casualties to prepare. Preparing adequately involves education and exercises for all levels of health care workers. Although nurses who are currently active in healthcare at all types of facilities are the primary workforce to target, inactive registered nurses are a group that must be considered, as these nurses will become the reinforcement necessary to maintain an effective response to disaster.

During and following a disaster, the NDMS section partners with the Federal Emergency Management Agency (FEMA) and the federal interagency community. As this partnership plans and implements a response, the NDMS section serves as the lead federal agency for health and medical services rendered within the Federal Response Plan (NDMS, 2004). Nurses in hospitals and other health care organizations should be familiar with the chain of command following a disaster and the official response system to facilitate adequate information and optimal response to a variety of events. This chain of command will involve a commander who may be outside of the agency or institution. All professional nurses should review the disaster response plan at regular intervals so that during a disaster, each role and its relationship to others, within and outside of the home agency, is automatic. Nonprofessional workers, as well as other professionals, will look to the professional nurse as a role model in responding to the influx of casualties. In addition, the protocols for obtaining supplies, pharmaceuticals, or additional staff should be readily available so that there are no unnecessary interruptions in patient management.

Resource Allocation

The release of biological or chemical agents requires rapid access to large amounts of pharmaceuticals and medical supplies. The Centers for Disease Control and Prevention's Strategic National Stockpile (SNS), formerly the National Pharmaceutical Stockpile (NPS), ensures the availability and rapid deployment of necessary pharmaceuticals, antidotes, medical supplies, and equipment to adequately respond to events involving nerve agents, biological pathogens, and chemical agents. These stockpile packages are stored in strategic locations around the United States, which enables rapid delivery anywhere in the country if the need arises. The stockpiles are designed to support local first response efforts, not as the primary first response tools, but rather to bolster the state's response over the time required to adequately respond (CDC, 2003a). See Chapter 3 for more information.

Bioterrorism Initiative

It is not enough to be reactive to terrorist events. Nurses must prepare proactively, so that an actual event is not the first time that protocols and procedures are enacted. In 1999, the CDC created a Bioterrorism Initiative. After the onset of the Bioterrorism Initiative, the CDC was designated to lead a collaborative project to upgrade the nation's public health capacity in mounting an adequate response to biological and chemical terrorism. This interdisciplinary team consists of governmental and nongovernmental allies. But it is not enough to know which governmental and nongovernmental agencies would be available to respond following the use of weapons of mass destruction (WMD). Each responder must know how he or she fits into the

---

BOX 6–1   Responsibilities of the Department of Homeland Security

- Provide a coordinated, comprehensive federal response to any large-scale crisis
- Mount a swift and effective recovery effort
- Prioritize citizen preparedness
- Educate families on the best ways to prepare their homes for disaster
- Provide suggestions for citizen's response to a crisis

Adapted from http://www.dhs.gov/dhspublic/index.jsp.

response plan and understand the relationships with other team members. Only then can the total response be coordinated and effective. The best plan in the world is ineffective if the key players are not comfortable with it. The plan should be available on each unit so that it can be reviewed during quiet times. Routine education about its implementation should be included within the educational opportunities held regularly for topics such as cardiopulmonary resuscitation (CPR), bloodborne pathogens, and safety regulations.

During and following mass casualty events, nursing staff must have both emergency and disaster preparedness and response skills that focus on preparedness, mitigation, response, and recovery in order to effectively respond while conserving valuable resources. Nurses must receive education about the meaning and interventions associated with each phase. Again, repetition will enable automatic response.

TRIAGE

Triage comes from the French word meaning "to sort." It is the continuous process in which priorities are reassigned as needed treatments, time, and condition of the victims change. Victims are quickly assessed and assigned a priority or classification for receiving treatment according to the severity of the illness or injury. It is a balancing of human lives with the realities of the situation, such as supplies and personnel. Professional nurses perform triage every day in every emergency room. Personnel assigned to triage are expected to function independently, yet as part of a coordinated effort. Several types of triage are explained below.

Three-Level Triage

In the past, the *Emergency Nurses' Association Manual* described several systems having three, four, and five category models for triaging casualties. The three-level system groups victims as:

- Category 1: Life threatening
- Category 2: Emergent
- Category 3: Stable, nonurgent

Research has suggested lower reliability and efficacy for this three-level model (Travers, Waller, Bowling, Flowers, & Tintinalli, 2002).

Five-Level Triage

The five-level model is generally thought to be safer and more stable than the three- or four-level model. It categorizes patients according to the Emergency Severity Index (ESI), and includes specific questions asked about the victim, with the answers fitting into an algorithm based on the acuity and resources needed to provide care (Travers

et al., 2002). In 2002, the Emergency Nurses Association (ENA) House of Delegates passed a resolution asking for the formation of a work group to compare and explore the National Five-Level Triage System with other tier levels. Currently, the ENA recommends the use of the five-tier triage system for the management of casualties.

START

Another form of triage is the Simple Triage and Rapid Treatment (*START*), which refers to a specific triage method to evaluate patient respiratory, circulatory, and neurological function and categorize each of them into one of four care categories (START, 2004). There is a commercially available belt that is designed for use with the START triage system. It uses four colors of survey tape in categorizing patients. The person who is triaging tears off the appropriately colored tape and ties it around the patients arm so that other responders know the condition of the patient. A small piece of tape the same color is placed on the side pouch of the belt. The triage officer can then track the number and severity of injury by looking at the pouch for a count of patients and their severity (*Conterra Triage Belt*, 2003).

Triage in Canada

Canadian EDs categorize patients and their potential needs to determine their acuity level, resource needs, and performance. This information is coupled with operating "objectives" or concepts (utility, relevance, validity). This acuity scale acknowledges that the community's demographic characteristics will not influence the typical presentation of a sentinel event, but will be significant variables in the different triage levels or case mix.

The objectives identify the maximum amount of time between nursing reassessments for categories of patients and will vary according to the triage level assigned to the victim. Level I or resuscitation patients, who can be nonresponsive, unstable, or in respiratory distress, require continuous nursing care. Level II, or the emergent category, includes patients with difficulties such as chest or abdominal pain, severe trauma, head injuries, or anaphylaxis who require reassessment every 15 minutes. Level III (urgent) and level IV (less urgent) patients should be assessed every 60 minutes, and level V (nonurgent) victims should be assessed every 120 minutes (Beveridge, Clarke, Janes, Savage, Thompson, et al., 1998).

Reverse Triage

The primary difference with the triage associated with a disaster is the magnitude of the event and the focus on saving the greatest number of people. Following a mass casualty event, nurses should expect an *upside-down triage*.

In a normal situation, severely injured or ill patients would be treated first, with less serious injuries or illnesses

TABLE 6–1. TRIAGE CLASSIFICATIONS: MASS CASUALTY EVENT

SURVIVOR CLASSIFICATION	TREATMENT NEEDS AND LOCATION
Class I	• Minor professional treatment • Handled in outpatient or ambulatory setting
Class II	• Injuries require immediate life-sustaining treatments • Moderately injured victims • Initial treatment requires minimum of time, personnel, and supplies
Class III	• Victims' definitive treatment can be delayed without jeopardy to life or loss of limb
Class IV	• Victims with wounds or injuries requiring extensive treatment beyond the immediate medical capabilities • Treatment of these jeopardize other victims. Victims need large amounts of supplies and personnel

treated afterwards. In a mass casualty event situation, this is reversed. Victims who are most severely injured—those who would require the expenditure of large amounts of supplies and provider time, with little chance of surviving—are treated last. After an event, victims are grouped into four classifications; see Table 6–1.

Nurses at each health care facility must be educated in that institution's triage procedures, enabling them to respond quickly and effectively should a mass casualty event occur, and to provide guidance to other personnel. The specific procedures for prioritizing patient needs must be familiar to them and readily available to all responders as wall charts, as well as portable or individual prompt or cue cards.

Triage After Disasters

Prior to 9-11, initial triage responsibilities, using the categories of immediate, delayed, minor, and dead/non-salvageable, were usually assigned to *first-in* responders at the scene, other than law enforcement officers. At the hospital, nurses triage patients again to determine any changes in condition. Nurses will be engaged in the triage process during and following a mass casualty event, and must be familiar with the differences in the triage process during such an event. The change in triage priorities results in different expectations for nurses, as they are expected to care for the less severely injured before those with more serious injuries and, consequently, a lower chance of survival. This conflicts with the routine guidelines used in daily nursing practice. Planning for this type of triage must include assistance and support for nurses as they incorporate this shift in priorities into their practice. Coupled with psychological support, education about the rationale for triage decisions enables the professional nurse to invest in the response plan and feel comfortable with its implementation.

There are several differences between the triage for the traditional disaster scenario and triage for a hazardous material incident or a chemical or biological terrorist event. Time demands, patient volume, and the personal protective equipment (PPE) worn by response personnel in the hot and warm zones may preclude normal lifesaving measures being rendered quickly, if at all. For example, verbal communication may not be possible because of the responder's PPE. A tactile examination may not be possible for the same reason. Additionally, the whole concept of traditional triage (treating the most seriously injured first) may not be applicable in a chemical or biological incident. Those walking around may need to be among the first to be decontaminated and evacuated from the site where the event took place (the hot zone, see below) because they have the best chance of survival. In some instances, when continued risk of injury or contamination is likely, it may not be desirable for victims to remain in place in the hot zone until they are examined and triaged. Rather, immediate evacuation occurs and the victims are directed towards the decontamination area.

Following a mass casualty event, the process of sorting the sick and injured on the basis of urgency and type of condition or triage takes priority. Interventions at ground zero are restricted to opening the airway, controlling severe hemorrhage, and elevating patients' lower extremities. All victims involved in the incident are to be quickly examined and tagged whether they appear injured or not injured. At the scene, there may be little time to indicate a patient's priority status on a triage tag, but it is important that all victims be tagged to assist in the identification of the injured and to help with later reunification of families and friends. Emergency personnel perform the basic triage examination, categorize the patient, and attach the appropriate tag in 60 seconds or less. The patient data recorded on a triage tag is at risk of getting defaced or blurred if the tag becomes wet during the decontamination process, so use a permanent marker.

Triage non-ambulatory casualties where they lie, unless they are in an unsafe area that requires their immediate movement. Ambulatory patients are separated from other wounded at the start of triage by short, simple directions such as, "Anyone who is able to walk . . . " followed by indicating an area to which the patients will walk. Triage tags are attached to casualties near the head. Give the removed portions of the tag to those determining resource requirements. Patients designated "red" are critical patients requiring immediate care. Patients designated "yellow" are urgent patients requiring evaluation and treatment as soon as possible. Patients designated "green" are non-urgent patients usually considered the "walking wounded." Patients designated "black" are patients who are deceased or dying in which medical treatment will not change the outcome. Patients tagged in the field should be reevaluated and reprioritized by triage nurses as appropriate. Misdiagnosis in the field or a change in condition is to be expected.

Casualties will be re-triaged on arrival at the treatment area; triage categories will be modified, if necessary, based on this examination. Following re-triage, treatment teams will provide stabilizing care and document actions and observations on the triage tag. Priority for transportation will be given to casualties tagged *immediate*, following evaluation and necessary stabilization in the treatment area, not delaying transport for stabilization. If the triage priority of the patient changes, remove the bottom portion of the tag, leaving the injury information and add a new tag identifying the new triage priority and the reason for change. Initial triage nurses and other medical personnel perform lifesaving procedures and move to the next victim. Minor casualties may be asked to assist with casualties needing critical treatment (e.g., maintain airway, maintain bleeding control). When all patients have been triaged, triage team members will be reassigned to other care and service areas.

The CDC (2003b) has developed a tool for rapid assessment of injuries. This instrument, coupled with the concise explanations for use, can facilitate rapid triage of casualties. See MediaLink.

Expanded Nursing Role

When large numbers of casualties arrive at the health care facility, requiring assessment and interventions simultaneously, disaster triage is not sufficient to effectively manage the situation. This situation may require the initiation or performance of independent diagnosis and treatment activities without a physician being present. In addition to requiring education for this role, there are legislative issues to be addressed prior to the actual event. Those professionals responsible for the development of the interagency response plans will also need to assume a leadership role in the development of an expanded nursing role plan, its treatment algorithms, and its initiation and implementation protocols. These professional nurses must be available to present the plan to persons with the authority to pass the appropriate legislation. Some of the possible scenarios for a mass casualty event should include information about illnesses and injuries that may be unfamiliar to nurses. Protocols for managing these situations must also be clearly delineated with posted algorithms to serve as reminders. Failure to do this may compromise the health and safety of staff and patients alike. Successful implementation of an expanded role plan requires the support of physician colleagues. Physicians and nurses must both adapt to the expanded role situation.

In addition to screening for appropriate skill sets, nurses who perform in this expanded role must be excellent practitioners, comfortable with the treatment algorithms, and able to provide leadership for less experienced nurses. Even with extensive education and practice, there will be psychological adjustments to the expanded role that should be addressed. As roles and responsibilities change, there may be an alteration of regular departmental structure and team assignments. Peers and colleagues may be required to assume a hierarchical relationship during a disaster response. This will be stressful, resulting in the development of an emotionally charged situation.

A disaster disrupts essential agency services, such as transportation and communication. Each agency should have alternative forms of communication as a backup if the usual system should fail. These may include traditional methods, cellular phones, satellite phones, and handheld two-way radios. When these systems are developed, each nurse must receive sufficient education in the primary and backup systems of communication so that during an event, communication within and between health care facilities proceeds without interruption. This education must be repeated at regular intervals.

Core Competencies

Core competencies exist for public health workers on how to effectively deal with a disaster (Gebbie and Qureshi, 2002). See Chapters 1 and 3. These competencies should become the foundation for educational programs at each facility. The response plan should outline how these skills and knowledge are incorporated into an educational program that culminates in regular exercises to evaluate each nurse's competency. In addition, the International Nursing Coalition for Mass Casualty Education (INCMCE) was formed to assist in the development of educational policies and competencies related to mass casualty events management. The educational plan recommendations looks at the preparation of nurses in categories of knowledge, competencies, role development, and professional values (Conway-Welch, 2002). See Table 6–2.

The nurses at each facility should be aware of how their institution interprets these competencies. Awareness of how the plan is to be implemented contributes to the safe and efficient management of large numbers of survivors. The specifics of role, supplies, and interrelationships with other agencies and providers must be defined on all shifts, including holidays and periods of staff shortages.

DECONTAMINATION

Following a mass casualty event, it may be necessary to decontaminate victims. When preparing nurses for their possible role during the decontamination process, time must be allotted for the classroom presentation of information and hands-on application in a controlled setting. This process must be carefully explained and demonstrated to all involved before practice exercises, so that nurses and staff become familiar with putting on protective gear and working in this cumbersome attire. If possible, HAZMAT experts should lead and coordinate this phase of preparation, or at least during some of the regularly scheduled practice sessions. An integral part of this drill is rehearsing the explanation to be given to victims as decontamination

TABLE 6–2. INTERNATIONAL NURSING COALITION FOR MASS CASUALTY EDUCATION (INCMCE) RECOMMENDATIONS

KNOWLEDGE	COMPETENCIES	ROLE DEVELOPMENT	PROFESSIONAL VALUES
• Health promotion	• Critical thinking	• Care provider	• Value-based behavior
• Risk reduction	• Communication	• Care designer	• Commitment to patient welfare
• Disease prevention	• Holistic assessment	• Care manager	• Altruism
• Disease management	• Synthesis of data	• Coordinator	• Autonomy
• Technologies	• Making judgments	• Professional	• Human dignity
• Ethics	• Technical skills		• Social justice
• Diversity	• Teaching		
	• Delegation		

Adapted from Conway-Welch, 2002.

BOX 6–2　Decontamination Triage

Decontamination Triage Procedure

Events involving massive numbers of victims require changing triage priorities to ensure the survival of the maximum number of patients. The command center will change triage modes based on the following:

- number of victims
- available decontamination equipment
- number of decontamination technicians
- availability of medications

The command center will contact the decontamination area and direct them to change triage priorities to what is called a **support mode.**

First priority will be victims exposed but not symptomatic.

Second priority will be victims exposed but minimal medical care required.

Third priority will be victims exposed requiring maximum medical care.

Final priority will be the deceased.

The **support mode** of triage requires establishing a temporary care area outside the hospital. Those awaiting decontamination will wait in the **support** area.

Reprinted with permission. J. Hamilton

---

occurs. As nurses gain comfort with the process and their role in the decontamination activities, the verbal explanation provides evidence of their understanding.

An important part of planning for disasters and possible decontamination needs is developing a process that will protect the hospital or agency itself from contamination during the care of disaster victims. Following a man-made, chemical, or radiological incident, many will self-refer to the hospital. Without a carefully developed plan that is rehearsed frequently, the sheer number of victims may limit the ability to effectively triage, decontaminate, and provide treatment. See Box 6–2. For example, in Tokyo, the nerve gas sarin was released in the subway system in 1995 by Aum Shinrikyo, a Japanese doomsday cult, killing 12 people and leaving 3,794 injured. Such a scenarios can potentially overwhelm an ED (Nakajima, Sato, Morita, & Yanagisawa, 1997).

Chemical disasters may result from industrial accidents including traffic accidents with industrial or nuclear accidents, transportation spills, radiation releases, police actions such as tear gas and pepper spray, and nuclear or terrorist activities and intentional releases (J. Hamilton, personal communication, May 14, 2003; Jagminas & Erdman, 2001). JCAHO and OSHA require emergency departments to prepare for hazardous material incidents. The plan must include the treatment of patients with chemical exposures, decontamination, and contingencies for contamination sources within the hospital and for ED evacuation. The hazardous materials plan often requires the professional input from medical toxicologists, hazardous materials teams, and industrial hygiene and safety officers (Jagminas & Erdman, 2001).

Decontamination protects the victims from further injury, the rescuers and health care workers from secondary contamination, and prevents hazardous materials from entering the hospital. Chemical contamination may be recognized by odors emanating from the victims; reports from the scene; or victims fainting, seizing, and complaining of eyes tearing and noses dripping. Additionally, one might witness multiple ill persons presenting with similar clinical complaints (point source exposure) seeking treatment at the same time and reporting exposure to common ventilation systems, and health care workers fainting after exposure to one or more patients. A quick decision must be made to protect the hospital from secondary contamination. Security must be notified to lock down the hospital. The contaminated patients are to be isolated to a single large room after removing nonessential and nondisposable equipment. Ideally, this isolation room will have a separate ventilation system to avoid further contamination of the hospital with recycled ventilation. This room would then be considered as a secure zone with yellow tape and only appropriately pro-tected individuals would be allowed to enter. In Israel, a yellow line is painted on the ground in the driveway leading to the emergency room to clearly demarcate the contaminated area and the decontaminated area. Contaminated persons must not cross this line. If clean or noncontaminated persons cross the yellow line, they are considered contaminated.

The site of the weapon release or where the contamination occurred is called the contamination zone or hot zone (Figure 6–1). Adjacent to the hot zone is the control or warm zone. This area is where decontamination and emergency treatment take place. The area adjacent to the warm zone is the safe or cold zone, where normal procedures occur. The cold zone is not considered as contaminated (J. Hamilton, personal communication, May 14, 2003).

Those who decontaminate victims exposed to hazardous substances should be educated at the first-responder operational level. This education should occur in a non-threatening environment and include both didactic and hands-on learning experiences (Figure 6–2).

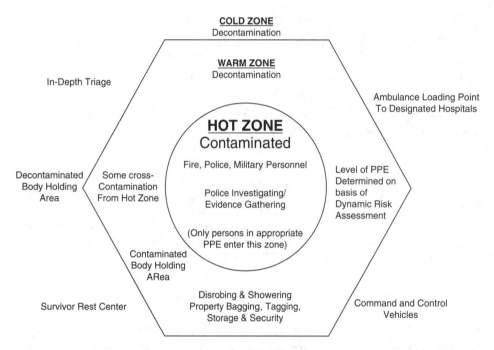

Figure 6–1. Contamination/decontamination zones. *Illustration by Rebecca Langan.*

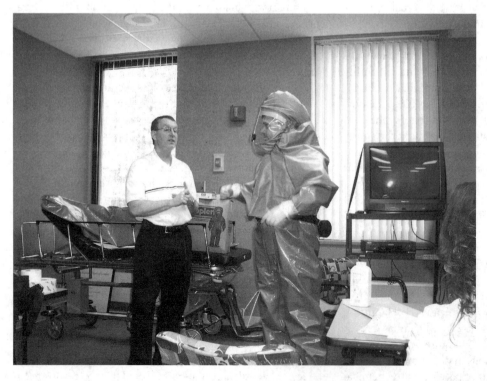

Figure 6–2. Classroom instruction on decontamination principles and donning personal protective equipment.

If the decontamination process is being completed in response to an unknown hazard, OSHA regulations require level B protection, which includes a positive pressure, self-contained breathing apparatus and splash-protective chemical resistant clothing (Jagminas & Erdman, (2001). (See Table 3–2: Personal Protective Equipment Levels.)

Gas masks are used in a broad range of industrial, military, and emergency situations to protect the user from hazardous dust, gas, or other aerosols. A gas mask may be considered as a high-performance respirator, usually equipped with both eye protection and air supply protection or treatment. A hood, helmet, or headgear is generally used to protect people from exposure to hazardous materials. Such devices generally protect the skin, eyes, airways, and respiratory systems against exposure to a range of hazardous substances. Protective clothing is made to guard against minimal exposure to mild irritants, to serious exposure to lethal materials. Some protective suits are disposable, meant for only one use. Others are made from multi-layer fabrics to provide strength and are completely impermeable and are reusable (Banthrax Corporation, n.d.).

It may be helpful to have all of the equipment necessary for an individual to dress in the decontamination gear stored in hanging laundry bags. In this way, avoiding the need to locate specific items saves time (Figure 6–3).

Decontaminating the Victim

If the patient requires immediate lifesaving interventions, these must be done either before or during decontamination. In Israel, highly skilled health care professionals in

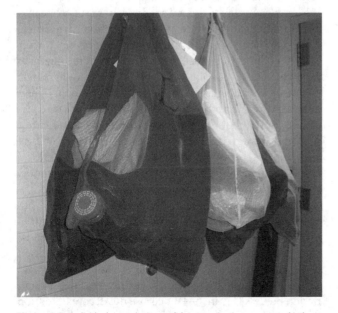

Figure 6–3. Individual, complete sets of decontamination gear stored in laundry bags for immediate use.

full PPE perform the intubation of patients. This is a very difficult task as manual dexterity is poor with thick rubber gloves in place. To prevent cross-contamination, the patient should be asked to perform as much of the decontamination as possible. The patient's clothes and jewelry as well as any other personal items are removed and placed in plastic bags. If water is available and safe to use, a head-to-toe wash is performed with soap and water. Agencies should keep bottled water in stock. The fire departments may have to use their pumper trucks to supply water for decontamination.

A detergent solution can be made of 0.5% detergent in lukewarm water (about three squirts of liquid detergent into a bucket of water) for the head-to-toe wash. The first rinse with this solution will remove particles and water-based chemicals such as acids and alkalis. The affected areas should be wiped with a wet sponge or soft brush. This first scrub helps to remove organic and oil-based chemicals that adhere to the skin (UK Resilience, 2003). However, it is important to avoid vigorous scrubbing to prevent breaks in the skin. Open wounds are to be decontaminated by irrigating with saline or water for an additional 5 to 10 minutes. Different sources recommend various times of flushing exposed areas with soap and water. Jagminas and Erdman (2001) suggest 10 to 15 minutes, while experts in Israel recommend a minimum 6-minute wash. Exposed eyes should be irrigated with saline for 10 to 15 minutes. Topical eye anesthetic may be required for effective eye irrigation to be performed (DeAtley, 2001). In the case of alkali exposures, eyes should be irrigated for 30 to 60 minutes. The skin under the fingernails should be cleaned with a scrub brush. If possible, collect the runoff water in steel drums (Jagminas & Erdman, 2001). Some experts, such as those in Israel, state that the runoff water does not need to be collected due to the dilution of the substance by the vast amounts of water which has been running constantly during the decontamination process and the sophisticated "cleaning" process done by large sewer districts. It has been "determined that if a chemical is diluted with water at the rate of approximately 2000:1, pollution of water courses will be significantly reduced" (Institute of Medicine National Research Council, 1998).

Warm Versus Cold Water in Decontamination

Many persons such as older adults, the frail, infants, and traumatized casualties are more susceptible to hypothermia. When possible, warm water should be used to reduce hypothermia. Advantages of cold water are that it is usually readily available, assists in rapid decontamination, and enhances vasoconstriction including the closure of pores in the skin thereby reducing chemical absorption. Disadvantages of cold water are hypothermia and thermal shock (UK Resilience, 2003).

Disadvantages of warm water are that it slowly increases the blood flow to the skin, thereby increasing the skin absorption of contaminants. Warm water does not

---

BOX 6–3   Gross Decontamination Procedure

Gross Decontamination Procedure (Strip and Rinse)

- Direct patient to the decontamination area (warm zone)
- Keep children with their parents or older sibling if possible, or a decon team member should assist the child
- Victim to wipe feet before entering decon area—use mat or remove shoes directly into bag
- Victim removes clothing
- Place clothing in plastic lined barrel—this clothing will be discarded

- Victim places valuables in zip-lock bag. Victim holds bag during decontamination[*]
- Victim or Decon team member writes name and birth date on bag with indelible marker
- Brush or wipe off particulate matter
- Victim steps into shower, eyes closed, mouth shut, arms raised above head
- Rotate twice, slowly
- Walk out of shower into technical decontamination area

Adapted with permission. J. Hamilton (2003); DeAtley (2001)

---

help to dissolve some chemical weapon materials, and it may not be readily available (UK Resilience, 2003).

Water may turn some compounds caustic. In these cases or where water is not available, dry decontaminants may be considered (UK Resilience, 2003).

Chemical Warfare Victims

Although the hope is that nurses will not be treating victims of chemical warfare agents (CWA), they must be aware of the possibility and be prepared. There are many commercial chemicals that are closely related to such agents. Cyanide is manufactured for industrial use and is shipped to users by truck and train throughout the United States. Phosgene is also manufactured in large quantities and is shipped across the nation. Nerve agents are not available outside the military, but are closely related to pesticides and insecticides that are sprayed on orchards. The effects of these compounds are similar to those of nerve agents; the medical therapy for them is the same (Sidell and Franz, 1997).

According to Jagminas and Erdman (2001) and Malone (2002), a 0.5% hypochlorite solution is the best universal liquid decontamination agent. This solution is prepared by diluting household bleach to one-tenth its strength or 9 parts water or saline to 1 part bleach. Hypochlorite solutions are safe for use on the skin and soft tissue injuries including open lacerations. It is not recommended for penetrating abdominal wounds, in the eyes, in open chest wounds, or in open brain or spinal cord injuries. Instead, these wounds should be irrigated with large amounts of sterile saline solution. All areas on which the hypochlorite solution was used should be flushed with sterile saline solution. Some consider the use of a hypochlorite solution controversial and unnecessary. Others recommend using dishwashing soap or baby shampoo, as the baby shampoo is not harmful to the eyes and can be used on children (J. Hamilton, personal communication, October 16, 2003).

There is a universal dry decontaminant known as M291. The military has access to this substance, which is available as pads packaged in small individual packets. "M291 resin is a dry black carbonaceous material that decontaminates by absorption and physical removal of the chemical warfare agents (CWAs) from the victim. M291 resin is used for spot decontamination of skin exposed to CWAs" (Jagminas & Erdman, 2001, p. 5).

Decontamination Procedure—Ambulatory and Nonambulatory Victims

Every victim with suspected exposure to an agent with a risk of secondary contamination to others must be decontaminated. Gross decontamination (strip and rinse) and technical decontamination (rinse, wash, rinse) procedures will be described. See Boxes 6–3 and 6–4.

Personal effects may be placed in a ziplock bag and labeled with identification, if the items are not soaked with a chemical fluid. If wet, they may need to be placed in a secure area to dry and off-gas. Depending upon the contaminant, the items may require disposal as hazardous waste. Some military installations take the exposed garments and hang them to off-gas where they are not upwind of any personnel. They usually air dry for at least 24 hours. Then, they are sometimes returned and worn again. HAZMAT teams have handheld devices or instruments that will measure the amount of hazardous chemical or off-gassing. They will let health care personnel know if they may return the items to clients or if they must be destroyed or left in a secure area to off-gas (B. Clements, personal communication, May 22, 2003).

It is important to keep in mind that nonambulatory patients may require airway positioning, suctioning, oxygen administration, spinal stabilization, and the IM administration of a lifesaving antidote. The extremities should be decontaminated before starting the IV for IV therapy. If patients are pulled out of the decontamination line to perform any of these procedures, they should remain in the decontamination area and return to the decontamination process (Figure 6–4). Because the decontamination process follows a type of reverse triage, getting the greatest number of the most able persons through quickly, CPR or

BOX 6–4   Technical Decontamination

Technical Decontamination Procedure (Rinse-Wash-Rinse)

- Give victim washcloth or soft brush and assist in washing from head to toe using dishwashing soap and tepid water; wash for 5 minutes when agent is non persistent or 8 minutes when persistent or unknown agent
- Ensure face, hair, axilla, creases, folds and genitalia are thoroughly washed
- Clean under fingernails with a scrub brush
- Use baby shampoo on children unable to close eyes
- Wash all open wounds gently. Do not abrade skin by washing too vigorously
- Discard wash cloths, brushes, sponges into nearby trashcan
- Rinse victim from head to toe with warmed water.

- Thoroughly rinse taking at least one minute to complete
- Swab ears and nose with cotton tipped applicator to remove contaminates
- Assist victim to dry thoroughly with towels. Place towel in linen discard barrel.
- Seat person, dry feet and swivel the chair to set feet down on clean mat or blanket, apply "booties"
- Place victim in gown and cover with blanket if needed
- Victim may now exit into hospital (cold zone) for rapid assessment, triage and assignment to a treatment area
- Antidote administration will be done via the IM route after cleansing the affected area
- Have backboards, stretchers or wheelchairs readily available for victims that deteriorate clinically and require immediate removal to non-ambulatory area

Adapted with permission. J. Hamilton (2003); (DeAtley, 2001)

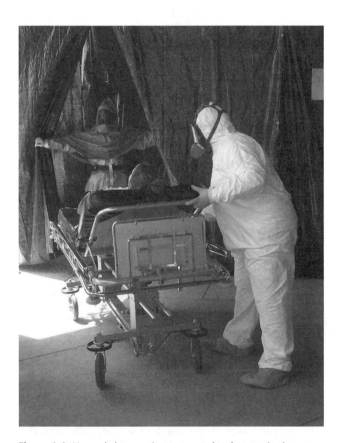

Figure 6–4. Non-ambulatory patient transported to decontamination area.

ACLS interventions should not be started unless there are no other patients awaiting decontamination. See Box 6–5.

As the patients leave the decontamination area, they should be guided to the appropriate triage treatment area. In Israel, colored signs are used above corridors to indicate the specific triage treatment area. Another suggestion is to have health care personnel wear colored vests and caps to indicate the specific triage team to whom they are assigned.

Special Considerations in Decontamination

Place eyeglasses in a ziplock bag as a valuable item unless the person cannot see without them. They must be washed and rinsed thoroughly during the decontamination process before being worn. Contact lenses should be removed and placed with other valuables in a zip-lock bag. If the contact lenses are permeable and it is likely that they have been contaminated, they will likely be discarded (DeAtley, 2001).

Patients may keep assistive devices, such as canes, with them, but these items must be decontaminated before they can be carried or used in the treatment areas or cold zone. Walkers can be used to support patients who are unsteady standing or walking as they go through the decontamination process. However, the walkers should be retrieved, decontaminated and returned to the front of the line to assist the next patient who may require it (DeAtley, 2001).

PICC lines and saline locks must be covered with Tegaderm or plastic wrap before the area is decontaminated unless the lines are contaminated. Contaminated PICC lines or saline locks should be removed before being decontaminated. After the area is cleaned, a dressing should be applied until the patient is in the treatment area where antibiotic ointment and a new bandage should be applied (DeAtley, 2001).

Hearing aids should be removed and placed in the bag with other valuables. If the patient must have the hearing aids due to deafness, the hearing aids may be cleansed with a 4 × 4 gauze moistened with saline, dried, and placed into a ziplock bag and handed to the patient.

BOX 6–5   Non-Ambulatory Decontamination

Decontamination Procedure (Non-Ambulatory)

- Place plastic sheet on cart, cover with sheet, place victim on sheet
- Remove all clothing, cutting if necessary
- Place clothing in plastic lined barrel
- Place valuables in ziplock bag for victim to hold or tape to body. Write name and birth date on bag with indelible marker[*]
- Brush or wipe off particulate matter
- Using hand held sprayer, rinse patient. Begin with face and airway then open wounds
- Close or cover victim's mouth, pinch nose shut when washing face
- Ensure axilla, genitalia, and the back are rinsed
- If a cervical spine injury is suspected and a C-collar is available, apply the collar as soon as possible
- Airway should be established and protected. Use non-rebreather mask or use bag-valve-mask
- Wash from head to toe using tepid water and dishwashing soap 5 minutes when agent is non persistent and 8 minutes when a persistent or unknown agent. Avoid rubbing too vigorously.
- Roll victim to side for washing posterior, use 2–4 personnel if available
- Wash and rinse creases such as ears, eyes, axilla, groin, rinse for about one minute
- Do not hold rinsing device too close to the skin to cause irritation
- Thoroughly dry patient and cover with a blanket
- Decon soap, brushes and sponges should be placed in a trashcan and not carried into the cold zone; oxygen materials should remain in the decon area
- Open wounds should be covered with dressings after decontamination is complete
- Transfer patient to clean backboard and exit into cold zone for rapid assessment, triage and assignment to a treatment area

Adapted with permission. J. Hamilton; (DeAtley, 2001)

BOX 6–6   Decontamination: Exit Procedure for Decon Team Members

- Walk through gross decontamination shower, rotating twice
- Enter technical decontamination area, dry suit
- Remove mask, hand to suit support
- Remove boots, hand to suit support, have clean socks, covered shoes ready (do not place clean feet on wet/contaminated surface/swivel chair to place feet on dry, clean area)
- Remove suit, hand to suit support
- Remove gloves, hand to suit support
- Proceed to rehabilitation area, weigh in, vital signs, rehydration

Suit Support
- Dry suit, boots, outer gloves, mask
- Wipe inside of mask with 1:9 dilution bleach solution
- Check suit and mask thoroughly for rips or tears
- Take equipment to ready room and assist oncoming technicians to suit up
- Check suit integrity before dressing technicians
- Tape all seams, boots and gloves
- Establish battery charging schedule
- Establish PAPR maintenance schedule
- Establish technician training schedule (at least annually)

(See Appendix C for Decontamination Post-Screening Form)

Reprinted with permission. J. Hamilton (2003)

Because hearing aids cannot be soaked with water, the cleaned hearing aid is not to be worn until the patient has completed the decontamination process and is in the treatment area. No decontamination is necessary for dentures unless the oral cavity is contaminated. If the oral cavity is contaminated, remove the dentures, place them into a zip-lock bag, and mark the bag with the patient's identifying information. The patient's mouth is to be decontaminated with mouthwash or saline. The patient should gargle and spit the solution into a biohazard bag. The dentures need to be decontaminated following the instructions of a dentist or the Poison Control Center (DeAtley, 2001).

The persons working in "suit support" may be those who are not able to tolerate the heat or the weight of the PPE or who have vital signs outside of normal limits during the prescreening (Boxes 6–6, 6–7). They serve a vital role as they ensure the integrity of the suits and tape all seams.

BOX 6–7   Lessons Learned about PPE and Decontamination

In Israel, a team of visiting health care providers donned the PPE. The temperature outside, where the decontamination area is located, was about 76 degrees Fahrenheit. Some sources recommend a maximum of one hour in the PPE. However, the person in the PPE may get very hot as the material is impermeable. Every 15 minutes the person performing the decontamination should be sprayed with cold water for cooling down. These persons must be monitored for the effects of the suit and fatigue. Hydration should be done before the persons don the PPE and rehydration is very important once the shift in decontamination is completed. It is also important to get baseline vital signs and weights on the persons participating in the decontamination process. The process is anxiety-provoking and blood pressures and heart rates may be elevated above what is normal for those involved.

However, decontamination personnel should be screened. If vital signs are not within normal limits before the PPE is donned, these persons should be assigned to alternative activities.

(See Appendix C, Decontamination Pre-Screening Form)

A universal signal such as tapping the top of the head should be adopted as a means of alerting others that one is having difficulty inside the PPE. Communicating is difficult inside the PPE; hearing and speech are muffled. The batteries on the PAPRs must be checked periodically to ensure that they are in safe working condition.

If the PPE is stored in a room on a level lower than the decontamination area, the mask and battery pack should not be placed until the person has mounted the stairs to the appropriate level. Excess energy is lost otherwise.

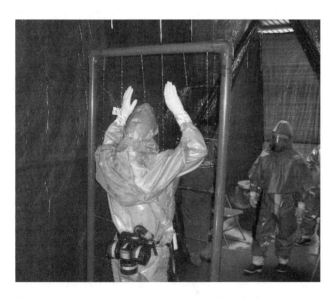

Figure 6–5. Decontamination personnel going through decontamination process before removing gear.

The seams to note are the areas between the sleeves at the wrist where the suit meets the gloves and at the ankle where the suit meets the boots. The front zipper and flap also need to be taped. Persons donning the PPE cannot properly wear the suits without assistance in the donning process. A laminated card with a visual of the order in which equipment should be donned, battery packs attached, and a means to indicate when the decontamination worker is "in trouble" or feeling poorly to a team member should be prominently displayed in the area where the PPE is donned. Assistance is also necessary in removing the PPE. See Figure 6–5.

A sample list of equipment and supplies to have readily available for decontamination follows (Box 6–8).

MANAGEMENT OF CASUALTIES

An important part of preparing nurses for a mass casualty event is providing education about the types and number of injuries that are expected, and the capacity of the facility. Knowledge and practice enable the nurses to maintain a level of control in a situation that may appear as chaos. When estimating the number of casualties to be expected, double the first hour's casualties for a rough prediction of the total *first wave* of casualties. If a building has collapsed, you can expect increased severity of injuries with a delayed arrival time due to difficulty in removing victims from the rubble (Leibovici et al., 1996). Generally, within 90 minutes of an event, 50%–80% of the acute casualties will arrive at the closest medical facilities (CDC, 2003c; CDC, 2003g). In addition to the seriously injured that are brought to the facility by emergency responders, less injured casualties may leave the scene before being seen by first responders and go by themselves to the nearest medical facility.

Although knowing the number of expected casualties is important, there are two other critical factors to consider when preparing for the arrival of victims. First, the agency should predict the severity of injuries for the casualties coming; and second, determine the agency's capacity to care for those critically injured. Following consideration of these factors, the agency is better able to implement an effective response. Generally, one-third of acute casualties will be classified as critical. This category includes those dead on the scene, those who die at the hospital, those who require emergency surgery, or those requiring hospitalization

BOX 6–8   Decontamination Equipment List

Sample List of Decontamination Equipment

Equipment	Quantity
Large barrels for clothing	2
Large barrels for linen	2
Plastic liners for barrels[*]	20
Plastic zip-lock bags for personal articles	100
Indelible marking pens to write on bags[**]	10
Towels	100
Washcloths	100
Gowns (pediatric to 3XL)	100
Sheets	25

Equipment	Quantity
Cotton tipped applicators	100
Fingernail scrub brushes	100
Dishwashing liquid	1 gallon
Baby shampoo	1 quart
Baby diapers	100
Bleach (1:9 dilution)	2 gallons
Spray bottles	4
Old wheeled carts	4
Plastic coverings for carts	4
Large scissors to cut clothing/tape	4

[*] Double bag all clothing.

[**] Marking pens must be thick enough to be held with heavy rubber gloves.

[***] Have a scale, blood pressure cuffs (regular and large adult sizes) stethoscope and pulse oximeter ready to get baseline readings, readings immediately following the shift in decontamination and readings 15–30 minutes after arriving in the decontamination team recovery area.

Reprinted with permission. J. Hamilton

(CDC, 2003d). Following the treatment of those who are critically injured, nurses can expect that two-thirds of the acute casualties will be treated and released from the emergency department or alternate treatment facility. This ratio can be changed by the use of manufactured weapons, explosions in a confined space, or collapse of a building or structure. These factors will increase the severity of injuries and subsequently the number of the critically injured.

When assessing a hospital's capacity for a given situation, knowing the number of available operating rooms is critical. It is not enough to take victims to a health care facility following a disaster. They must be taken to a facility that has the resources to provide adequate treatment in a timely manner. If the number of predicted or actual casualties exceeds the number of operating rooms available, consideration must be given to transferring or diverting critical casualties to other hospitals (CDC, 2003d). This decision, as well as who is authorized to make it, must be clearly defined in the disaster response plan. The institution's response plan is part of state or regional planning. Generally, officials in authority for the incident will monitor the capacity of all institutions and coordinate the distribution of casualties.

Knowing the number of available surgery suites is not sufficient to determine an institution's capacity, however. When considering the capacity to care for noncritical casualties, the capacity of the radiology department is a major factor. Each casualty exposed to a blast will probably have a chest X ray to screen for fractures, foreign bodies, or *blast lung* (see below). Each X ray will take approximately 10 minutes. Therefore, the radiology department can see approximately six patients per hour per machine (CDC, 2003d). Again,

those in authority at each facility should consider transferring or diverting casualties when the number of casualties exceeds the capacity to treat in a timely manner.

Emergency Medical Treatment and Active Labor Act (EMTALA)

In addition to the assessments previously discussed, consideration is given to the Emergency Medical Treatment and Active Labor Act (EMTALA). EMTALA has had a significant influence on the emergency management and admission of patients to hospitals in the United States. Hospitals may not deny treatment and admission to individuals regardless of their ability to pay. The Department of Health and Human Services has recommended the following during a mass casualty event:

- The use of community-based Emergency Medical Service (EMS) protocols does not violate EMTALA.
- In the event of bioterrorism or a threat of bioterrorism, EMTALA does not apply to those hospitals directly affected.
- Where hospitals follow a community-based, regional, or CDC-directed protocol, EMTALA does not apply.

(CDC, 2003d)

Patient Flow

Planning for large numbers of casualties must also include the internal and external traffic flow and control patterns. To effectively manage large numbers of victims, the flow must be uninterrupted as much as possible. Certain areas of the hospital are prone to bottlenecks or slowing of transfers due to the time taken to perform procedures or assessments. These include departments that perform X rays, CT scans, ultrasounds, laboratory testing, airway management, table thoracostomy, blood transfusion, and any area in which there is a lack of staff preparation.

The *traffic* that can be anticipated during a response to a large-scale disaster will include patients walking or moving via wheelchairs and gurneys. Consideration should be given to designating specific routes or hallways for patients categorized according to the severity of their injuries. To facilitate movement, especially when staff and/or volunteers may not be familiar with the geography of the facility, managers should determine what types of signage or markings will be used as guides. Some institutions use the familiar color-coded lines on the floors or walls to correctly guide patients and staff. Another economical alternative is small, window-shade flags mounted above doors and along the corridors that can be lowered during an event, and remain out of sight for day-to-day functioning.

Hospitals or traditional health care facilities may not be the best site for the management of all casualties. Plans should be made to move less severely injured victims to alternate sites for assessment and treatment. In addition, patients who can safely be discharged must be moved to less acute areas in order to free space in departments required for the management of the critically injured. It may be impossible to use traditional methods of movement, such as ambulances. In addition to identifying spaces and modes of transportation, facilities must also identify personnel responsible for leading or guiding those identified for discharge or transfer to designated areas.

Staffing Needs

When a mass casualty event is announced or suspected, supervisors or designated nurse managers must begin the process of determining staffing needs. This process begins with the confirmation of exactly how many nurses are currently on duty, as well as their type and skill level. Nurse managers should then begin the relocation of staff according to the response plan. After determining the number of staff reporting to the ED, it is time to begin the call-up of needed staff that are not currently on duty (Newberry, 2002). Throughout the day and on all shifts, specific nurses should be identified as authorities. Staffing assessment and relocation is a procedure that can be managed effectively with a tabletop exercise, a theoretical situation where the response plan is implemented around a table, or on paper only, with no physical response.

Identifying all nurses according to teams or color facilitates their movement or admittance to the hospital during a disaster. The *classification* of individual nurses is based on their skill level, such as intensive care nurses, outpatient setting nurses, and operating or emergency department nurses. Logically, those nurses accustomed to caring for critically injured or unstable patients would be assigned to the areas where the patients would initially be seen and stabilized. Nurses will be sent to the emergency department who do not routinely work there. Consequently, it is important for these nurses to become familiar with the location of equipment and basic protocols of care that are a part of the response plan. If possible, during regular and unannounced exercises, nurses should have an opportunity to become comfortable with the basic setup of the emergency department, and provided with a mentor or resource person.

Nurse managers should evaluate the skill sets of nurses from various departments. Nurses from ICUs will have shorter periods of adaptation to the emergency department than nurses from less acute units, yet all nurses can make a valuable contribution to patient care. During a mass casualty event, nurses from less acute units should not be placed in areas in the emergency department or triage, where seconds count in locating equipment and medications. Their nursing skills can be used in the treatment of mild and moderately injured victims, as well as some of the more stable patients in the ICUs, thus freeing up emergency department nurses and staff to care for the critically injured victims. All nurses should know their role in a disaster, especially if it involves relocating to a different department or location.

Attention must be given to meeting the needs of staff and nurses currently on duty. Logically, these nurses may experience anxiety related to the status of their families. To reduce the stress and worry of staff currently on duty, permit one telephone call for each staff person to family or friends (Newberry, 2002). Making arrangements for the safety and care of family enables the staff to concentrate more fully on the tasks at hand.

In addition to the phone call to family members at home, agencies should consider providing support services to their staff. These include the establishment of a child care area, perhaps staffed by volunteers or reserve staff. This would permit nurses to come to work without the worry about their children. Additional consideration should be given to those families caring for aging parents or grandparents. Perhaps in the United States, attention should be given to establishing an elder care area to address this issue. Another topic of discussion should involve assessing the staff's need for care for those with special needs, medical or psychological.

Mobilization of Resources

As soon as the disaster has been announced, and casualties are anticipated, nurses should begin the relocation of supplies to the designated triage and decontamination areas. These supplies should be dedicated to disaster response only, not used as a backup supply reservoir for individual units. To familiarize nurses with the amount, location, and type of supplies and medications on the carts, staff nurses should share the responsibility of checking the content of the cart and rotating supplies with an approaching expiration date to the general stock and replacing them with newer stock.

Assignment and Rotation of Nursing Staff

It may be difficult for necessary employees to get to the hospital or clinic due to traffic congestion or interruption. Develop a plan for these necessary employees, such as *pickup* points located throughout the area, and van services to transport employees to the agency. Each employee must be aware of the gathering place, and the approximate time to be there. Designate a telephone line for notification and contact purposes. The main agency switchboard may be overwhelmed with calls and thus unreliable as a notification method.

Communicate frequently with staff members, updating them with accurate knowledge about what the disaster is, how many patients may be coming, and when they will start to arrive. A television placed in a lounge provides contact with the outside and news about what is happening. During the 9-11 disaster, Queens Hospital Center in New York set up an e-mail system to notify staff at least twice a day about the disaster and the hospital's role in responding (JCAHO, 2001b).

At the time of a mass casualty event, there must be a coordinated use of staff to ensure their continued availability for the duration of the crisis. One method of assessing currently available nurses and other health care workers is the use of a staging area for clinical staff. In this area, the clinical personnel are matched with specific areas of need. JCAHO recommends that prior to the need, each agency answer key questions to assess their level of readiness. The use of tabletop exercises as supplements to management exercises will make these assessments quicker and easier to calculate. The questions include:

- At what point would you request assistance from other health care organizations?
- How can the plan be integrated into overall community planning?
- Will you use unsolicited volunteers?
- How will you ensure minimum credentials (license)?
- How will you orient clinical staff from other agencies?
(JCAHO, 2001b)

As previously mentioned, victims may be *re-triaged* upon arrival at the hospital or clinic. This occurs outside the hospital if decontamination is necessary, for example, following a chemical event. Patients whose conditions have deteriorated or who need immediate lifesaving procedures, such as intubation or chest tube insertion, are sent to a station for these procedures prior to decontamination. This station is outside the hospital and staffed by professionals wearing PPE. In normal situations, patients trans-ferred to the general care floors are relatively stable. During a disaster, patients will be given initial treatments and moved to the floors or alternate treatment sites to complete their care. Therefore, it is important that all staff are comfortable in the assessment and care of the more severely injured. The expanded authority of the nurse discussed earlier in the module will occur in the triage and emergency departments rather than on the patient care floors.

Agency Protection

In addition to secondary injuries incurred while caring for casualties from the event or agents used in the event, agencies must protect themselves against direct attacks. During and after 9-11, transportation within the immediate and adjacent areas to the twin towers was interrupted, initially due to recovery efforts, and later, security measures. Needed health care staff responded to this critical situation by meeting patients at central locations and escorting them to the agency site. Access to the agency remained restricted for a period of time, so the response plan must include plans for patient and staff movement.

If a chemical agent is suspected and decontamination is anticipated, all staff coming in contact with victims before they have been decontaminated must wear PPE. This includes impermeable clothing, gloves, boots, and a gas mask. Performing critical procedures while wearing this attire is difficult and requires practice. Education for nurses must incorporate time for practice in donning the PPE, and should be a part of the disaster exercises held by each agency and community.

Managers must evaluate the practicality of using nurses for the decontamination procedure. Consider assigning unlicensed personnel or nursing students who, with training, may be used outside to decontaminate the more stable victims. This frees the nursing staff to address the more complex care issues inside the hospital, where unlicensed personnel would be unable to assist.

Chemical weapons are classified according to their mode of action or time that they remain active in the environment or persistence, and lethality (Evison, Hinsley, & Rice, 2002). The characteristics of a chemical weapons attack as compared to routine hazardous materials exposure is that the chemical weapons attack results from an intentional act with potentially more toxic substances. There is a greater risk to EMS personnel, and those at hospitals or agencies will be faced with large numbers of worried well, and may encounter mass hysteria and panic (Henretig, Ciedslak, & Eitzen, 2002). The chemical weapons can act in a variety of ways, so health care providers must be aware of symptom groups suggestive of classes of agents. Inhalation of a nerve agent vapor results in the first clinical symptoms being respiratory, with dimming of vision, and miosis. Blister agents, such as sulphur mustard, are accompanied by a faint odor of mustard or garlic, and the development of large blisters (Evison et al., 2002).

As agents are suspected or confirmed, the specific protocols are initiated. For example, if symptoms of cholinesterase poisoning (e.g., pinpoint pupils, dyspnea, local or generalized sweating, fasciculation, copious secretions, nausea, vomiting, diarrhea, convulsions, or coma) are observed, initiate a nerve agent protocol. Nursing staff must be prepared to administer common antidotes to the agents (CDC, 2003h) (Table 6–3).

If a chemical agent is suspected, it is important to identify it as soon as possible. The CDC offers decontamination and treatment protocols by agent, and these can be downloaded from its website. See MediaLink.

Organizing these valuable resources in a binder on each unit provides an educational resource that can be studied during less busy periods. The protocols also serve as a guide to ensure that adequate and appropriate supplies are available for use following chemical exposure (CDC, 2003i). One of the challenges in remaining prepared is the development of new threats from terrorists. Assistance in remaining current is available from the CDC through a subscription update service. The CDC Clinician Registry for Terrorism and Emergency Responder Updates and Training Opportunities is another resource available through the CDC.

It is important that nurses are knowledgeable about the appropriate treatment to avoid unnecessary expenditure of resources. Most chemical agents can penetrate clothing and are rapidly absorbed through the skin. Therefore quick and effective decontamination is vital. A significant reduction in exposure to the toxic chemical can be achieved by simply undressing victims. A chemical in its liquid or solid form requires people to remove their clothing and thoroughly wash exposed skin. With exposures to chemicals in a vapor form, people need only to remove their clothing and leave the source of the toxic vapor (HHS, 2003; Henretig, Cieslak, & Eitzen, 2002). If clothing cannot be removed over the head to avoid contact with the mouth, eyes, and nose, it may have to be cut off. Eyeglasses, contact lens, or other items in contact with the body must be decontaminated. Containers and markers for these and other items must be available on the mobile supply carts. Nursing staff must be comfortable with procedures that will protect and maintain control of the environment during a suspected or confirmed biologic attack. EPA (1998) recommendations in Box 6–9 can serve as a guide when planning educational programs for protecting nurses and other staff members during a biologic attack. Each recommendation can be accompanied by specific procedures and protocols that provide consistency and control in a potentially chaotic situation.

It is important to differentiate a biological weapons attack from a natural infectious disease epidemic. A weapons attack is an intentional attack, in which the diagnosis is delayed because the agent is often exotic, thereby placing the health care providers at greater risk. At the hospital or agency, there will be many worried well who may panic when seeking help. There will be high infection rates in a compressed time frame, with more respiratory forms of disease than would naturally occur (Henretig et al., 2002). When large numbers of casualties flood emergency departments and health care settings, it is confusing and nurses will be caring for victims before a final diagnosis has been made about the cause of their distress. There are general symptom groupings that can suggest the type of agent that is causing the illnesses. See Table 6–4. These groupings will enable the nursing and medical staff to begin preliminary treatment while awaiting the final laboratory diagnosis.

Each facility must adopt procedures and education that provide knowledge and protection to their workers. There are various products available commercially that may assist in this process and should be explored to determine their fit within the organization. The *Biological Terrorism Response Manual* (Rega, 2000) introduces "Bio-Terry" as a method of preparing for and managing potential bioterrorism incidents. Specific syndromic descriptions associated with each agent can be found on each Bio-Terry page. See Figure 6–6.

TABLE 6–3. COMMON ANTIDOTES FOR NERVE AGENTS

COMMON ANTIDOTES	EFFECT/SYMPTOMS
Anticholinergics	Antagonize muscarinic effects
Oximes	Reactivate inhibited acetylcholinesterase and antagonize nicotinic effects
Prophylactic anticonvulsants	Prevent seizures

From "Chemical Weapons" by D. Evison, D. Hinsley, and P. Rice, 2002, British Medical Journal, 324, (7333), pp. 332–335.

BOX 6–9   Recommendations to Maintain Environmental Control

- Establish control measures to reduce viral contamination on fabric, clothing, & bedding
- Clean and disinfect reusable equipment
- Maintain cleaning and appropriate reprocessing of medical instruments
- Clean and decontaminate large environmental surfaces
- Regulate medical waste containment, treatment, and disposal
- Become familiar with indications for decontamination of air space in rooms and vehicles

Adapted from Work Practice Controls, EPA (1998)

TABLE 6–4. AGENTS AND GENERAL SYMPTOM GROUPINGS

AGENT TYPE	SYMPTOMS
Nuclear	Fatigue
	Non-healing burns
	Fatigue
Biological	Elevated temperature
	Headache
	Fatigue
	Progression to respiratory failure in days
	Rash → pustular vesicles
Chemical	Nausea/Vomiting/Diarrhea
	Choking
	Blisters & erythema
	Dyspnea
	Gastric emptying
	Convulsions/coma
	Pinpoint pupils
	Increased salivation

Adapted from: Joint Commission on Accreditation of Healthcare Organizations. (2001a). Joint Commission Perspectives, 21 (12).

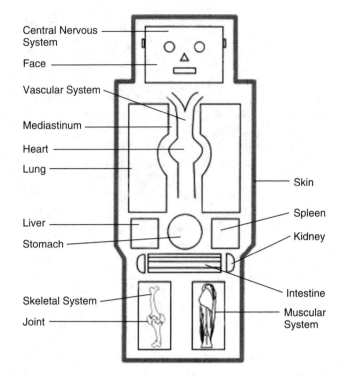

Figure 6–6. Bio-Terry. (Rega, 2000)

BOX 6–10   Nuclear Contamination

Suspicion of Radiation or Nuclear Contamination

If radiation or nuclear contamination is suspected and detection equipment is available, perform head to toe sweep (passing radiation detection wand over entire body) **before** exiting technical decontamination area.

Perform second technical decontamination procedure if elevated radiation levels are detected.

Perform a second sweep. An elevated second reading suggests incorporated radiation. A third decontamination procedure is not indicated.

The victim may now exit into the hospital (cold zone).

(J. Hamilton, personal communication, May 14, 2003)

In the event of a nuclear or radiation event, it is important to quickly move people who are near the incident away, while protecting the nose and mouth with a filter-equipped mask. Unfortunately, people may not be aware of the incident until considerable exposure has occurred. All who have been exposed should be decontaminated by removing clothing and washed with soap and water prior to entering the hospital. See Box 6–10.

Security

Security must be prepared to provide protection to the staff and agency. To perform efficiently and effectively, nurses must feel secure and protected. Protection will include effective crowd control, as people will flood the facility for medical care or in search of family and friends. It is vital to secure access and egress to the facility, and to ensure that decontamination occurs prior to entrance if this is indicated. Complicating the situation is the fact that terrorist events result in ground zero also becoming a crime scene. All necessary facility employees must be properly identified. To maintain security, nurses must have a recognizable identification. It is also helpful if the identification includes an indication of the *call-in* status of the nurse. This allows security, police, and fire personnel to assist needed staff in reaching the facility. At present, plans are underway by the American Red Cross and other agencies to use a *universal identification card*. This will permit the verification of credentials at a time when urgency is not a concern, and will speed the integration of volunteer nurses within the response team.

CASUALTY ASSESSMENT

One of the initial assessments required for victims of disasters is a comprehensive head-to-toe examination of the body. This brief systematic assessment provides valuable information. Gloves and eye protection should be used until the cause of the event is determined.

The examination begins with the neck to detect spinal injuries and serious injury to the trachea. The necessary observations can be categorized under four words: look, feel, listen, and smell. If at the scene of the event, begin by kneeling at the side of the patient's head to perform the following steps:

Look

- Observe color changes, deformities, wounds, penetrations, or unusual chest movements.
- Inspect for wounds and trauma. Note point tenderness.

Feel

- Palpate for deformities, tenderness, pulsations, spasms, temperature.
  - When the victim is unconscious, assume that there is a spinal injury.
  - Begin stabilization with a cervical collar. Observe for obvious injury.
  - Inspect the scalp without moving the head.
  - Do not remove a wig or hairpiece, to avoid restarting bleeding.
  - Gently palpate the skull and face for deformities and depressions.
  - If there are no burns, cuts, or injuries examine and open the patient's eyes.
  - Observe pupils for the size, equality, and reactivity. Note the presence of contact lenses.
  - Inspect the ears and nose for the presence of blood or clear fluid.

Listen

- Assess breathing patterns or sounds.
  - Evaluate for airway obstruction.
    - Reposition if needed according to American Heart Association guidelines for CPR.
  - Look for a medical identification necklace, deviations from the midline, bruising, or deformities.
  - Observe for distention of the jugular vein.

Smell

- Note unusual odors
  - A fruity smell indicative of diabetic coma or prolonged nausea and vomiting.
  - Petroleum odor indicative of ingested poisoning.
  - Alcohol odor indicative of possible intoxication.
    (*Integrated Publishing, 2003*)

An assessment instrument for mass trauma is available from the CDC (2003b). This instrument was adapted from a tool used at the World Trade Center and can be modified for specific agencies or events. Explanatory notes are also available; both of these tools can be downloaded through the CDC website and will provide a foundation to promote consistency in responding to disasters.

In addition to assessment tools for physical status, the CDC offers a mental health survey tool with explanatory notes (CDC, 2003e). The complexities of assessing the person's psychological status are discussed in Chapter Four.

Assessment and Management of Hemorrhage

Patients with injuries causing severe blood loss should be quickly assessed to determine whether a tourniquet was applied at the scene, or whether immediate intervention is needed to save lives. Staff should be comfortable with the principal points on the body where hand or finger pressure can be used to stop hemorrhage. These skills can be incorporated within the education program and reviewed at regular intervals. This information may also be available in diagrams on walls or laminated cards attached to the staff identification card.

Each victim must be evaluated for shock and measures taken to prevent and control it. These skills must be incorporated within orientation programs and continuing education for the professional nurse. Be alert for the early signs of developing shock, such as restlessness and apprehension. The degree of symptoms can be correlated with estimated blood loss. Assess the victim's skin, pulse, blood pressure, and mucous membranes. As you assess the peripheral pulse, remember that it may be absent with severe hypotension. The rate may be rapid in hemorrhagic shock or slowed in neurogenic shock.

Shock

Blood pressure may be low in moderately severe shock, with a systolic pressure below 100 mm Hg, and a pulse above 100, due to the peripheral vasoconstriction as the body tries to compensate for circulatory fluid loss. This process can maintain blood pressure at near normal levels despite a moderately severe loss of blood volume. This compensatory mechanism cannot be maintained indefinitely. At some point, even a small additional loss results in a sudden fall in blood pressure. Nurses and other providers must be aware of significant signs of volume loss, such as nausea and vomiting, dry mucous membranes, thirst, and decreased urinary output.

Shock may result from different causes. In hemorrhagic shock, whole blood is lost. The lowered blood volume causes a decreased cardiac output and decreased peripheral circulation. Perfusion of major organs is reduced, as well as the transport of wastes from the cells. This alteration in circulation cannot continue indefinitely without altering cellular function. An attempt at compensation results in fluid from body tissues entering the circulation, with a resultant decrease in hematocrit and red cell count. Burn shock presents with a different clinical picture. In this case, there is an increase in hematocrit and red cell counts due to hemoconcentration as plasma is lost via the burn area. Neurogenic or vasogenic shock occurs when there is a disruption of the autonomic nervous system control over vasoconstriction. Neurogenic shock can result from increased fluid loss, central nervous system trauma, or emotional shock. A common form is seen in fainting or syncope. A temporary pooling of the blood causes loss of consciousness, and fainting occurs, at which time blood rushes to the head and solves the problem. It can occur with stressful wartime experiences. The onset of most forms of shock results in vasoconstriction. Normally, the autonomic nervous system maintains partial contraction of the veins and arteries; but this cannot be maintained indefinitely, and eventually the vessels dilate, expanding the volume of the circulator system and causing a drop in blood pressure (Integrated Publishing, 2003).

Cardiogenic shock results from the inadequate functioning of the heart that causes inadequate circulatory pressure in the presence of normal circulatory volume. Shock develops as the pressure falls. Septic shock typically develops 2 to 5 days following the injury. It may occur following penetrating abdominal wounds or contaminated injuries. Vasodilation occurs, followed by increased permeability of the blood vessels and escape of fluid into the tissues. Anaphylactic shock occurs following exposure to a substance to which the victim is sensitive (Integrated Publishing, 2003).

Treatment for shock involves intravenous fluids. Ringer's lactate is appropriate, although normal saline can be used while waiting for blood. The electrolyte solutions replace the blood volume, as well as the extracellular fluid. In addition to these treatments for shock, it is important to maintain the airway, control blood loss, reduce pain and conserve body heat (Integrated Publishing, 2003).

Pneumatic counterpressure devices, such as medical anti-shock trousers or military anti-shock trousers (MAST) are tools that may be used to treat shock. These correct or counteract certain internal bleeding conditions. They may be used with systolic pressure less than 80 mm Hg, systolic pressure less than 100 mm Hg with symptoms, and fractures of the pelvis or lower extremities. MAST treatment is not indicated in the presence of pulmonary edema, congestive heart failure, heart attack, stroke, pregnancy, or major traumatic injuries. After being applied, the garment is inflated to maintain the systolic pressure at 100 mm Hg. It is important to have oxygen available, together with appropriate administration devices such as mask, nasal cannula, and endotrachial tube. Suction devices are necessary to maintain the airway. If the airway cannot be maintained with these devices, a cricothyroidotomy or emergency tracheotomy may be necessary. This procedure involves an incision into the cricothyroid membrane beneath the skin between the thyroid cartilage and the cricoid cartilage. This area can be located by hyperextending the neck so that the thyroid notch or Adam's apple becomes prominent, then the correct area is palpated with a finger (Integrated Publishing, 2003).

Wounds

Wounds are categorized according to which skin or tissue is broken. The six types of wounds are as follows:

- **Abrasions**   occur when the skin is rubbed or scraped off. It can become infected when dirt and germs become embedded.
- **Incisions**   are made with sharp cutting instruments. Incisions tend to bleed freely because the blood vessels are cut cleanly with little surrounding tissue damage.
- **Lacerations**   are torn wounds with torn tissue underneath. They are made with blunt objects. Bomb fragments can cause lacerations.
- **Punctures**   occur when objects penetrate into the tissues, leaving a small surface opening. They do not bleed freely, but larger wounds may cause internal bleeding.
- **Avulsions**   are the tearing away of tissue from a body part. Bleeding typically is heavy. The torn tissue may be reattached, so place the tissue in a sterile dressing in a cool container. Take care not to freeze the tissue or submerge in water or saline.
- **Amputations**   are traumatic or nontraumatic removal of limbs from the body. Shock will develop, and a tourniquet is often necessary.

(Integrated Publishing, 2003)

Wound closure may have to be delayed due to contamination. As wounds are cleaned and dressings applied, tetanus status of the victim must be investigated and treatment initiated as indicated.

Etiology of Injuries

Knowing what caused the injury is helpful when planning care. In wartime or terrorism, the velocity of bullets or shrapnel is an important variable. Low-velocity bullets damage only the tissue they contact. High-velocity bullets can result in enormous damage as they force the tissues and body parts away from the track.

Bombs and explosions result in unique injuries that are seldom seen outside combat. Due to the blast, multisystem and life-threatening injuries occur simultaneously to many persons. The severity and pattern of the injuries are dependent on the composition and amount of explosives used, the environment, delivery method, distance between victim(s) and the blast, and barriers that may have absorbed some of the energy (Wightman & Gladish, 2001).

The CDC has developed a primer to prepare health care providers to become proficient in dealing with casualties caused by explosions. When considering bombs, understanding the ways in which damage results is helpful for anticipating the possible types of injuries. Explosives are grouped under two categories: high-order explosives (HE) or low-order explosives (LE). High order explosives produce a defining, supersonic, overpressurization shock wave. Some types of explosives in this category are C-4, Semtex, nitroglycerin, and dynamite. Low-order explosives result in a subsonic explosion without the overpressurization wave. Explosives in this group include pipe bombs, gunpowder, and pure petroleum-based bombs, such a Molotov cocktails (CDC, 2003f).

Bombs are also categorized according to their source, for example manufactured with an implied standard or improvised, in which a substance is utilized outside its traditional use. The transformation of the solid explosive into gas generates a highly pressurized wave of air that propagates radially from the site of the explosion, at the speed of sound, and is succeeded by a wave of negative pressure. The leading front of the massive air movement is the blast front, which is responsible for the peak of high pressure that at different intensities will cause different types of damage.

Injuries from blasts are grouped under four types (primary, secondary, tertiary, and quaternary) based on the mechanism of the blast. The classifications consider the anatomical and physiological changes from the direct or reflective overpressurization force impacting the body's surface. A distinction should be made between the blast wave, or over-pressure component and the blast wind, or forced super-heated airflow (CDC, 2003f).

Primary blast mechanisms occur only with high-order explosives. Gas-filled structures within the body are affected most frequently, such as the lungs, GI tract, and middle ear. In the lung, pulmonary barotraumas occur, also known as blast lung. The tympanic membrane can rupture in the ear, and causing middle ear damage. In addition, abdominal hemorrhage can occur, globe or eye rupture, and concussions without the physical signs of head injury.

In the secondary category, injuries result from flying debris and bomb fragments. Any part of the body can be affected, and injuries range from penetrating ballistic (fragmentation) to blunt injuries.

Tertiary injuries result from individuals being thrown by the blast wind. Fractures, traumatic amputations, and open and closed brain injuries can occur. Finally, in the quaternary category, all injuries not fitting into the previous three categories are grouped. It may include exacerbations or complications of existing conditions affecting any part of the body. Injury types include burns (e.g., flash, partial and full thick-

ness), crush injuries, asthma, COPD, respiratory problems, angina, hyperglycemia, and hypertension (CDC, 2003b).

Low-order explosives lack the high-order overpressurization wave. Most of the injuries due to low-order explosives result from fragmentation or ballistics, blast winds, and thermal.

Internal soft tissue injuries can result from either type. Although some injuries are obvious, others may not be easily seen, and you must rely on your assessment skills and observations. Some of the visible indicators of internal soft tissue injury are:

- Hematemesis: vomiting bright red blood
- Hemoptysis: coughing up bright red blood
- Melena: excretion of tarry black stools
- Hematochezia: excretion of bright red blood from the rectum
- Nonmenstrual vaginal bleeding
- Hematuria: passing of blood in the urine
- Epistaxis: nosebleed
- Pooling of blood near the skin surface

(Integrated Publishing, 2003)

Frequently, there are no visible signs of injury and more subtle clues will have to be used, such as:

- Pale, clammy skin
- Lowered body temperature
- Rapid, thready pulse
- Decreasing blood pressure
- Dilated pupils that are slow to react
- Ringing in the ears or tinnitus
- Syncope
- Thirst
- Yawning, air hunger
- Anxiety, restlessness with feelings of impending doom

(Integrated Publishing, 2003)

Once suspected, treatment is initiated according to institutional protocols for shock or hemorrhage. Lung injuries or blast lung is caused by the overpressurization wave; it is the most common fatal injury among initial survivors. Symptoms are often present at the initial triage, but may occur as late as 48 hours. Lung injury is characterized by the clinical triad of apnea, bradycardia, and hypotension. The injury to the lung varies from scattered petechae to confluent hemorrhages. Suspect blast lung with victims with dyspnea, cough, hemoptysis, or chest pain after an explosion. The diagnosis can be confirmed with a chest X ray showing the characteristic "butterfly" pattern. Care must be taken before general anesthesia or air transport. Many experts recommend a prophylactic chest tube or thoracostomy.

Post explosion, injury to the ear results in significant morbidity. The type and extent of the injury is dependent on the orientation of the ear to the blast. Tympanic membrane perforation is the most common injury. Symptoms include hearing loss, tinnitus, otalgia, vertigo, bleeding from the external canal, TM rupture, or mucopurulent otorrhea. Following an explosion, those exposed should have an otologic assessment and audiometry.

Gas-containing sections of the GI tract are vulnerable to the effects of the blast. The effect can result in immediate bowel perforation, hemorrhage, mesenteric shear injuries, solid organ lacerations, and testicular rupture. Suspect blast injury when victims present with abdominal pain, nausea, vomiting, hematemesis, rectal pain, tenesmus, testicular pain, unexplained hypovolemia, or other symptoms of an acute abdomen.

Air embolism is common following these injuries. Nurses and other health care providers must maintain a high index of suspicion when patients present with stroke, myocardial infarction (MI), acute abdomen, blindness, deafness, spinal cord injury, or claudication. Be aware of the option to use hyperbaric oxygen therapy if this chamber is available.

Following an explosion, the primary blast waves can result in a concussion or mild traumatic brain injury (MTBI), when no evidence of head injury can be seen. Evaluate victims complaining of headaches, fatigue, poor concentration, lethargy, depression, anxiety, and insomnia. The symptoms of this brain injury can be similar to symptoms of posttraumatic stress disorder.

A mass casualty or terrorist event may result in large death tolls. This is magnified when advance planning has not included management of bodies. Planning must include decisions on temporary morgues. Since most agencies have limited refrigerated space, plans may include arrangements to use area facilities such as walk-in coolers, refrigerated trucks, or ice rinks.

LOGISTICS

Patient Tracking

Communication within and between agencies about victims provides a method for friends and relatives to locate their loved ones. The patient record is a vital source of information during a disaster. During and following September 11, 2001, various methods of managing the patient record have been proposed. This process is likely to become more complex due to enactment of the Health Insurance Portability and Accountability Act (HIPAA) law. Some agencies have records remain with patients at all times as they move throughout the agency. This provides a challenge to keep the record updated, accurate, and with the patients as they are moved between departments. In addition, standard triage tags take time to apply and are difficult to write on once in place. Some hospitals initially use a simple number system to track victims. All clothing, requisitions, and charting pages are marked with the same number. As time permits, identifying information is added, as well as the name, once identity has been confirmed.

A newer technology offers the familiar bar code as a method of patient identification and tracking. The bar

coded bracelet is applied as the victim enters the health care system. This may be at the site of the disaster, or in transit to an agency. Accompanying the bracelet are numerous tags with the same bar code. Patient information is entered using a handheld computer, and is updated throughout the patient's contact with the health care system. Information can be read using a handheld scanner, much like that used by commercial delivery services. Patient privacy is protected by a password access system. This system requires the implementation of the scanner system for accessing the information, and therefore incurs additional financial expenditures.

Another system for tracking patients within the hospital involves the use of tracking sheets in each treatment area. For example, each room contains a clipboard near the door. As patients are being moved, a number or bar-code sticker is placed on the page, with a notation about the destination. This process continues throughout the acute treatment phase. Whichever system is adopted, nurses must be included in the plan development and provided an opportunity to become familiar with the system prior to its implementation.

Activating Inactive Nurses

It will not be enough to rely exclusively on the nurses currently working at health care facilities. The increased need for nurses during a disaster coupled with the nursing shortage demands that nursing managers and administers think creatively about how to increase the workforce during a crisis. The current nursing workforce can be supplemented with professional nurses not currently active within nursing. The establishment of a reserve workforce, adequately trained and educated in appropriate response techniques, will be the foundation of an adequate response effort following a disaster (AHA, 2000).

Consideration should be given to the development of a community-wide concept of "reserve staff," identifying physicians, nurses, and hospital workers who are retired, have changed careers, or work in areas outside of direct patient care. This reserve staff would have to be classified according to skill level and expertise. This concept would work only if adequate funding is available for regular education and updates. Another concept involves adapting licenses so that nurses and physicians in one state could work in another.

Many physicians, nurses, and support personnel work at more than one hospital. When individual agencies are counting their potential available personnel, there is a real possibility of double counting personnel. It is important that agencies work together to provide an unduplicated estimate of available personnel.

In addition to the listing of reserved or retired staff, consideration should be given to expanding this to include medical, nursing, or allied health students in programs affiliated with the agency. Consider also the use of first responders once the initial scene is stabilized. Care should be taken to cycle staff on and off, to maintain accurate assessment and intervention skills and provide psychological support. All staff members should know if they are on the first group of responders to the agency, or the second, for example, at the 12-hour mark.

Vendors

If the communication systems are interrupted, agencies may not be able to contact vendors to secure additional supplies and equipment, such as ventilators. Prior to the need, agencies should discuss with vendors the locations of additional supplies so that alternate plans can be made in case airports are closed or roadways destroyed. Nurses must be educated in the protocols for acquiring additional supplies and the chain of authority for ordering additional supplies during a disaster.

Worried Well

One of the most challenging services required during and following a disaster is the development and implementation of a system to assist in the reunification of victims with family and friends following a disaster. It is important that they not be entering the decontamination and triage area, thereby obstructing the flow and delaying treatment. Designate an area or entrance for them, or perhaps an adjacent building, such as a school or hotel. This area should be staffed with personnel sensitive to the trauma experienced by these people and skilled in talking with persons experiencing severe emotional trauma, such as counselors, social workers, or nurses. Security staff must also be included, to provide protection for staff and others, since grief reactions can take many forms, some of them violent.

Telephone lines and computer communication is important so that staff in this area can be kept current on the victims being treated at that, and perhaps other, agencies. Consider developing a database to be used that would include traditional identification characteristics such as name and address, but also physical descriptions, clothing descriptions, and marks on the body. These may be the only way to locate and identify victims. Some agencies are utilizing digital photography of all victims. These images are stored on the computer and when a match is made on description parameters, the staff would verbally prepare the family to look at the picture and make a positive identification. Plans must be in place as to how remains are to be claimed or family united with victims. An escort may be necessary as victims are identified and family members reunited.

As your agency prepares to manage large numbers of victims, be sure that the planning and education is documented and reviewed on a regular basis. All staff should be regularly updated on its contents because the best plan is worthless if it remains unknown. Consider developing a manual that is readily available on each unit. This manual should include a comprehensive plan for meeting increased demand for services. A detailed index permits rapid access to vital information and plans. Topics may include:

- Opening remarks or the philosophy of the agency CEO
- Line of authority during an event (before and after an incident command system is established)
- Explanation of manual use
- Definitions of terms
- Scope of responsibility for different types of employees
- Plans for different shifts or times when the event occurs
- Call-up protocol with phone numbers identifying specific persons or job types, and their response role
- Departmental response plans (e.g., nursing, surgery, laboratory, blood bank, security, housekeeping, transportation)
- Maps and schematics of traffic flow internally and externally
- Plans for dealing with families
- Plans for dealing with the media

This manual should be examined and revised if necessary at designated intervals.

Once developed, your response plan will not cover all scenarios. Plan for the unexpected, and do not plan in a vacuum. Collaborate with area health care agencies and civil authorities. Know who is the ultimate authority, and follow instructions from that person or agency. Expect a period of time requiring your agency to be self-sufficient and independent before federal assistance arrives. Thorough planning in advance results in efficient handling of the victims, and protection of the health care providers. Each person should understand the whole plan, and react confidently when challenges arise.

PERSPECTIVES OF A U.S. EMERGENCY ROOM NURSE

In the past, emergency staff experienced in disaster situations were accustomed to providing essential emergency care to the majority of the victims of trauma. In addition to the larger scale of a disaster, another concern is the increased risk for toxicological or biological incidents and the minimal experience of most emergency workers in this area. Incidents that reach beyond the experience of emergency staff need to be identified and training needs to be planned, rehearsed and automatic. This makes the importance of clear plans of action and drills a necessity. JCAHO has minimal standards in place for hospitals that seek accreditation. At Saint Louis University Hospital, drills are organized according to threat level. If the potential for a biological, chemical, or radiological event is identified, the hospital drill will be focused on that potential incident. Debriefings are scheduled following the drill and particular needs or weaknesses are identified and retested. Policies, procedures, and protocols need to be firmly in place prior to an event. Emergency staff are the backbone of the hospital during disasters and staff should be able to work from short, simple, and specific protocols appropriate to the incident.

The following information will identify the pitfalls and practices related to traditional disaster plans prior to 9-11 and focus on the enhancements to include chemical, biological, or radiological emergencies. Many emergency departments have activation plans based on the number and acuity of incident victims coming to their facility in addition to the present emergency department volume, acuity, and bed availability at the time of the incident.

Some hospitals have tiered responses in which activation involving small numbers of victims is limited to on-call emergency personnel. It is important for leadership staff in the ED to know how to activate the disaster response 24 hours a day. At Saint Louis University Hospital, the ED charge nurse is a key player, as well as the ED attending physician on duty. They evaluate the incident from the information available and activate the system accordingly. To error on the side of the patient is the practice and if the activation was deemed not necessary after the fact, re-education is implemented.

Incidents usually occur without warning, so time is of the essence. Many emergency departments have developed checklists for leadership staff in the event of an incident. The checklists are utilized during drills so that staff are familiar with the process when the actual event occurs. For example, our emergency department has a disaster cart which contains personal protective equipment readily available in the department. In addition, we have six bags pre-packaged with level C suits in various sizes, chemical-biological facemasks, boots, and other personal protective items necessary for decontamination. Once a disaster is activated, this cart and bag system will provide enough equipment for decontamination until the large decon cart arrives via protective services.

The code D cart contains resources regarding the following:

- Code D Disaster policy
- Patient decontamination
- Self-decontamination
- Biological protocols
- Chemical protocols
- Nuclear protocols
- Geiger counter
- Emergency patient tracking system (EPTS) scanner
- Disaster tags (EPTS)
- Combined MD/RN disaster documentation forms
- Disaster vests and hats

Each drawer is clearly marked and restocked after each event. All documentation forms associated with disaster preparedness are located on this cart.

Incidents that are most challenging are those that occur after normal business hours when resources and services are not at full capacity. Most hospitals are supervised by nursing house supervisors during these times. When a disaster alert is activated, the house supervisor becomes the administrator on duty and has the responsibility to manage hospital-wide operations until additional administrators arrive. Direction of situations requiring full disaster activation resulting in dissemination of staff via the personnel pool should be delegated by the house supervisor to the most available senior nurse on duty. Assigned areas within the hospital are designated according to acuity using the universal, color-coded disaster tagging system. Assigning staff to appropriate areas depends on the staff members presently available and their level of experience. At our facility all critical care nurses are assigned to the "red patient area" located in the emergency department to care for critically ill patients. Medical-surgical nurses are assigned to the "yellow" urgent patients requiring assessment and intervention as soon as possible. Non-clinical nurses and student nurses are assigned to the "green" patients, which are those with minor injuries. Student nurses can also be of great value as decon staff.

Emergency department nurses are assigned as team leaders of each team. They are designated by the appropriate color hat and titled vest. The purpose of color identification assists float staff in locating assigned areas and leaders. Physicians are also designated in the same manner.

During times of extreme emergencies, when crowd control keeps people from responding to their assigned area, a badge system is used.

Available staff sign in under designated specialty areas that specify the location of their assignment. The person in control of the personnel pool assigns badges. To physically enter the assigned area, staff must show their badge. If they are in the correct area, they are allowed to enter. Staff without badges are not allowed in the emergency treatment area. This keeps staff and unidentified visitors from entering before officially signing in. In this way, all staff can be accounted for.

The disaster plan in the emergency department must include who is in charge, disposition of patients currently in the ED, and identification of the triage site and treatment areas, including decontamination, patient flow, staffing, and supply needs. The persons in charge in the ED are usually the designated charge nurse on duty and the ED attending physician. Decisions are made collaboratively.

It is important to keep in mind that the triage area is not a treatment area but an area in which patients are sorted and classified according to acuity. Attempting to treat patients in the triage area will result in a backflow of patients that can jeopardize the entire system.

The great challenge of the 21st century in emergency care is triaging and decontaminating disaster victims at the same time. Many facilities are not equipped to decontaminate multiple patients in a timely fashion. Decontamination of both ambulatory and stretcher patients have to be considered. In addition, critical patients who are contaminated must be decontaminated prior to entering the facility. Critical care may have to be instituted during decontamination procedures. Allowing decontaminated patients into the ED will result in the shutdown of the ED and loss of an area that was providing lifesaving care.

Patient flow may be a straightforward plan or altered if decontamination is added. Decon capabilities require additional staff and additional space. There should be a designated dirty triage RN and MD, as well as a clean triage RN and MD. Staffing and supply needs will depend on the volume and acuity of patients, the need for decontamination, the extent of the disaster, and the time frame in which victims arrived. Duplicate supply and linen carts should be available both in the clean and dirty decon areas. Staff working in "dirty triage" should have additional staff to care for life-threatening injuries while the triage team continues to prioritize patients. Supplies should be readily available and separate from the clean triage area to avoid contamination.

In conclusion, your plan will only be as good as the educational investment in your staff. Long, detailed plans may be conclusive, but if they are not easy to use, they are impractical. Thankfully, mass casualty incidents are infrequent, but this also lends to inexperience. Drills and identifying areas of strengths and weakness are the keys to a successful ED plan. Our efforts toward the future could be summarized by President Lyndon Johnson, "Yesterday is not ours to recover, but tomorrow is ours to win or lose."

PERSPECTIVES OF AN ISRAELI NURSE

Early preparations for mass casualty events are mandatory to increase the survival of those injured and to decrease the potential devastating impact on society. It is of utmost importance that the proper educational measures are taken in order to prepare the medical, prehospital, nursing, and paramedical staffs for any and all possibilities. Adequate preparation of the medical teams will decrease the chaos associated with mass casualty events, and increase patient survival and social durability (Shemir & Shapira, 2001).

Data collected from the recent years of Israel-Palestinian conflict by the Israel Center for Disease Control identify differences between injuries caused by explosion and those resulting from all other mechanisms of trauma. Terrorism caused more severe injuries, reflected by the higher injury severity score (ISS) of patients admitted to the hospital following terrorist attacks (30% with ISS >16 versus in all other trauma admissions) and consequently also increased mortality. In-hospital death among

terror victims (6.2%) was double that of all other trauma victims combined. Surgical interventions, especially procedures related to the musculosketelal system, were preformed significantly more frequently in survivors of bomb explosions than in casualties of all other kinds of trauma. The length of hospital stay and the need for intensive care were also significantly increased for bombing victims.

Death from Bombing

When conspicuous injuries are found in explosion fatalities, it is easy to determine the cause of death, but sometimes no distinctive injuries are identifiable. It is postulated that in some victims without obvious external injuries, cardiac dysrhythmias or air emboli caused cardiac arrest and eventual death. This type of injury is related to the effect of the blast generated by the explosion. In most victims, death from explosion is the aftermath of combined blast, ballistic, and thermal effect injuries. Only after recognizing the differing death patterns in such victims and understanding the underlying mechanisms can research and management of explosion injuries be realized (Mellor & Cooper, 1989).

Four Components of Knowledge

We have identified four components of knowledge as critical to master by medical terms intending to treat victims admitted following explosions.

- **Detonation:** the physics of the explosion, and the potential for complications from such injuries
- **Wound ballistics:** understanding the resultant injury patterns
- **Triage:** the art of sorting patients according to the severity of injury
- **Medical concerns:** treating multiple patients with multidimensional injuries and special injury patterns

Detonation and Explosion

The explosive being used for mass casualty can be military, commercial, or homemade. Often terrorists add metal particles of various shapes to the explosive to increase its wounding potential. These include steel balls, nails, and nuts.

Wound Ballistics

The primary blast injury results from the blast wave passing through the human body. Spalling, implosion, inertia, and pressure differences are the putative mechanisms by which blasts induce damage in the tissue. The human body suffers damage in relation to the elastic properties of the involved tissues and their density and composition, resulting in different patterns of injury for different organs. The most deadly pathological hallmark of blast injury is the appearance of air emboli that fill the pulmonary vessels and the coronary blood vessels. This is most likely the leading mechanism of death in the blast victim.

Triage

Triage, the art of sorting patients according to the severity of their injury, is the key for successful management of MCEs. It is preformed in the field and in the emergency department. Field triage identifies critically injured patients who need immediate care, provides lifesaving procedures, and transfers patients to suitable surrounding hospitals. Immediately after the explosion the chaos phase starts, when family members, bystanders, and passing vehicles evacuate 6% to 10% of the injured to the nearest hospital. When trained medical personnel reach the scene, the medical command phase starts and triage principles are employed in the management of the remaining injured.

The hospital triage officer, a well-trained surgeon, sorts the patients according to their severity of injury. Surgery for the injured from bomb explosion is challenging. Damage control surgery is the most commonly acceptable and logical concept governing the treatment of these patients. This strategy enables surgeons to deal with physiological derangements and anatomic damage in a timely manner.

After the acute triage stage is over, a tertiary survey of all patients admitted is crucial. Missed injuries after bomb explosions are not uncommon. Physical trauma is our primary concern. Some of the injured will also suffer post-traumatic reactions that should be managed by specialized teams, and these symptoms can be identified by the nurse. Physicians and nurses should be instructed on post-traumatic reactions and their symptoms (Kluger, 2003).

All nurses currently working in high trained areas as emergency and intensive care should also undergo specific training. An ED nurse should be trained in trauma as well as intensive medicine. The intensive care nurses should pass a trauma course. The majority of the nurses working today in ICU and the recovery room at Hadassah have been specially trained in intensive care (a 9-month course with national boards at the summation), as well as a specialized course in trauma medicine. Therefore, when a mass casualty occurs, the nursing staff is fluid. The specially trained ICU nurse can easily rush to the ED when a MCE occurs. After the initial rush of patients have arrived, been triaged and undergone X ray, angiogram, CT scan, and admitted into the operating theatre, these nurses can return to their original department. Many emergency room nurses, at home when a MCE occurs, arrive at the hospital to give assistance. After a few hours the emergency room empties and the recovery room and intensive care departments start to overflow.

In times of mass casualty, the recovery room at Hadassah Ein Kerem becomes the center of the hospital, with the most severely injured arriving after surgery, or embolization in angiogram. Terrified families wait for the surgeon for some word of their wounded relatives. While these patients are in the operating room, the nurses in the recovery room get acquainted with the anxious families. They take the time to offer water and a few comforting words while waiting for the operation to finish. We have found that the number of people in the waiting room is usually overwhelming. When a mass casualty occurs, people who are barely acquainted with the injured, appear at the hospital to support, to be a part of the tragedy. It is quite common for a visitor to appear at the recovery room door who doesn't know what the injured person looks like. The visitor may have known the patient long ago or only by phone conversation. There is an appealing effect, to some people, in slightly knowing someone injured in a mass casualty.

Simultaneously, the administration of the hospital stops all elective surgeries for that day and clears the emergency room by discharging or transferring patients to another hospital. All patients currently hospitalized who can be released from the hospital are discharged. Patients in intensive care (who have had no room in the departments for days before) are quickly released, and somehow, an empty bed has been found. The bedside areas are thoroughly cleaned and prepared for the quick admissions. In addition, two nurses (a midwife and a teacher in the nursing school) automatically arrive at the hospital when a mass casualty occurs. They have been trained to identify the victims. They check each victim who is unconscious or in shock. They check children for identifiable markings, clothes, birthmarks, and other outstanding markings that can be relayed to the information center and waiting relatives. These two nurses are responsible for the communication of the seriously wounded as well as the deceased to the information center.

A social worker is responsible for opening the information center whenever a mass casualty event occurs. Volunteers answer the switchboard of the hospital. The telephone numbers are announced by all radio stations within minutes of an event. The social worker collects all the details concerning the victims and ultimately concentrates this information in order to relay it all to the hospital spokesman, administration, and concerned parties.

Approximately 10% of the victims arriving at the emergency department are not physically injured. They were at the scene of the event and their personal security has been thrown off balance. They feel that they need to be seen by a physician, even though they have no physical injury. The ambulance squads are fully aware of this phenomenon and after they have distributed the wounded to the various hospitals, they always ask if anyone else would like to go to the hospital. These patients arrive at the emergency department, are checked by a physician and the emergency room psychiatrist for early post-traumatic stress disorder and are discharged.

The operating room nurses who are not currently on duty arrive without being called. When an injured victim arrives in the operating room, the nurses do not know what they are about to see or do. The surgeons are anxious and they also do not know what they will find. Many times a vascular surgeon is called in the middle, or a plastic surgeon or another specialist when they open the wounded and meet with the unknown. There have been many occasions when the specialist was busy in various rooms and there was no one to spare.

How Can The Hospital Admit So Many Patients At One Time?

In the Hadassah Medical Organization, the entrance halls of the hospitals are transformed into auxiliary emergency and admitting departments. Extra stretchers are removed from storage and quickly set up. Staff is positioned and patients are triaged to this area if their wounds are less severe, or if they have been checked first in the main, primary emergency room.

The recovery room has 10 stations. Each station is equipped with a monitor and has the capability for mechanical ventilation. This is the area where patients are admitted after primary diagnosis has been made, after X ray, CT, and/or preliminary surgery has been preformed. This will be the area for the most severely injured. All nurses in recovery are experienced in trauma nursing and they have learned how to work under great pressure. They have also been trained to look for secondary injuries that were overlooked during the primary diagnosis period and have experience in talking with hysterical and anxious families. They have the knowledge gained by hindsight. They know that in time, the injuries will heal. They take things one at a time. They discuss what will happen in the next hour, or 8 hours. "Let's just see that Debbie remains stable, she might develop a fever, but let us hope for stability." The nurses help the families keep things in perspective. The ground rules of visitation hours, who can visit, and who will be the designated caller are all set up at the initial meeting. Once families know what is going to happen, and what everyone's job is, they calm down and settle in. As long as the information keeps flowing and the communication channels are kept open, everything can be controlled. Although a rare occurrence, a security guard can be summoned for a combative individual.

The recovery room nurses work overtime, eight and nine shifts a week during the period following a mass casualty event. It is expected. Sometimes the recovery is overflowing for a number of weeks following a MCE. There have been occasions when seriously wounded patients have been transferred from other hospitals to Hadassah, after that hospital was over capacity. In other hospitals, nurses from other intensive care units are called to the recovery room for assistance. The first day after a MCE, elective surgeries commence as scheduled and the recovery room works at 200% capacity. Nurses in the recovery room work overtime for weeks after the initial mass casualty.

SUMMARY

The foundation for the preparation of professional nurses is education and exercise. The chaos of a mass casualty event demands nurses respond confidently, and confidence comes with knowing that preparation has been thorough. Staging interdisciplinary exercises fosters a sense of camaraderie that is essential for functioning as a team. Preparation is not an economical solution, but the alternatives will be more expensive.

The discussions in this chapter are often based on the ideal, a situation where adequate intensive care and general medical beds are available in adequate numbers, and where physicians and nurses can be reached by telephone and are available to come to the hospital. In addition, a caveat must be given that the chapter also assumes that civic infrastructure is intact. This includes telephones, water, gas, electricity, transportation, sanitation, and roads and bridges are unaffected and functioning. During the regularly scheduled preparedness exercises, scenarios must be created that assume the loss of one or more of these services. Only by planning for these contingencies can the health care system remain functioning. The responsibility for staging and evaluating these situations is part of the responsibility of the professional nurse functioning as a member of the interdisciplinary team preparing each community and setting for the unthinkable.

CASE STUDY

Decontamination

John Jones is a member of Springfield Community Hospital's decontamination team. He received the call to report to the decontamination preparation area as the hospital expected to decontaminate 30 individuals who were saturated with a suspicious liquid product. It is mid-July and the temperature outside is 95° Fahrenheit. Mr. Jones has gained 15 pounds in the nine months since his last decontamination training and drill. He dons the decontamination gear, mask, and battery pack on the lower level of the hospital and climbs the flight of stairs to reach the decontamination area outside of the emergency department. He feels light-headed as he reaches the top of the stairs, but continues to decontaminate victims for the next one-half hour. The person working next to John in the gross decontamination area sees John sway and fall to the ground unconscious.

1. What measures could have been taken to anticipate John's light-headedness?
2. How could the fatigue he experienced at the top of the stairs be prevented?
3. What signal should Mr. Jones have used to indicate distress?

4. How will Mr. Jones be treated now that he has collapsed?

5. Would Mr. Jones receive priority treatment as a member of the hospital's decontamination team or will he be triaged with the incoming victims?

TEST YOUR KNOWLEDGE

1. Identify two responsibilities of the Department of Homeland Security.

2. Identify the key difference between triage in times of peace and triage in times of mass casualty events.

3. Following a mass casualty event, you can expect that _____ of the victims will be critical, and _____ of the victims will be treated and released from the hospital.

4. Describe a method of assessing an institution's capacity to handle victims of a mass casualty event.

5. During and following a terrorist event, application of the EMTALA standards must be followed.
   A. True
   B. False

6. If decontamination of victims is necessary during the winter or in cold weather, plans must be made to move the decontamination stations inside the hospital.
   A. True
   B. False

7. Knowing about the ways in which bombs cause injuries helps the nurse anticipate the types of injuries. High-order explosives cause a _____ _____ that results in injuries to _____.

8. Explain a method to increase the availability of health care workers during a time of emergency.

9. Discuss methods for handling the family and friends of victims, or victims who are not severely injured.

10. Explain methods to identify the teams that are formed to handle various types and severity of injuries.

EXPLORE 🌐 MEDIALINK

Interactive resources and an audio glossary for this chapter can be found on the Companion Website at http://www.prenhall.com/langan. Click on Chapter 6 to select the activities for this chapter.

REFERENCES

American Hospital Association. (2000). Hospital preparedness for mass casualties. Summary of Invitational Forum. *American Hospital Association, 3*, 8–9.

Banthrax Corporation (n.d.). *How to handle hazardous materials.* Retrieved June 6, 2003 from http://www.banthrax.com/Haztech.html

Beveridge, R., Clark, B., Janes, L., Savage, N., Thompson, J., Dodd, G., Murray, M., Jordan, C. N., Warren, D., & Vadeboncoeur, A. (1998). Implementation guidelines for the Canadian Emergency Department Triage & Activity Scale (CTAS). Retrieved on May 15, 2003 from http://www.caep.ca/002.policies/002-docs/ctased16.pdf

Centers for Disease Control and Prevention (CDC). (2003a). *National Pharmaceutical Stockpile.* Retrieved May 6, 2003, from http://www.bt.cdc.gov/stockpile

Centers for Disease Control and Prevention (CDC). (2003b). *Overview of instrument for rapid assessment of injuries and other medical conditions.* Retrieved May 6, 2003 from http://www.cdc.gov.masstrauma/response/rapid assessment.htm

Centers for Disease Control and Prevention (CDC). (2003c). *Mass trauma casualty predictor.* Retrieved May 6, 2003 from http://www.cdc.gov/masstrauma/preparedness/predictor.htm

Centers for Disease Control and Prevention (CDC). (2003d). *Predicting casualty severity and hospital capacity.* Retrieved May 6, 2003 from http://www.cdc.gov/masstrauma/preparedness/capacity.htm

Centers for Disease Control and Prevention (CDC). (2003e). *Overview of mental health survey instrument.* Retrieved May 6, 2003 from http://www.cdc.gov/masstrauma/response/mhsurvey.htm

Centers for Disease Control and Prevention (CDC). (2003f). *Explosions and blast injuries: A primer for clinicians.* Retrieved May 6, 2003 from http://www.cdc.gov/masstrauma/preparedness/primer.htm

Centers for Disease Control and Prevention (CDC). (2003g). *Mass trauma preparedness and response fact sheets.* Retrieved May, 6, 2003 from http://www.cdc.gov.masstrauma/factsheets

Centers for Disease Control and Prevention (CDC). (2003h). *Emergency room procedures in chemical hazard emergencies: A job aid.* Retrieved May 6, 2003 from http://www.cdc.gov/nceh/demil/articles/initialtreat.htm

Centers for Disease Control and Prevention (CDC). (2003i). *Sarin (GB).* Retrieved May 6, 2003 from http://www.bt.cdc.gov/agent/sarin/index.asp

Conterra triage belt. (2003). Retrieved May 15, 2003 from http://www.buyemp.com/dept.asp?dept_id=1051707

Conway-Welch, C. (2002). Nurses and mass casualty management: Filling an educational gap. *Policy, Politics and Nursing, 3*(4), 289–293.

DeAtley, C. (2001). *Patient decontamination procedure.* Retrieved June 6, 2003 from http://www.hazmatforhealthcare.org/download/doc/misc/Patient_Decontamination_Procedure-complet.doc

Department of Health & Human Services (HHS). (2003, February 28). Chemical agents: Facts about personal cleaning & disposal of contaminated clothing (Draft).

Emergencies and disasters. (2003). Retrieved May 15, 2003 from http://www.dhs.gov/dhspublic/theme_home2.jsp

Environmental Protection Agency (EPA). (1998, June). Work practice controls, SHEMP operations manual for laboratories. Retrieved June 21, 2004 from http://www.epa.gov/ProjectXL/nelabs/Chapterf.pdf

Evison, D., Hinsley, D., & Rice, P. (2002). Chemical weapons. *British Medical Journal, 324*(7333), 332–335.

Gebbie, K. M., & Qureshi, K. (2002). Emergency and disaster preparedness: Core competencies for nurses. *American Journal of Nursing, 102,* 46–51.

Giorgianni, S. J., Grana, J., & Scipioni, L. (Eds.). (2002). Health system preparedness: Fine tuning communication, coordination, and care in a new era. *The Pfizer Journal, 6,* 4.

Henretig, F. M., Cieslak, J.J., & Eitzen, E.M. (2002). Biological and chemical terrorism. *The Journal of Pediatrics, 141*(3), 311–326.

Institute of Medicine National Research Council. (1998). Improving civilian medical response to chemical or biological terrorist incidents. Interim report on current capabilities. Washington, DC: National Academy Press.

Integrated Publishing. (2003). Objective examination. Retrieved April 21, 2003 from http://www.infodotinc.com/corpsman/124.htm

Jagminas, L., & Erdman, D. P. (2001). *CBRNE-Chemical decontamination.* Retrieved June 6, 2003 from http://www.emedicine.com/emerg/topic893.htm

Joint Commission on Accreditation of Healthcare Organizations (JCAHO). (2001a). Using JCAHO standards as a starting point to prepare for an emergency. *Joint Commission Perspectives, 21*(12), 4–5.

Joint Commission on Accreditation of Healthcare Organizations (JCAHO). (2001b). Talking to each other in a crisis. *Joint Commission Perspectives, 2* (12), 16–17.

Kluger, Y. (2003, April). Bomb explosions in acts of terrorism. *Israel Medical Association Journal, 5,* 235–240.

Leibovici, D., Gofrit, O. N., Stein, M., Shapira, S. C., Noga, Y., Heruti, R. J., & Shemer, J. (1996). Blast injuries: Bus versus open-air bombing: A comparative study of injuries in survivors of open-air versus confined space explosions. *Journal of Trauma, 41,* 1030–1035.

Malone, M. V. (2002). Mass casualty decontamination. In P. M. Maniscalso & H. Christen (Eds.), *Understanding terrorism and managing the consequences.* Upper Saddle River, NJ: Pearson Education.

Mellor, S. G., & Cooper, G. I. (1989). Analysis of 828 servicemen killed or injured by explosion in Northern Ireland 1970–84: The Hostile ACTION Casualty system. *British Journal of Surgery, 76,* 1006–1010.

Mobilizing America's health care reservoir. (2001, December). *Joint Commission Perspectives, 21,* 1–23.

Nakajima, T., Sato, S., Morita, H., & Yanagisawa, N. (1997). Sarin poisoning of a rescue team in the Matsumoto sarin incident in Japan. *Occupational and Environmental Medicine, 54*(10), 697–701.

National Disaster Medical System (NDMS). (2004). Welcome to NDMS. Retrieved July 1, 2004 from http://www.oep-ndms.dhhs.gov

Newberry, L. (2002, September). Practical suggestions for helping emergency nurses handle mass casualties. *DMR: Disaster Management & Response* (pp. 15–17).

Rega, P. P. (2000). *The Biological Terrorism Response Manual.* Retrieved May 15, 2003 from http://bioterry.com/

Shemer, J., & Shapira, S. C. (2001). Terror and medicine: The challenge. *Israel Medical Association Journal, 3*(11),

Sidell, F. R., & Franz, D. R. (1997). Overview: Defense against the effects of chemical and biological warfare agents. In R. Zajtchuk (Ed.), *The textbook of military medicine. Part I. Warfare, weaponry and the casualty: Vol. 3* (pp. 351–360).

Simple Triage & Rapid Transport (START). (2004). START. Retrieved on March 30, 2004 from http://www.sortteam.org/START_TRIAGE.pdf

Travers, D. A., Waller, A. E., Bowling, J. M., Flowers, D., & Tintinalli, J. (2002). Five-level triage system more effective than three-level in tertiary emergency department. *Journal of Emergency Nursing, 28*(5), 395–400.

UK Resilience. (2003). *The "rinse-wipe" method of casualty decontamination.* Retrieved September 7, 2003 from http://www.ukresilience.info/cbrn/appendixb.htm

U.S. Department of State. (2003). *Responding to a biological or chemical threat: A practical guide.* Retrieved September 30, 2003 from http://www.ds-osac.org/inc/documents/biochem.pdf

Wightman, J. M., & Gladish, S. L. (2001). *Explosions and blast injuries.* Annals of Emergency Medicine, 37, 664–678.

CHAPTER

Management and Preparation for Battlefield Casualties

Michelle R. Mandy

LEARNING OBJECTIVES

1. Discuss the past, current, and future initiatives of battlefield nursing care.
2. Explain how the roles of military nurses during war improve battlefield casualty care.
3. Differentiate and evaluate the basic components of the military expeditionary medical services concept for battlefield nursing care.
4. Analyze a civilian scenario and suggest ways to improve nursing disaster preparedness using military lessons learned.
5. Apply military training principles to the civilian nursing training environment.

MEDIALINK www.prenhall.com/langan

Resources for this chapter can be found on the Companion Website at http://www.prenhall.com/langan. Click on Chapter 7 to select the activities for this chapter.

CHAPTER OUTLINE

Know Your Terms
Audio Glossary
MediaLink Applications

GLOSSARY

Aeromedical Evacuation (MEDEVAC). An available transportation option when the medical needs of a patient exceed the resources available in the local medical department or when medical needs can be better met at another military treatment facility (MTF)

Aeromedical evacuation team. A five-person team consisting usually of a medical crew director, a flight nurse, a charge medical technician, and two aeromedical evacuation technicians whose primary work center is the cabin or cargo hold of an airplane flying several miles high. This team supports the critical care air transport teams

Bunker. An underground defensive position with a fortified projection above ground level for gun emplacements

Combatant. A person or a combat vehicle that takes part in armed strife

Convoy. A group, as of ships or motor vehicles, traveling together with a protective escort or for safety or convenience

CONUS. Continent of the United States

Critical Care Air Transport Team (CCATT). A three-person team consisting of a doctor, critical care nurse, and cardiopulmonary technician who provide critical expertise and capability to monitor and manage patients in transit to definitive care destinations. They enhance the aeromedical evacuation team in transferring critically ill patients who require continuous stabilization and advance care during transport to the next level of care. Primary work is to keep the critical patients stabilized during the flight to a higher-echelon medical facility

Detainee. A person held in custody or confinement

Expeditionary Medical Support/Air Force Theater Hospital (EMEDS/AFTH). EMEDS Basic refers to the operational medical support required to provide medical care to a single bed-down with a population at risk (PAR) of 500–2,000. It provides forward stabilization, primary care, force protection, and preparation for aeromedical evacua-

tion. Additional increments of the EMEDS/AFTH include EMEDS + 10 Bed AFTH for PAR of 2,000–3,000/52 staff and EMEDS + 25 Bed AFTH for PAR of 3,000–5,000/86 staff. These two increase the diagnostic capability and the inpatient bed capacity

Military Operations Other Than War (MOOTW). Operations that encompass the use of military capabilities across the range of military operations short of war. These military actions can be applied to complement any combination of other instruments of national power and occur before, during, and after war

MOPP gear. A chemical protective suit known as mission-oriented protective posture. It is a standard military two-piece charcoal lined overgarment that is designed to protect the user from chemical, biological, and nuclear agents. A gas mask, overboots, and butyl rubber gloves are also part of the ensemble

INTRODUCTION

Nurses have performed care on the battlefield for years, and this history has greatly influenced the way nursing care is delivered today. There are many similarities between battlefield nursing and civilian nursing during a disaster. In this chapter we will review the history of preparedness and the management of battlefield casualties utilizing lessons learned from past wars and some of the changes likely to result from the current right sizing of the U.S. military forces. We will point out the differences and similarities in the management of civilian and battlefield casualties, unique features of military nursing, and its preparation for disaster response. In addition, we will review how military and civilian interactions can provide optimal care during disasters, and explore some visions of the future.

Battlefield nursing has not only made an impact on the way military nursing is provided, but on civilian nursing practices as well. To understand the influence of battlefield nursing, it is essential to understand how actions of the past have helped define present day nursing. A nursing lesson learned today is a new nursing technique applied tomorrow.

INNOVATIONS IN NURSING CARE FROM THE BATTLEFIELD

Crimean War—1854–1856

Florence Nightingale introduced ideas of sanitation and humane nursing care to the battlefield during the Crimean War, where nurses cleaned the patient areas, instituted procedures for sanitary waste disposal, replaced dirty clothes, and improved nutrition of the soldiers. Nightingale convinced army engineers to redirect a sewage canal that ran beneath the field hospital, and had her nurses scrub the walls and floors of the sick room (Bullough, 1978). These changes, together with the art of nursing care

and dietary treatment, reduced the death rate from 420 to 22 per thousand (Strachey, 1918).

Great Battle at Solferino—1859

Henri Dunant, a Swiss-born businessman from Geneva, traveled to Italy to discuss a business venture with Napoleon III and witnessed the bloodiest battle of the 19th century (Nobel, 2002). Being familiar with Nightingale's work, Dunant noted that preparations to care for the wounded had not changed since the Crimean War 5 years earlier (Trends, 1996). Dunant received approval from the National Congress to set up the International Committee of the Red Cross in 1863, which led to the birth of the Treaty of Geneva in 1864. This treaty, known today as the Geneva Convention, was signed by 16 countries who agreed that military hospitals were to be respected by all armies as zones of safety, and their staffs of doctors and nurses were to be regarded as neutral, serving the wounded of any nationality without prejudice (Jamieson, Sewall & Suttrie, 1996). It was during this time that the concept of the red cross on a white flag was accepted as the symbol identifying field hospitals.

Civil War—1861–1865

The battlefield was split during this war, but disease ravaged both sides. Battle wounds were more severe, and going to the hospitals often meant death. The nursing care provided by the Union army (North) and by the Confederate army (South), was remarkably different.

The Confederate nurses had little or no formal training, and provided nursing care in dangerous battlefields and ill-equipped, unsanitary environments of the military hospitals. Their duties included bathing patients, changing dressings, assisting surgeons with treatments, distributing food, administering medications, and beating and airing out straw mattresses (Megmeister, 2003). Theses nurses made great contributions to battlefield nursing by changing the stereotype of nursing from a profession for the lower socioeconomic classes to being a respectable profession for all classes of people.

Union army nurses were volunteers trained and organized by Dorothea Dix of Boston. They served on battlefields, at the front lines, on troop transport trains, and at numerous field and general hospitals, but they were not allowed to assist with surgical procedures (Megmeister, 2003). There were more deaths from communicable disease than gunshot wounds. This took a toll on the Union nurses, emotionally and physically. Nurses wondered what took more courage—a man stepping onto the field of battle, or a nurse about to step onto a smallpox ward (Megmeister, 2003).

Clara Barton, the "Angel of the Battlefield," was the pioneer of battlefield nursing in the United States. She brought nursing care to the battlefield during the Civil War in 1850 during a time when the United States was unable to cope with overwhelming numbers of wounded soldiers. Barton brought aid behind enemy lines to troops of opposing armies. She practiced exclusively on battlefields, experiencing firsthand the horrors of war on 16 different battlefields (Women in History, 2002). Barton dressed wounds, fed soldiers, and wrote letters for those too badly injured to write (Cobb, 2003). She fought to bring the Red Cross Treaty of Geneva to America just as Durant did in Europe. In 1882, many years after the war, the Treaty of Geneva was ratified by the United States.

Spanish-American War (1898)

This was the first war fought under the Geneva Convention with the relief efforts of the American Red Cross. Graduates of an approved nursing school were appointed under a contract to provide nursing care on the battlefield. The nurses cared for the wounded and treated those suffering from the typhoid fever epidemic, malaria, and yellow fever. These nonbattle-type diseases turned the spotlight on the issue of communicable disease, and prompted the nursing community to consider including this content within nursing education. The outstanding care provided by the nurses during the Spanish-American War resulted in the formulation of the Army Nurse Corps in 1901, followed by the Navy Nurse Corp in 1908 (Furey, 2001).

World War II (1941–1945)

During World War II, increased numbers of nurses allowed more care to be provided to the soldiers with a lower patient/nurse ratio. There were approximately 57,000 nurses who served in the Army Nurse Corps and 11,000 in the Navy Nurse Corps (Gendergap, 2001b).

Three new changes occurred for nursing during this war: (1) a new role of flight nursing, (2) immediate post operative care, and (3) combat readiness training for nurses.

On November 30, 1942 the army made a nationwide appeal for commercial airline hostesses (who were all graduate nurses at the time) between the ages of 21 and 35 to volunteer for the air evacuation units of the Army Nurse Corps (Gendergap, 2001). The ability to rapidly transport patients to higher levels of care saved lives and decreased permanent injuries. The use of the fixed-wing aircrafts for evacuation helped; the new flight nurses posted a remarkable record of only five deaths in flight per 100,000 injured (Mientka, 2003).

During World War II nurses' skill level was raised and intensive care nursing skills began as the doctors performed damage control surgery. In addressing these advanced skills, a nurse wrote, "Nurses had to assume a lot of responsibility . . . as there were not enough doctors to supervise every case at every stage" (Tomblin, 1996). As the nurses' skills increased, so did the medics' skills: They had to perform some of the nurses' duties (such as passing medications and starting intravenous lines). By assisting in technical advances in the field of nursing, army nurses developed the concept of recovery wards for immediate postoperative nursing care and gained a greater understanding of the process of shock, blood replacement, and resuscitation (Mientka, 2003). See Box 7–1.

As the war progressed, nurses were given combat readiness training, an intensive four-week training program during which they went on 20-mile hikes wearing combat boots and four pound steel helmets while carrying a 30-pound pack, a mess kit and gas mask. They learned to pitch tents, dig foxholes, chlorinate water and extinguish incendiary devices. They trained in camouflage and learned to identify different poison gases and lethal chemicals. They went through a tear gas chamber and crawled on their stomachs through a 75 yard infiltration course pitted with trenches and strung with barbed wire while dynamite charges went off around them and machine gun bullets sprayed overhead. Some trained in 108 degree desert heat; others crawled through snowdrifts or swamps. They learned to setup, make operational and dismantle a 500-bed field hospital in a matter of hours (Gendergap, 2001b).

Although World War II was the most violent war to date, the added changes for nurses, such as air evacuation and progressive combat military training, resulted in fewer

BOX 7–1   Damage Control Surgery

It's important to understand the meaning of damage control surgery in order to understand the care nurses provided for these types of patients on the battlefield. The central tenet of damage control surgery is that patients die from a triad of coagulopathy, hypothermia, and metabolic acidosis (Brohi, 2000), and the goal is to interrupt that process. Damage control surgery, also called staged surgery or staged laparotomy, is performed in stages, with the first stage principle being control the hemorrhage, prevent contamination, and protect from further injury (Brohi, 2000). After the initial rapid lifesaving technique, procedure, the patient is sent to the intensive care unit until stabilized and then sent back to the operating room for definitive resection and reconstruction (Zacharias, Offner, Moore, & Burch, 1999).

This concept was developed by the U.S. surgeon general during World War II and was adopted by the U.S. Army, which obligated a surgeon to perform a colostomy for any colon wound (Mattox, 1997). Surgeons used this approach to effectively care for multiple trauma patients during war. In 1968, hepatic packing was explored again in a case study in which a patient with bilobar hepatic injuries survived after his injury was treated with gauze packing that was removed 6 days later (Zacharias, et al., 1999). Damage control surgery continues today and has been adopted by some civilian surgeons.

---

than 4% of all U.S. soldiers—who received medical care in the field or were evacuated by air—dying from their wounds or disease (Gendergap, 2001b). The role of the military nurse became important and worthy of holding high ranks.

Korean War (1950–1953)

During the Korean War, nurses were also sent forward with mobile army surgical hospital (MASH) units and placed with evacuation hospitals, where wounded were air evacuated to hospitals. The hospital and MASH units were close to the front lines. Nurses also served aboard a new type of mobile hospital—ships (Department of Defense, 2000). Nurses proved to others how valuable their skills and talents were on the battlefield. They helped pioneer many new surgical techniques, such as renal dialysis, disposable supplies, MASH units, and the use of shock treatment centers made possible by the improved air mobility via helicopter (Mientka, 2003).

Vietnam War (1964–1975)

There were no direct front lines in the Vietnam War. Instead, the army checkered the countryside with many base camps that could become a battlefield at any time. The mobile hospital concept from World War II and the Korean War became more stationary and did not follow the advancing army units (Neel, 1991). This allowed the field hospital to acquire more sophisticated stationary equipment (such as ventilators and Stryker frames). The hospitals needed more advanced equipment to care for patients undergoing damage control surgeries, which meant nurses performed more intensive care nursing in the field.

For most of the nurses, Vietnam was the only period in their professional lives when they experienced such collegiality with the physician and professional autonomy. They filled leadership positions and served as assistants during the evacuation procedures, and in the times of rocket or mortar attacks (Megmeister, 2003). They also understood and prepared for early air evacuation because patients could be mobilized earlier due to the rapid closures of their wounds.

During the Vietnam War, the body of knowledge on air evacuation procedures and skills was developed. The Army Nurse Corps developed intensive care and trauma care specialization units that expedited the *chain of evacuation* of wounded from the battlefield to nearby army hospitals to state-side hospitals, in as little as three days (Mientka, 2003).

Operation Desert Storm (1991)

During the Persian Gulf War, the concept of deployable medical systems (DEPMEDS) was utilized, sparking the idea for highly mobile and smaller medical units.

Somalia, 1993 Humanitarian Mission in Mogadishu

This humanitarian mission taught many lessons, primarily that the battlefield can develop during a peacetime mission. The military troops, as part of the UN food relief mission, disarmed local warlords to ensure adequate distribution of the food and supplies. The mission turned into a day-and-night battle. When two black hawk helicopters were shot down, the humanitarian mission became urban combat. The streets were filled with heavily armed military, making it difficult to evacuate the wounded from the helicopters. The hospital was set up approximately 2 miles from the battle site and staffed as a hospital for humanitarian relief. When the urban combat began, the medical personnel were quickly overwhelmed. The nurses had to perform at a higher level (Figure 7–1). At one point, they made decisions about care because the physicians were in surgery with breaks only between cases.

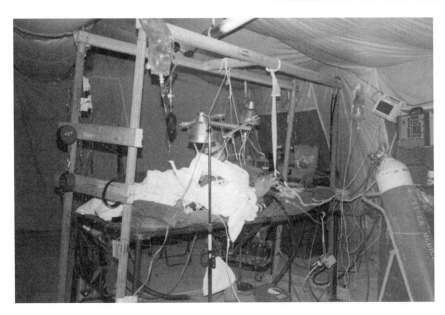

Figure 7-1. Traction frame, 86th evac hospital, Somalia, 1993.

Following is an example of doctor's orders as they were written on a patient's chart in the ICU on October 3, 1993.

- Keep the fresh whole blood going while he is hypotensive.
- Draw an ABG and fix the vent.
- Use any drug in the pharmacy as appropriate.
- Give some pain meds.
- I'll be back in an hour.

(J. Holcomb, personal communication, 2001)

Dr. John Holcomb, director of the Joint Trauma Training Center, Ben Taub General Hospital, Houston, Texas, stated, "If the nurses can accept these orders, then they are ready" (2001). The nurses were ready. They survived the battle and returned with more lessons learned.

Operation Iraqi Freedom (2003)

During this war the nurses were part of the new expeditionary medical teams. In the army, they were stationed in combat support hospitals and forward surgical teams throughout the battlefield. Navy nurses were aboard the *USNS Comfort* hospital ship, a well-equipped level III trauma center in the sea near Iraq and forward surgical team close to the front lines. The air force nurses were on different expeditionary medical support (EMEDS) teams, which included mobile forward surgical teams (MFST), **critical care air transportation team (CCATT)**, and aeromedical evacuation crews. These teams were located throughout the war zone. The EMEDS concept will be discussed in detail below.

Battlefield Casualty Management in the 21ˢᵗ Century

The wartime mission of the military expeditionary medical services is to support the line commander by conserving the fighting strength so that he or she may accomplish the military mission. The mission encompasses the following objectives: (1) Save lives; (2) clear the battlefield of casualties; (3) provide state-of-the-art care; (4) return a soldier to duty as rapidly as possible or evacuate him or her to a higher echelon of care for more definitive treatment; and (5) provide the most benefit to the maximum number of personnel (Davis, Hosek, Tate, Perry, Hepler, & Steinberg, 1996).

To accomplish its mission, the military expeditionary medical service identified the essentials of early resuscitation and early evacuation to save lives through lessons learned from past wars. The early resuscitation includes, but is not limited to, (1) securing an airway and intravenous access, (2) volume resuscitation and hemodynamic stabilization, (3) immobilization of spine and extremities if fracture is suspected, (4) protection from hypothermia, (5) surgery, and (6) early evacuation. In addition to early resuscitation, military expeditionary medical service identified the need for early evacuations to higher levels of care accompanied by critical care personnel. They also identified the need to reduce the incidence of disease and non-battle injury (DNBI) through preventive medical support to the troops (Davis, et al., 1996). Finally, they identified the need for trained personnel to be rapidly placed in the right location at the right time.

The concept of a critical care air transport team (CCATT) is a part of the new **Expeditionary Medical Support (EMEDS)** care concept. EMEDS is the term used in the air force, primarily designed to support the Expeditionary Air Force as the first echelon of medical support during contingency operations (Purificato, 2001). All services utilize this concept that brings medical surgical care to the front lines of the battlefield and provides stabilizing care so patients can be moved to a permanent facility with more resources. Studies have shown that lives are often lost in the battlefield due to hemorrhage and delay in treatment. "Crowley's Golden Hour" is the standard used by all military—and civilians—as the critical window of time to meet.

One major concern when caring for patients is a delay in care due to a chemical or biological environment. The air force has introduced new technology to assist medics in rapidly detecting biological agents. This system, the Global Expeditionary Medical System (GEMS), is a worldwide medical surveillance network that detects trends in symptoms and diagnosis among thousands of deployed military patients (Meridith, 2001).

Additional challenges in taking care of battlefield injuries are time, resource constraints, environment, and being under fire. Consequently, the military is bringing health care closer to the front line to overcome these issues and to eliminate preventable deaths. The expeditionary medical service also has some of the most sophisticated portable equipment approved for air evacu-ation, such as handheld ventilators, intravenous pumps, and ICU parameter monitors. The EMEDS have also been used during a civilian disaster, for example, the Houston flood, a result of Tropical Storm Allison in June 2001. During that situation, the air force was able to gather real data to compare the old medical responses of air transportable hospitals (ATH) with the new EMEDs. In comparing their medical disaster response to Hurricane Andrew in Florida to their medical disaster response to Tropical Storm Allison in Houston, one could clearly see how the new expeditionary forces were truly exceptional (Figure 7–2). It took the air force medical service 17 days to become operational for Hurricane Andrew and only 36 hours for Tropical Storm Allison (P. Carlton, personal communication, August 15, 2001). See Box 7–2.

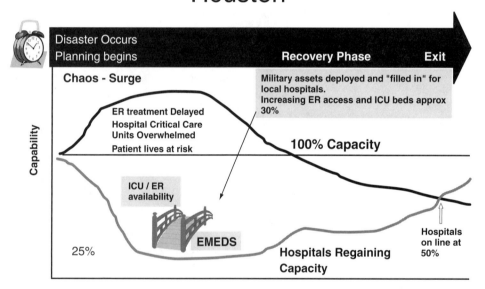

Figure 7–2. EMEDS in Houston schematic. (Adapted from Missouri Air National Guard)

BOX 7–2   Expeditionary Medical System (EMEDS) Capabilities

Lt Col John L Binder, USAF

Introduction

In 1999, the U.S. Air Force revolutionized its ability to deploy medical capability into the field. Integrating new medical, information management, and other technologies, a new expeditionary medical support (EMEDS) was created. The EMEDS is lighter, leaner, and more lifesaving than the previous air transportable hospital. EMEDS, staffed by Air Force nurses, and technicians is now deployed around the world supporting humanitarian, civil defense, disaster response, and peacekeeping forces. See Figure 7–3.

Aims

In an expeditionary military environment, both weight and cube are important in determining what equipment can and will be deployed in support of combat force. Since 1994, the USAF Medical Service has conducted an extensive overhaul of its deployable medical capability by developing modular, incrementally built and mission-tailorable deployable medical systems to

(continued)

BOX 7–2   (continued)

Schematic Modular Build of EMEDS
SPEARR/EMEDS/AFTH

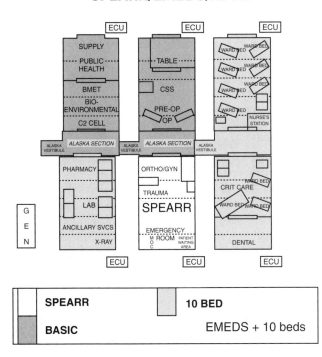

Figure 7-3. Schematic modular build of EMEDS.

replace the older, airlift intensive air transportable hospital. See Figure 7–4.

Methods

Using a multidisciplinary team approach, the U.S. Air Force, in a short period, crafted, scientifically validated, implemented, and deployed EMEDS throughout USAF Medical Service.

Results

The EMEDS provides a medically robust, highly adaptable, and better approach to deployed medical and dental care which places trauma care at the front of the queue. The net result is a lower burden on the strategic and tactical transportation system, and a smaller "footprint" (which in turn requires less support itself). The EMEDS can be tailored in terms of medical specialties represented and consequently has a readily adaptable range of contingencies including humanitarian assistance, disaster response, and homeland defense. A growing

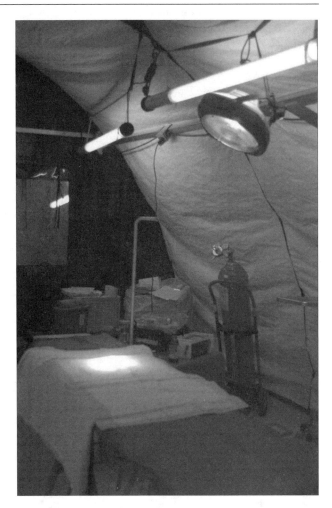

Figure 7-4. EMED OR.

number of examples validate its utility in these settings. The EMEDS concept also incorporates the latest in technological advances to increase capability while reducing or holding the line on transportation requirements. Diagnostic and therapeutic improvements including information management/information technology systems and telemedicine are added to the system.

Conclusion

EMEDS has established its role in the expeditionary air force of the century and continues to improve with enhanced adaptability and capability. It has become the "gold standard" for deployable medical treatment within the USAF and the U.S. Department of Defense (Binder, 2002).

Unique Features of Military Nursing

The practice of military nursing is the root of nursing practice, as it has developed over time and is the basis of trauma nursing as we know it today. Today the military nurse's scope of practice exceeds any state's nurse practice acts. Nursing care performed in the wartime environment could be explained as nursing based on a mass production basis, often in a hostile and resource-limited environment. In a sense, the nurse becomes accustomed to the concept, "provide the best care you can with what you have" for the survival of the patient.

When we think of battlefield care we commonly envision the critical, multiple injury patient; but the reality is that the types of injured patients on the battlefield include pediatric, obstetrical, nonbattle diseases, and trauma. This is why the military nurses must be multitalented. Specialty nurses in obstetrics, pediatrics, and critical care are trained in resuscitation care, and they can care for urgent and emergent-type casualties. Nurses and medics must act independently in order to save lives and must be trained to do so. Colonel Quinn stated the following during a memorial ceremony honoring military nurses in Weymouth, Massachusetts, in November 1987.

The nurse must be armed to fight just as the soldier, sailor, or marine. The nurse's weapons are knowledge and skills that can be employed to wage war on disease and injury wherever these calamities have laid low a man, woman, or child. (Army Nurse Corps History, 2003)

Nurses are assigned to mobility teams during wartime and to military treatment facilities (MTFs) during peacetime. Most Department of Defense MTFs are not involved in trauma care, which is the military core responsibility. This poses a problem in maintaining critical skills needed for deployment. Working in the MTFs allows nurses to maintain basic clinical skills while caring for active duty personnel, dependents, and retirees, but for critical trauma skills they are sent to trauma training sites. When nurses are deployed, they are part of small groups and must be familiar with everyone's job. One nurse during World War II addressed this issue and said,

Nurses had to be rotated in the operating room, for we feared the day might come when something would happen to those in charge and we'd be left stranded without operating room nurses. "Girls," I told them, "you've all got to take a turn at it so we won't be left high and dry one of these days." Every nurse must become familiar with every job, so that if any thing should happen to some of us, the others will be able to carry on. (Archard, 1945, p. 416)

The military has a multidisciplinary approach to care that permits a variety of perspectives and gives the nurses input into the decision making for the care of the patients.

They are designated as officers in the United States military and are required to keep their professional military education current. This allows them to grow administratively and to be prepared for and promoted into supervisory positions because they never know when they might be put in charge. A young novice nurse, an ensign who is only 23 years old, is in the casualty receiving areas on the USNS Comfort. She supervises four corpsmen who are dealing with emotional issues of caring for young soldiers who are their peers. She now has to deal with the responsibilities of being an officer as well as a nurse (Boivin, 2003b). The nurses also work with the medical staff, administration (command), lab, and respiratory, among other specialties, to coordinate standards of resuscitative care and air evacuations.

Nurses play a significant role in the medical aspects of disasters and are trained in triage, treatment, administrative management, and processing techniques in mass casualty or disaster situations. To understand triage and the military nurse's role, one must first understand the definition of triage during war versus triage during peacetime. The ultimate goal for the military nurse to understand during war, as succinctly stated in the *NATO Emergency War Surgery Handbook*, "is the return of the greatest number of soldiers to combat and the preservation of life and limb in those who cannot be returned." Do the most good for the greatest number with the assets available (Taft, 2003). Triage is a vital concept to military medicine, and it needs to be consumed, regurgitated, and discussed at all levels, with as much input from as many sources as possible, and at regular intervals (Swan & Swan, 1996). Four triage categories have been adapted for use by both U.S. and NATO forces (Taft, 2003). The categories used are immediate, delayed, minimal, and expectant. Sometimes the military adds a fifth category called "contaminated." These are summarized as follows:

T1: Immediate. Patients requiring emergency lifesaving surgery. Minimal operating time. Expected good quality survival such as respiratory obstruction.

T2: Delayed. Patients badly in need of time-consuming major surgery. Life not jeopardized by delay. Stabilization minimizes effects of delay.

T3: Minimal. Patients with relatively minor injuries who can effectively care for themselves or receive care from untrained personnel.

T4: Expectant. Patients having serious and often multiple injuries, requiring time-consuming and complicated treatment with a low chance of survival. Treatment consumes considerable personnel or resources. (Taft, 2003)

By using the acronym MEDIC, one can easily remember all five patient categories (Mattox, Feliciano, & Moore, 2000). In addition to sorting casualties for care on the battlefield, the nurse begins to set evacuation priorities as well. The military nurse's role is to assist the physician, usually the surgeon, in guarding against overcommitting resources by communicating with command and logistics for restocking.

In the battlefield there are no level I trauma centers with the capabilities of computed tomography imaging scans, neurosurgeons, and magnetic resonance imaging. Instead, there are tents where damage control surgeries are performed, and patients are prepared to be air evacuated by critical care teams to a higher level of care and eventually back to the **continent of the United States (CONUS)**. Within these tents, nurses have to deal with dirt, darkness, extreme temperatures, unlimited numbers of patients, chaos, and varying levels of nursing experience. The outside environment is usually hostile and living conditions can be harsh without the physical comforts of civilian communities. The nurse understands the art of war on the battlefield and maintaining the strength of the fighting force to have a successful outcome. They must be aware of the Geneva Convention and provide care to the enemy prisoners of war.

SIMILARITIES IN MANAGEMENT OF CIVILIAN AND BATTLEFIELD CASUALTIES

Military forces have been cut by 34% since peaking in 1987 (from 2.1 million to 1.4 million), and major overseas deployments have increased dramatically during this period (by more than 300% since 1989) (Eisenstadt, 1998). The decrease in available resources and the increase in operations tempo have forced the military to do more with less, resulting in retention problems. Therefore, there is a shortage of nurses both in the military and in the civilian communities.

Nurses are considered the single largest population in health care with a 24/7 mission; and military and civilian health care agencies cannot operate without them. A diverse group of nurses ranging from the novice to the highly experienced serve in the military, and they range in age from 20 on active duty to 50 on reserve, which is similar to the civilian community. "Fifty percent of the reserve nurses in all three branches of the military are older than 45, which is similar to the statistics being reported in the civilian sector" (Boivin, 2003). The challenge to military and civilian nurses is the preservation of professional nursing practice in an era when outside forces are in the process of trying to change its scope and practice under the rubric of cost-containment (Ray, 1996). "Everyone—even the military—has to work harder to get the nurses they need," said Brigadier General Barbara Brannon, the assistant air force surgeon general for nursing, "but things may be looking up." The air force staff of 2,300 reserve nurses is only 140 members short, rather than the 400 projected (World, 2002). The nursing shortage can be summarized by the fact that there are now over 120,000 open positions for registered nurses nationwide (Stahl, 2003).

During resuscitation, the nurse's role is the same in caring for civilian and battlefield casualties. Many of the resuscitative techniques used in civilian trauma centers were learned during war while caring for patients on the battlefield. The use of sophisticated nursing tools (such as handheld ventilators and parameter monitors) has allowed more highly skilled nursing care to be provided in the field

setting. In general, the intensive care nursing utilized to care for critically injured patients, whether civilian or military, is essentially the same.

The military nurses provide intensive care in the air similar to civilian nurses. The air evacuation ambulances and civilian EMS air ambulance both are routinely staffed with nurses and medics and have high-technology medical equipment. All the medical equipment found on modern ground ambulances can now be found in the air.

DIFFERENCES IN MANAGEMENT OF CIVILIAN AND BATTLEFIELD CASUALTIES

The nursing care provided on the battlefield to trauma patients is not the same as nursing care provided in the civilian environment. Advance trauma life support, basic trauma life support and prehospital trauma life support, although worthy programs, were never designed for use on the battlefield (Allen & McAtee, 1999). In combat medicine, care of the patient must be modified to fit the situation on the battlefield (Allen, 1955). When faced with unusual situations, the nurse must improvise, adapt, and overcome to meet the need of the patient.

A key difference between battlefield nursing and civilian nursing is that civilian caregivers are able to draw on a broad set of clinical skills, support personnel, equipment, and supplies. They are usually focused on providing trauma care to small numbers of patients with potentially unlimited amounts of resources. The arrival time from the scene to the hospital for these patients is usually less than 30 minutes. In battlefield care, there are limited numbers of caregivers and resources for potentially unlimited numbers of patients. Sometimes the lag time between the wounding and hospital presentation is of such duration that those who temporarily survive the initial impact of their injury are no longer salvageable (Bowen & Bellamy, 1988). The nurses use reverse triage (treating the least injured first) during battle to maintain fire superiority. Therefore, the nurse must balance the care and minimize delays in interventions and treatments to those who need it. These unusual circumstances make the military/battlefield nurses mindset in caring for patients different from that of the civilian peacetime mindset. This mindset causes the military nurse to learn to be strong and compassionate, to turn off facial expressions, and sometimes emotions, when faced with patient suffering, the goal to relieve pain and suffering of his/her fellow comrades.

On the battlefield, the surgeons, emergency and critical care physicians, nurses, and medics have a close, cooperative working relationship. The air evacuation nurses carry the same equipment as the EMEDS nurses have in the tent, which allows for a seamless transfer of equipment. The surgeon may show trust by handing the nurse suture materials and giving instructions to finish closing the patient while he attends to another patient. The surgeon and emergency physician determine which patient is the next surgical candidate. At times, the one who was in the *next* status may change to *expectant* while awaiting surgery. In some civilian hospitals, there may be battles over who is in charge of the patient and who should provide specific care for the patient. This occurs when the emergency physician and the trauma surgeon both feel they should be in charge of the patient in the emergency room. The emergency nurse's equipment may be completely different from that of the air evacuation and/or unit nurse's equipment. This causes a delay in patient care while they transfer out all the equipment.

Most nurses in the civilian community are specialized and do not respond to traumas and/or codes. These are managed by a limited group of emergency department and intensive care nurses. This does not occur with the military nurse; they are all trained in resuscitation, have multiple specialties and are cross trained. This is especially helpful when a nurse needs to fill a mobility spot and/or backfill an area due to deployments. Some nurses on the USNS Comfort during the war in Iraq were pediatric nurse practitioners, certified nurse-midwives, and neonatal ICU nurses in peacetime. Their wartime mission, however, was to care for adult patients in the medical/surgical units (Boivin, 2003). Nurses caring for patients outside of their specialty in the civilian community may result in more resistance. The civilian nurses may be concerned about their licenses and the fact that they are not experts in that area. The military nurses are not as concerned during battlefield conditions. Instead, they jump in and care for patients outside of their specialties with no resistance, being in the mindset, "It's my job, I'm a nurse, let's save lives".

Military nurse training is intense and includes exercises covering clinical and patient flow and command, control, communication, intelligence, logistical demands, and contamination procedures (Mattox, 2002). The nurses in the military also care for patients who have undergone damage control surgeries. This type of surgery has not been adopted by all civilian surgeons. Therefore, most civilian nurses have not had the opportunity to care for these types of patients.

The military has a list of skills that all nurses must be competent in performing prior to deployment. The Readiness Skills Verifications Program (RSVP) is maintained through attendance in formal training programs, ongoing clinical practice, and individual study. This checklist is filed in the nurse's record. If the nurse joins another unit during a mission, others will know the nurse's competency level. Civilian nurses have competency training, but some programs are not as comprehensive as that of military nurses.

After the tragic events of September 11, 2001, one civilian nurse wrote the following in regards to preparedness.

But we were clearly not prepared to respond to a major community disaster in which the health care system—and nurses—would be a vital resource to be mobilized. Although many nurses receive basic education in first aid, epidemiology, and outbreaks of infectious disease, and perhaps some facility-based training on disaster plans related to fires, multiple vehicle accidents or train/plane crashes, few (if any) educational institutions or health care facilities provide any courses or electives on mass casualties or disasters of this scale. (Orr, 2002)

There is a saying in the civilian community that discharge begins on admission; therefore, the civilian nurse is focused on discharge. This differs for the military nurse whose focus is on returning military members back to duty. In other words, the nurses on the battlefield do not have to deal with insurance issues for the casualties. Many of their patients are non-American civilian casualties and prisoners of war. Discharge planning is a minimal, or nonexistent, concern on the battlefield.

MILITARY/CIVILIAN INTERACTION AND ROLE OF THE MILITARY WITH THE CIVILIANS IN A DISASTER

Military hospitals and staff can be a very useful resource for civilian medical communities before and during a disaster, as many principles of military nursing will be exercised during a disaster.

Before a Disaster

Two ways to utilize the military hospitals before a civilian disaster are information sharing and planning and organizing exercises. "We must share our knowledge and learning experiences with our civilian partners to save lives in the current environment," said Air Force Surgeon General Lt. Gen. (Dr.) Paul K. Carlton Jr. "The concepts of medical modularity are applicable in any mass casualty environment and need to be shared" (Bouchard, 2002).

Information sharing occurs in the area of nuclear, biological, and chemical (NBC) warfare. The military has many experts in the area of NBC warfare and is better prepared as a group to care for these types of casualties than the civilian sector because of ongoing training. The knowledge of these individuals is valuable and must be shared. The military has full-time personnel whose job is to organize and plan these types of training events. These people can help local communities coordinate disaster planning events. Currently there is little communication between civilian staff nurses and military staff nurses. Sharing nursing expertise, training, resources, and future ideas of working together in times of emergencies would be a good way to start. See Nursing Vignette 7–1.

"Lessons learned" is another type of information sharing that the military can provide to the civilian community. For example, the military has learned that when nurses, medics, and physicians wear protective suits during simulated biological warfare environments, between 4% and 10% of participants terminate the exercise because of psychological symptoms (predominantly claustrophobia,

NURSING VIGNETTE 7–1   Lessons Learned: Military/Civilian Interaction a Vision for the Future.

One trauma surgeon had a vision and began to ask the question, "Who does the emergency medical system call when they are overwhelmed with a disaster? In other words who's the 911 for the 911?" Colonel (Dr.) Michael E. Hayek, MD was the Missouri State Air Surgeon for the Air National Guard, and his vision was that the air national guard would be the 911 for the 911. He was a strong proponent of the development of the air force expeditionary medical support (EMEDS) concept as an asset to serve both the civilian and the military roles in disaster preparedness.

Being a trauma surgeon at a St. Louis hospital, medical director for the Bi-State EMS, and the initial medical director of the Missouri-1 Disaster Management Team (DMAT), Hayek knew the limitations of the civilian community in time of a disaster. He was aware that the emergency room volume had increased by approximately 50%, the emergency room had replaced the physician's office for primary care, and the intensive care units were full or near capacity every day. Therefore, he knew if a disaster was to happen and stress was placed upon the already "stressed" system of emergency medical care, that there could be potential lives at risk by delayed medical care.

As a member of the military air national guard, he also knew its resources and capabilities. He began advocating for the EMEDS to become part of the air national guard units as well as the active duty bases. Therefore, his vision was to develop a way to bring the military and the civilian communities together seamlessly during a disaster.

He suggested that the military and the civilian community interact in the following way: During a disaster, the ANG EMEDS will serve as a bridge or 'RED WEDGE' until the civilian facilities can take back over, generally thought to be from 5 hours to 7 days. This could be from days to months if needed, although it is more likely that the Federal Military Assets would be used. In addition, all of the units do not have to be used during the entire time, only the assets that are needed. The State and Federal Command and Control, Governors/TAG's, Federal Emergency Management Agency (FEMA) directors and beyond, in partnership with military authorities will dictate what the need is and how the ANG can provide that need. Once the need has been fulfilled and the local hospitals are back functioning, the unnecessary modules of the EMEDS can stand down or be used to rest civilian response workers (Figures 7–5a, b, c).

He began by giving briefings on reorganization of ANG Medical to the air national guard bases under his command and then to four other states in FEMA Region 7 (Iowa, Nebraska, Missouri, Kansas).

Dr. Hayek proposed a regional approach for responding to disasters using the expeditionary medical support (EMEDS) concepts. He suggested air national guard bases meet with their army counterpart and discuss their mission/capabilities and assets. He explained that the army guard could be very helpful by providing patient retrieval and transportation issues. After explaining how the army could be utilized, Dr. Hayek suggested that there should be a civilian and military exercise to help bring the two agencies together and that the army should be included in the training as well.

Therefore, Hayek organized and planned an exercise to put his "Homeland Medical Response" vision to a test. His mission was to validate the use of the EMEDS model in a civilian setting. The exercise was called "Care 02" and held in Alpena, Michigan, August 2002. It was a joint exercise which involved the following: two Missouri ANG bases, 131st FW from St. Louis and 139th FW from St. Joseph, Missouri, DMAT headquartered in St. Louis, Civil Support Team from Ft. Leonard Wood, Critical Care Air Transport Team (CCATT), and an Aeromedical Evacuation (A/E) Crew.

The exercise was intended to provide realistic training in the following areas:

A. Promote and assess interoperability of the EMEDS, DMAT, and CST personnel during critical in-state disaster.

B. Rehearse mass casualty care resulting from a domestic terrorist attack in a civilian setting.

C. Further develop the medical proficiency of the Missouri Air National Guard (MOANG) medical personnel with the air force expeditionary medical support + 10 (EMEDS+10) field hospital system.

D. Provide a cooperative training environment between civilian emergency response teams and military medical and support units.

E. Determine and refine as applicable, command and control issues that arise between civilian and military entities.

The intense preparation and planning over a 5 month time frame paid off and the "Care 02" exercise was a success. The interoperability between

(continued)

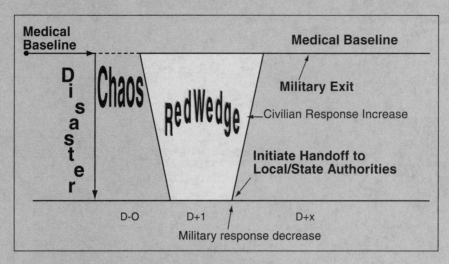

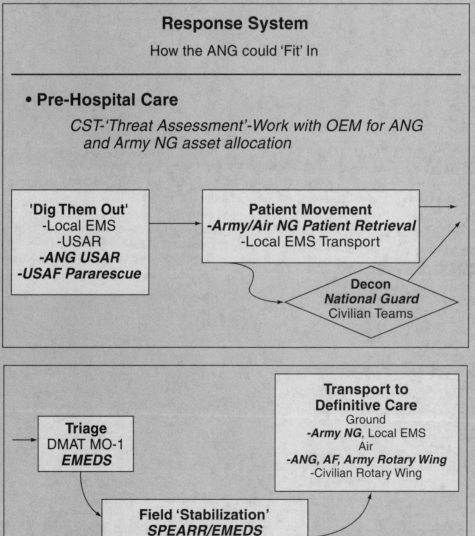

Figure 7–5a–c. Red wedge response system series, three illustrations.

the military, DMAT, and CST worked well and opportunities to improve the working relationships were discovered (Figure 7–6). The following are a few of the lessons learned: (1) The EMEDS platform is superb for homeland security; (2) it fully integrates the National Guard into the EMEDS program; (3) it streamlines a pathway from the requirement to execution at state and local levels; (4) it establishes communication channels between DMAT and EMEDS personnel; and (5) it identifies local force protection requirements from on-scene medical personnel (M. Hayek, personal communication, February 2002).

This was not Dr. Hayek's first vision; he also saw a deficit in trauma skills within the air national guard. His vision was to provide guardsmen with trauma skills by training in civilian trauma centers. Therefore, he suggested that the military and civilians collaborate in providing a 2-week trauma training refresher course for the military medical professionals to improve medical readiness. This vision led to the establishment of the Center for Sustainment of Trauma and Readiness Skills (CSTARS) St. Louis, which was supported by the USAF surgeon general and initiated in 1998.

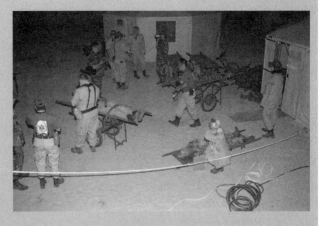

Figure 7–6. Collaboration between the military and DMAT.

Unfortunately, Hayek died in August 2002 but his vision continues. The C-STARS-STL program is quite successful and has trained over 200 military and civilian doctors, nurses, physician assistants, medics, medical students, nursing students, and physician assistant students since January 2003. The air national guard has adopted the EMEDS concept and Readiness Skills Verification program standards for competencies.

anxiety, or panic) (Mattox, 2000). This is valuable information for the civilian community whose care providers typically do not train to care for patients in protective clothing. Learning from the military may help them prepare for the potential of care providers taking off their suits prematurely and contaminating themselves.

Planning and Organizing Exercises

Planning and organizing exercises is another area where the military is very resourceful. A key in planning is to know whom to contact for military assistance and for developing an agreement with them before a disaster strike, and including this communication in an exercise. If military nurses are needed to augment civilian nursing staff, they must be activated via the Federal Emergency Management Agency (FEMA) and through the Department of Defense. The nurses in the Department of Defense, Veterans Affairs, and Health and Human Services have begun working on a National Disaster Medical System (World, 2002). The military can also assist civilian communities in setting up exercises that address communication, triage, decontamination, and the use of **mission-oriented protective posture (MOPP)** gear. The MOPP gear is readily available for the military and possibly could be used in an exercise to give civilians the protective gear experience. See Figure 7–7.

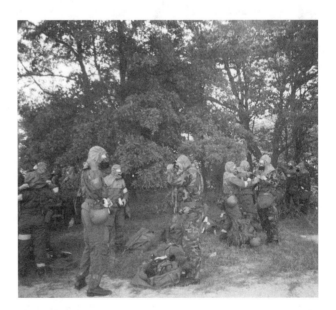

Figure 7–7. MOPP gear training.

During a Disaster

The military can offer valuable resources and play an important role in a disaster situation. To understand the military's resources, one must be aware of the military's limitations and capabilities in order to get the maximum support.

Limitations

Prior to Operation Iraqi Freedom in 2003, the military medical services were not well prepared for trauma. This is surprising to some civilians because they believe the military to be the best in caring for trauma patients. This was true until the wartime missions decreased and right sizing during peacetime began. With right sizing, the priorities of the medical missions changed to meet the needs of supply and demand. The mission changed to maintain a healthy workforce and care for dependents of active duty members and retirees.

This change in focus during peacetime has prompted concern for future military care. The military right sizing resulted in full inpatient hospitals being decreased to outpatient clinics and emergency rooms being decreased to urgent care centers. In 2003, the military had two level I trauma centers.

The military medical system has worked well during peacetime, but has caused great concern for the future wartime mission. With the lack of trauma experience and the decrease in inpatient critical care units, military medical personnel skills have decreased. Many ICU nurses have been put into case management and infection control while being kept on the **CCATT** mobility team. Many operating room nurses and technicians have not only become accustomed to elective surgeries but their experience with emergency multiple trauma cases is also rare. Nurses are in short supply and those employed have been groomed in the current system of "minimal trauma." The active duty component of the military nurse corps is young and at the novice skill level.

The military has acknowledged these limitations and has created trauma training centers in several urban level I trauma centers. The goal is to send military personnel for trauma refresher training before being deployed overseas. The rotations vary from 2 to 4 weeks and provide training for surgeons, anesthesiologists, nurses, physician assistants, and medics. The training includes medical simulations with battlefield scenarios, EMEDS equipment familiarization, didactics, and clinical rotations in the intensive care units, emergency rooms, operating rooms, civilian air ambulances and fire department emergency medical services. The training centers for the air force are in Baltimore, St. Louis, and Cincinnati and are called Center for Sustainment of Trauma and Readiness Skills (CSTARS). The army also has a similar program in Miami and the navy has one in Los Angeles. See Figure 7–8.

See Nursing Vignette 7–2.

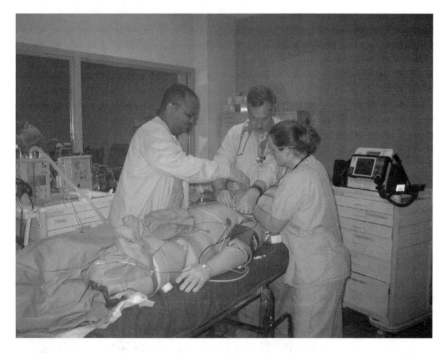

Figure 7–8. Training on HPS at CSTARS.

NURSING VIGNETTE 7–2

CSTARS is a new concept, unfamiliar to many. The air force senior nursing staff asked the following questions in preparation for the 2003 Senate testimonial. The answers are provided by Major Michelle R. Mandy, USAF, NC, Clinical Branch Chief, CSTARS-STL.

1. How does your course/program provide/improve wartime clinical readiness training for nurses?

Our program improves wartime clinical readiness by providing didactic and hands-on trauma training. The nurses are provided the opportunity to refresh their trauma skills in a level 1 trauma center. Many of the guard nurses have jobs other than bedside nursing and the ones who do bedside nursing have not cared for a level 1 multiple trauma patient. These nurses at the beginning of the 2 weeks expressed fear in caring for emergency room and critical care patients—fear that their skills are not as sharp as they once were. By the end of the course they express confidence in their refreshed trauma skills and feel they can fulfill their wartime mobility positions.

So, how do we do this? Our program allows the nurses the opportunity to try their skills out on a human patient simulator (HPS) before caring for a live patient. They start IVs, draw blood using the updated needleless system, etc. They are introduced to the equipment (triple channel infusion pump, impact ventilator, ISTAT, Life Pack 12 defibrillator, ICU parameter monitor etc.) in the EMEDS, which many of them are not familiar with. They are taught how to operate them and then they actually use them on the HPS (Figure 7–8).

They are given the opportunity to assess a patient with a tension pneumothorax, pericardial tamponade, pelvic fractures, femur fractures, etc., through our wartime trauma scenarios. They are taught how to needle decompress, apply traction splints, and insert a chest tube, just to name a few skills.

After the simulation they get the pleasure of caring for these types of patients in the ER and ICU. An example of their clinical experience is they may get a gunshot victim in the ER then follow the patient to the OR, where they will scrub in with the trauma surgeon, then they will follow the patient to the intensive care unit. This allows them the opportunity to witness and care for the patient through the continuum.

2. How many nurses did you train in 2002?
In 2002, we trained 47 medical personnel and 5 nurses. We moved to Saint Louis University in January 2003 and from then to February 9, 2003 we have trained 11 military medical personnel, 5 nurses, and 22 civilian nursing students.

3. What kind of feedback have you received from your nurses on this training?
When the students leave we ask them the following question, "How did this course help you to improve your skills as a health care provider?" The following are a few statements written by the students who attended class during fiscal year 2003:

- *Excellent chance to resuscitate cognitive and procedural skills relevant to my wartime tasks in my air force*

specialty code (AFSC) that are not always used in my current practice.
- *It refreshed previously used skills, added new trauma skills, provided familiarization with EMEDS equipment, and allowed recertification of ACLS.*
- *The hands-on really helped me. It reinforces the old saying, "If you don't use it, you lose it." I really benefited from this rotation.*
- *It helped me to refresh my respiratory therapy skills since as an RN I do not use my RT training very much.*
- *It allowed me to see how I would work or respond in a trauma setting.*
- *I have more confidence in trauma.*
- *Better understanding of trauma.*
- *Great opportunity for hands-on experience with multiple traumas, great instruction by the military trauma surgeon and the rest of the C-STARS staff and an excellent working relationship with the surgical residents, ER and ICU staffs at Saint Louis University. I've been in many hospitals over the last 20 years and Saint Louis University is one of the best, probably the best overall considering physical facility, staff, working environment, cleanliness, etc.*
- *This is far and away the greatest training program I have been able to attend in the Air Force/ANG, even better than flight surgeon's school.*

4. What kind of changes have you made to your program based on this input?
We have provided more time in the hospital and less on didactics. We are also expanding to allow clinical in the level 1 burn center. We are going to be offering Advance Trauma Nurse Course certification along with the physicians ATLS course, and ACLS will be available during the course for those who need recertification, and a suture course will be available. Our goal is to give them more bang for their buck during the time spent away from their units (M. Mandy, personal communication, March, 2003)

The military may not be on par in dealing with acute trauma patients compared to their civilian counterparts, but the resources are there. They have facilities and personnel who can help decompress trauma centers by taking care of less injured. The military EMEDS was successfully deployed for the first time stateside during the Houston floods that occurred as a result of Tropical Storm Allison in June 2001. "Wilford Hall Medical Center at Lackland Air Force Base, Texas deployed their mobile field hospital with 87 staff in three buses with six trucks of equipment. The unit was fully functional within 12 hours of deploying. The hospital saw more than 1,000 patients in 10 days and eased the strain on Houston's recovering hospital network." (Bouchard, 2002)

SUMMARY

The war experiences have taught the military and civilian communities that improvement of field resuscitation, increased efficiency of transportation and aggressive treatment of war causalities proved to be a major contributing factor to saving lives. Military nurses have been on the battlefield for many years caring for patients and improving their survivability by the *art of nursing* itself. By using lessons learned from past wars, battlefield nursing care has continued to evolve.

Over time, throughout the history of the battlefield nursing, nurses have acquired some of the following skills/roles that have brought them to where they are today: advanced clinical skills, quick thinking in emergency situations, difficult decision making, leadership and supervisory skills, sense of professional competency, physician trust, team playing, emotional stability, combat readiness, patriotism, survival skills, physical endurance and agility. On the battlefield today, it has become more technical with the use of sophisticated nursing tools, like handheld ventilators and ICU parameter monitors that are also compatible for the air evacuation system.

Civilian and military nursing care is similar yet different, due to their mission. The military nurses trauma experiences are dwindling due to right sizing and can benefit from clinical time in civilian level I trauma centers. The military nurses undergo intense training to ensure they are combat ready and ready for deployment. The Readiness Verification Program is the Air Force's way of ensuring nursing competency prior to deployment. Trauma training programs have been developed to help nurses accomplish these skills.

During times of disaster, the military nurses can augment civilian nursing staff if activated via the Federal Emergency Management Agency (FEMA) and through the Department of Defense. Rapid medical capability now exists within the Department of Defense and is available if local and critical care capacities are overwhelmed. Once the military system has been approved, they can be operational within six hours plus flying time. The military can tailor their response using *buildings of opportunity* which means only personnel and equipment would be needed. In comparing Hurricane Andrew to Tropical Storm Allison, it is evident that the new expeditionary forces, is truly exceptional. It took the Air Force medical service 17 days to become operational for Hurricane Andrew and only 36 hours for Tropical Storm Allison.

Looking at the past, one can learn valuable lessons to improve the overall nursing care for both civilian and military patients. Civilian nurses who have been called to duty return to their civilian jobs with newly acquired practical skills, which is a great benefit for all.

CASE STUDY

Under Attack

On April 4, 2004, U.S. troops were attacked in Baghdad by rockets. Fifteen rounds hit the airport and one landed near the expeditionary medical support (EMEDS) + 25 beds air force theater hospital (AFTH) but did not detonate. All the staff and patients hurried to the **bunkers** where they stayed for 5 hours. Later that night a convoy was ambushed and they received as many patients as there were EMEDS staff (approximately 52). They worked for the next 9 days at 100% to 300% capacity. They ran out of beds.

The staff of five doctors (two surgeons, two flight doctors, one internist) and the rest of the EMEDS medical service personnel worked as long as they could stay awake and those who needed to sleep slept until the next multiple traumas arrived. They went one entire evening without a nurse because none could remain standing anymore.

Everyone in the EMEDS stepped out of their comfort zones. The public health officers became expert radiology technicians. The biomedical environmental technician became an OR circulator. The dentist began drawing arterial blood gases. The supplies began to disappear faster than expected and there were more patients than the EMEDS had equipment for.

All of the patients survived.

1. What type of triage should be used in this situation?
2. What can the staff do to improve the bed situation?
3. How can the EMEDS staff better prepare for this type of situation?
4. What can the staff do about the lack of supplies?

TEST YOUR KNOWLEDGE

1. MEDIC is the acronym of the five NATO and military categories. List and define each category.

2. All of the following are effective strategies that military nurses use to ensure coverage during wartime except

   A. Multiple specialties
   B. Intense training
   C. Maintaining a large nursing reserve force
   D. Working 8-hour shifts

3. What is the name of the modular lightweight deployable medical units?

4. A casualty's first encounter with nursing care on the battlefield is in

   A. Mobile forward surgical team (MFST) units
   B. European hospitals
   C. Navy ships
   D. Air evacuation planes

5. Who is the American nurse known as the "Angel of the Battlefield" from past wars?

6. During war nurses do not have to care for prisoners of war.

    A. True
    B. False

7. What's the name of the Treaty that requires nurses to care for enemy prisoners of war?

8. During times of disaster, the military nurses can augment civilian nursing staff if activated by the

    A. Local EMS and mayor
    B. Overwhelmed hospital and local EMS
    C. Department of Defense and FEMA
    D. Active duty base commander and mayor

9. Which of the following is not a current or future concept for the military battlefield care?

    A. Global expeditionary medical support (GEM)
    B. Expeditionary medical support (EMEDS)
    C. Readiness Skills Verification Program (RSVP)
    D. Air transportable hospitals (ATH)

10. Which of the following is not a way military and civilian nurses can interact together?

    A. Information sharing
    B. Planning and organizing exercises
    C. Lessons learned
    D. Financial support

See Test Your Knowledge answers in Appendix B.

Explore MediaLink

Interactive resources and an audio glossary for this chapter can be found on the Companion Website at http://www.prenhall.com/langan. Click on Chapter 7 to select the activities for this chapter.

References

Allen, G.W. (1955). *Solitary singer* (p. 288). New York: The Macmillan Company.

Allen, R. C., & McAtee, J. M. (1999). Pararescue medication and procedure handbook. Washington, DC: USAFP.

Archard, T. (1945). *G.I. Nightingale: The story of an American army nurse*. Binghamton, NY: Vail-Ballou Press.

Army Nurse Corp History. (2003). *The mixed blessings of combat nursing assignments: Major Mary C. Quinn, ANC, Chief Nurse, 71st Evacuation Hospital, Pleiku*. Office of Medical History, OTSG. Retrieved May 20, 2003, from http://history.amedd.army.mil/ancwebsite/anchhome.html

Binder, J. L. (2002, November 27–29). *The United States Air Force Expeditionary Medical System (EMEDS) Capabilities*. Paper presented at 43rd Annual Indian Society of Aerospace Medicine Conference Abstracts. Retrieved April 10, 2003, from http://www.isamindia.org/events/programslist.shtml

Boivin, J. (2003a). At home and abroad, reserve RNs answer call to duty. *Nursing Spectrum, 4*(5).

Boivin, J. (2003b). Floating hospital a welcome berth for the war wounded. *Nursing Spectrum, 4*(5).

Bouchard, B. (2002, May 29). Medical training offers civilians insight. *Air Force News*. Retrieved 2003, from http://www.af.mil/news/may2002/n20020529_0869.shtml

Bowen, T. E., & Bellamy, R. (1988). *Second United States revision of the emergency war surgery NATO handbook*. Washington, DC: United States Government Printing Office.

Brohi, K. (2000). Damage control surgery. *Trauma Org, 5, 6*.

Bullough, Y. L. (1978). *The Care of The Sick: The Emergence of Modern Nursing*. New York: Prodist.

Cobb, K. (2003). *Clara Barton: Learning to give*. Retrieved April 19, 2003, from http://www.learningtogive.org/papers/people/clarabarton.html

Davis, L. M., Hosek, S. D., Tate, M. G., Perry, M., Hepler, G., & Steinberg, P. S. (1996). *Army medical support for peace operations and humanitarian assistance*. RAND Publication. Retrieved April 19, 2003, from http://www.rand.org/publications/mr/mr773/index.html

Department of Defense: Korean War 50th Anniversary. United States of America Korean War Commemoration. Women in the Korean War. (2000). Retrieved April 10, 2003, from www.Korea50.mil/history/factsheets/women.shtml

Eisenstadt, M. (1998). U.S. military capabilities in the post cold-war era: Implications for Middle East allies. *Middle East Review of International Affairs (MERIA) Journal, 2*(4). Retrieved March 12, 2003, from http://www.ngdc.noaa.gov/seg/hazard/resource/soc/medical.html

Furey, J. A. (2001). *Her military. Women Sustaining the American spirit*. Retrieved May 20, 2003, from http://hermilitary.com/militarywomen3.htm

Gendergap. (2001a). *American women and the military*. Retrieved May 25, 2003, from http://www.gendergap.com/military/usmil3.htm

Gendergap. (2001b). *World War II: 1941–1945*. Retrieved May 25, 2002, from http://www.gendergap.com/military/usmil6.htm#ww2

Jamieson, E. M., Sewall, M. F., & Suttrie, E. (1996). *Trends in Nursing History*. Philadelphia: W.B. Saunders.

Mattox, K. (1997). Introduction, background, and future projections of damage control surgery. *Surgical Clinics of North America, 77*(4), 753–759.

Mattox, K., Feliciano, D., & Moore, E. (2000). *Trauma* (4th ed.). New York: McGraw-Hill Companies, Inc.

Megmeister, M. (2003). *Historical nursing: Nursing's role in selected American wars*. Retrieved May 1, 2003, from http://hometown.aol.com/ksurn/page

Meridith, M. (2001, January 26). Medical "watch dog" protects deployed forces. *Air Combat Command News Service*. Retrieved May 1, 2003, from http://www2.acc.af.mil/accnews/jan01/01028.html

Mientka, M. (2003). Army nurse corps celebrates centennial news highlights. *U.S. Medicine*. Retrieved April 19, 2003, from http://www.usmedicine.com/dailynews.cfm?dailyID=23

Neel, S. (1991). *Medical support of the U.S. Army in Vietnam 1965–1970*. Washington DC: Department of the Army. Office of Medical History, OTSG. Retrieved April 19, 2003, from http://history.amedd.army.mil/booksdocs/vietnam/medicalsupport/chapter4.htm

Nobel e Museum. (2002). *Henri Dunant-Biography*. Retrieved April 19, 2003, from http://nobel.se/peace/laureates/1901/dunant-bio.html

Orr, M. (2002). One year later: The impact and aftermath of September 11: Ready or not, disasters happen. *Online Journal of Issues in Nursing*, 7(3), Manuscript 2. Available from http://www.nursingworld.org/ojin/topic19/tpc19_2.htm

Purificato, R. (2001). Brooks EMEDS team supports Houston flood recovery effort. *Discovery*, 25(12), 1, 5

Ray, M. (1996). Econometric analysis (studies I, II) of the Nurse-Patient Relationship. *TriService Nursing Research*. Retrieved May 13, 2003, from http://www.usuhs.mil/tsnrp/funded/fy1996/ray.html

Stahl, L. (2003). Nursing shortage in critical stage. *60 Minutes*. CBS News. Retrieved March 12, 2003, from http://www.cbsnews.com/stories/2003/01/17/60minutes/main536999.shtml

Strachey, L. (1918). *Eminent Victorians*. New York: Harcourt Brace & Co.

Swan, K. G., & Swan, K. G. Jr. (1996). Triage: the past revisited. *Military Medicine, 161*, 448–52.

Taft, Dave. (2003). *Triage concepts*, Retrieved August 15, 2003, from http://www.vnh.org/fleetmedpocketref/triage.html

Tomblin, B. B. (1996). *G.I. Nightingales: The army nurse corps in World War II*. Lexington, KY: University Press.

Women in History. (2002). *Clara Barton biography*. Lakewood Public Library. Retrieved May 19, 2003, from http://www.lkwdpl.org/wihohio/bart-cla.htm

World, H. (2002). On the front lines, reserve nurses come away from their battlefield experiences with cutting-edge training, and bring this new expertise back to their civilian workplaces. *Nurse Week.com*. Retrieved March 12, 2003, from http://www.nurseweek.com/news/features/02-09/reserves.asp

Zacharias, S. R., Offner, P., Moore, E. E., & Burch, J. (1999). Damage Control Surgery. *AACN Clinical Issues Advanced Practice in Acute and Critical Care, 10*(1).

Preparing Community Health Nurses and Nurses in Ambulatory Health Centers

Dotti C. James

LEARNING OBJECTIVES

1. Identify the groups of people or unique locations that require special consideration during a mass casualty event.
2. Explore disaster response plan development in schools and on campuses.
3. Discuss the role of the school or campus nurse.
4. Discuss the unique needs of the elderly during and after a mass casualty event.
5. Identify ways in which to prepare businesses to protect their employees before, during, and after a mass casualty event.
6. Explore the role of the parish nurse during a mass casualty event.
7. Discuss the role of the correctional facility nurse during a disaster in protecting those who are incarcerated and the community.

MEDIALINK www.prenhall.com/langan

Resources for this chapter can be found on the Companion Website at http://www.prenhall.com/langan. Click on Chapter 8 to select the activities for this chapter.

CHAPTER OUTLINE

Know Your Terms
Audio Glossary
Web Links
    Business Resources
    School Resources
MediaLink Applications

GLOSSARY

Contextual vulnerabilities. The building's proximity to other targets or its designation by the Department of Homeland Security that render the building more attractive to attack

Crisis management plan. Organized response for agencies and institutions involving local emergency preparedness agencies, law enforcement, and fire, health, and mental health agencies. Addresses first phase of a disaster

Mitigation. The last phase of the emergency management model, during which sustained activities are undertaken to prevent or minimize the negative impact of an event. It describes interventions to either prevent or reduce morbidity and mortality, and ease the economic and social impact of the event on the affected community

Operational vulnerabilities. The dynamic building-specific characteristics that motivate a terrorist to select a specific building. These include governmental offices or embassies

Preparedness. Activities that assist emergency responders in rescuing and protecting students and faculty

Recovery. Period during which activities address issues including a plan to facilitate the return to routine activities

Risk reduction matrix. Schematic representation

Structural vulnerabilities. Characteristics inherent within a building that could be exploited by terrorists. Include things such as sprinklers, air ducts, and the blast resistance of the structure

Threat level. System for estimating the risk of attack

INTRODUCTION

In addition to groups of people who can easily be placed within age or condition categories, there are other groups who require special accommodations or management because of the location in which they live or work. First responders must plan carefully for situations that would require evacuation, rescue, or medical assistance, for these locations pose unique risks to the providers as well as to those who work or live in them. Some of these locations include:

- Elementary and high schools
- College campuses
- Residential centers
- Prisons
- Businesses
- High rise buildings

Exploration of these unique situations will highlight their vulnerabilities and methods of protecting the area.

Events of primary concern related to terrorism include biological (viruses, fungi, bacteria, toxins), chemical (everyday or military chemical compounds), and radiological (radioactive materials). When the release of these agents is threatened or actual, appropriate and prompt response by those in authority and those charged with the protection of health is imperative. Bombs are a frequent weapon chosen by terrorists. They can be disguised to look like routine items. Preparation for the management of suspicious packages or items should be a routine part of orientations and yearly educational reviews in all settings where people assemble. Continuing education is critical since what we know today will change tomorrow.

EDUCATIONAL SETTINGS

Elementary and High Schools

Nurses working in elementary and high schools will have a key role in the planning efforts for schools. As experts in the health care and protection of students, they offer valuable information as the response plan is developed, and can coordinate health care efforts within the school with first responders and providers from outside the school. In addition to preparing the school for a terrorist event, the school nurse may be involved in preparing the school building to double as a treatment center for less severely injured victims outside the school itself. These secondary centers will work in conjunction with public health agencies to respond to a mass casualty event. Those in authority (incident command system) will determine whether additional surge capacity for patients should be accommodated using

nonacute care facilities for preventive, diagnostic, minor medical and supportive care.

Position Statement
The National Association of School Nurses (NASN) issued a position statement in 2002 defining its position on the role of the school nurse in bioterrorism emergency preparedness. More than 61,000 school nurses working in private and public elementary and secondary schools are identified as front line responders in many states. In June 2002, the NASN adopted the position that school nurses should be recognized as first responders for mass casualty events, including bioterrorism. They further recommended that they receive education about this role and the collaborative efforts needed during a disaster (NASN, 2002).

Schools become another vulnerable population due to the large numbers of students at one location. Several important considerations related to the idea of *school* as a location will be discussed in this chapter; children as a separate population are covered in Chapter 10.

American Red Cross Guidelines
The American Red Cross (2003a) has developed guidelines for schools to use when planning their disaster response and protection of students. The initial recommended analysis looks at the most common natural threats to the school, such as tornadoes. Then the attention focuses on whether the school has instruments and tools to clear debris if necessary, and basic supplies should students be forced to remain inside for a period of time, such as if a shooting occurs. Secondly, school should make some planning assumptions based on where the students come from, specifically looking at the distance, bridges, and viaducts. This influences

whether students could possibly be stranded for a brief or extended period. For example, if you believe that students will be picked up by parents within one day, half of the remainder within a day, and the remainder within another day; you should stock supplies for 100% for day 1, 50% for day 2, plus 25% for day 3. Also factor in the number of staff and other adults who may be on campus.

The second largest area for consideration is the storage of these supplies. Each classroom should have some supplies in addition to a larger storage area for the entire school. If a school's biggest threat is earthquakes, then persons should consider an area outside of the primary building for storage of the main supplies. For economical reasons, use large, waterproof wheeled trash cans for storage. Be sure that anyone who could possibly need to use the supplies is aware of their existence and how to access them. These supplies should be in areas that are not likely to be deeply buried during an earthquake. Consider a garage or equipment shed, rather than the basement. To ensure safety, incorporate regular checks of supplies and their expiration dates.

The Red Cross (2003a) also recommends asking each student to bring in a personal kit of supplies containing toiletries, a few nonperishable food items, water, a space blanket or large plastic trash bag, a nontoxic chemical light stick, and a letter or photograph from home. These kits, while helpful, require time and supervision to assemble. If incorrect items are brought, or the student cannot afford to bring items, the school must have a plan so that each student has a kit. Kits for the entire classroom are also needed to cover times when the central supply cache is unavailable or unreachable. See Box 8–1 and Table 8–1.

Crisis Management Plan

Highlights of the plan include the importance of each school partnering in the development of a crisis management plan with local emergency preparedness agencies, law enforcement, and fire, health, and mental health pre-

paredness agencies. The plan should address traditional emergencies, such as fire, school shootings, and accidents, as well as biological, radiological, chemical, or other terrorist-sponsored activities. This crisis management plan should be reviewed regularly, especially the components related to terrorist events, and integrated with exercises and practice sessions. The individual school plan, together with a separate plan for each school building, must be a component of the larger school district crisis plan and address any unique circumstances and needs occurring in the individual schools. The plans must address prevention and mitigation, preparedness, response, and recovery. In March 2003, U.S. Secretary of Education Rod Paige and U.S. Secretary of Homeland Security Tom Ridge announced a new section on the U.S. Department of Education's Website designed to be a one-stop shop to help school officials plan for any emergency, including natural disasters, violent incidents, and terrorist acts (U.S. Dept. of Education, 2003a, 2003b). See MediaLink.

The disaster response plan must also cover how the parents will be notified and where the teachers and students will go should evacuation be necessary. Additionally, the nurse must plan for *sheltering in place* should that be necessary. Is there enough food and water for several days? What about medical supplies? There must be regular exercises to rehearse the plan. If the plan remains on a shelf, it will not work in a crisis. Ideally, these exercises are conducted quarterly, or at least every semester.

Prevention and mitigation include an individual building assessment to identify areas of increased risk for occupants. They also include the development of a plan for reducing the risks, previously identified, to faculty and students. These risks may include fuel storage areas, geographical barriers such as steep hills or inclines, and fences. In addition, it is necessary to conduct an analysis of the access and egress to buildings and surrounding traffic patterns to identify potential obstacles to a safe evacuation.

BOX 8–1   Classroom Supply Kit

- Work gloves, leather
- Latex gloves, 6 pr.
- Safety goggles, 1 pr.
- Small first aid kit
- Pressure dressings, 3
- Crow bar
- Space blankets, 3
- Tarp or ground cover
- Student accounting forms, blank
- Student emergency cards
- Buddy classroom list
- Pens, paper
- Whistle

- Student activities
- Duct tape, 2 rolls (for sealing doors & windows)
- Scissors
- Suitable container for supplies (5-gallon bucket or backpack)
- Drinking water and cups – stored separately
- Toilet supplies (large bucket, used as container for supplies and toilet when needed, with 100 plastic bags, toilet paper, and hand washing supplies)
- Portable radio, batteries or other communication system
- Flashlight, batteries
- Push broom (if classroom includes wheel chairs)

American Red Cross (2003a). Model Emergency Response and Crisis Management Plan. http://www.redcross.org/disaster/masters/supplies.htm

TABLE 8–1. SUPPLIES FOR THE WHOLE SCHOOL: WATER, FIRST AID, SANITATION, TOOLS, FOOD

Water:
- ½ gallon per person per day times three days, with small paper cups

First Aid:
- 4 × 4" compress: 1000 per 500 students
- 8 × 10" compress: 150 per 500 students
- Elastic bandage: 2-inch: 12 per campus 4-inch: 12 per campus
- Triangular bandage: 24 per campus
- Cardboard splints: 24 each, small, medium, large
- Butterfly bandages: 50/campus
- Water in small sealed containers: 100 (for flushing wounds, etc.)
- Hydrogen peroxide: 10 pints/campus
- Bleach, 1 small bottle
- Plastic basket or wire basket stretchers or backboards: 1.5/100 students
- Scissors, paramedic: 4 per campus
- Tweezers: 3 assorted per campus
- Triage tags: 50 per 500 students
- Latex gloves: 100 per 500 students
- Oval eye patch: 50 per campus
- Tapes: 1" cloth: 50 rolls/campus; 2" cloth: 24 per campus
- Dust masks: 25/100 students
- Disposable blanket: 10 per 100 students
- First aid books 2 standard and 2 advanced per campus
- Space blankets: 1/student and staff
- Heavy-duty rubber gloves, 4 pair

Sanitation Supplies: (If Not Supplied in the Classroom Kits)
- 1 toilet kit per 100 students/staff, to include:
- 1 portable toilet, privacy shelter, 20 rolls toilet paper, 300 wet wipes, 300 plastic bags with ties, 10 large plastic trash bags
- Soap and water, in addition to the wet wipes, is strongly advised.

Tools per Campus:
- 3 rolls barrier tape 3" × 1000"
- Pry bar, pick ax, sledge hammer, shovel, pliers, bolt cutters, hammer, screwdrivers, utility knife, broom, utility shut off wrench, 1/utility

Other Supplies
- 3' × 6' folding tables, 3-4
- Chairs, 12-16
- Identification vests for staff, preferably color-coded per school plan
- Clipboards with emergency job descriptions
- Office supplies: pens, paper, etc.
- Signs for student request and release
- Alphabetical dividers for request gate
- Copies of all necessary forms
- Cable to connect car battery for emergency power

American Red Cross (2003a). Model Emergency Response and Crisis Management Plan. http://www.redcross.org/disaster/masters/supplies.html

---

BOX 8–2   Preparedness Activities

- Prepare maps for each building
- Identify multiple evacuation routes and meeting points
- Practice all parts of the plan regularly
- Develop a communication plan
- Inspect all needed equipment and become familiar with its operation
- Develop a plan for discharging students
- Identify a secondary person for each child
- Collaborate with law enforcement officials and emergency preparedness agencies

---

Adapted from: Emergency Planning for America's Schools (U.S. Department of Education, 2003a)

Preparedness

Preparedness encompasses activities that assist emergency responders in rescuing and protecting students and faculty. Box 8–2 summarizes these activities. One component is described in the response portion of the crisis management plan, which is the command structure for responding to a crisis. All stakeholders must be identified and all persons involved—educators, law enforcement and fire officials—must be familiar with their defined roles and how they relate to other responders.

In the recovery component, the issues to be addressed include a plan to facilitate the return to routine activities and teaching and learning. Some of these activities are the provision of mental health services by credentialed mental health professionals (U.S. Department of Education, 2003b). In addition, the U.S. Department of Education (2003c) adapted a response model from the San Diego School District to facilitate decisions made by schools during a disaster situation (Figure 8–1). This decision tree assists in focusing on the specific criteria for action.

Work done in the Seattle public school system (McEvoy & Reineke, 1997) suggests needs that must be met to effectively manage a disaster in the school setting. The first need, *everyone must speak the same language*, addresses the issue of collaborative efforts between those at the school and those responders within the community. Precise communication speeds the handling of emergency calls. Secondly, the emergency response system must adjust itself depending on the specific emergency. Rather than having multiple crisis-specific plans, consistent response teams should be identified that can be activated as a situation develops. Third, the model should be equally manageable at the central school office and at the individual schools. The model should allow for easy education of faculty, staff, and students. Finally, the model must allow for evaluation. Using a model similar to this permits all involved agencies to feel that their needs are being met, and encourage collaborative efforts in preparing for emergencies.

When students are physically or mentally challenged, special care must be taken to identify their particular needs related to communication and evacuation. The U.S. Department of Education's model school safety plan contains recommendations on planning for these students. The plan must specifically address the deficit areas, such as speech, hearing, mobility, or cognitive delays.

If a school receives a terrorist threat, it is imperative to remain calm. The students, faculty, and staff are at increased risk of harm if panic and hysteria are present. Students will look to faculty and staff for direction and reassurance. During and after terrorist acts, it is important to maintain the crime scene so that the perpetrator can be identified. This is made difficult if panic ensues. If the threat is made in writing or by a package, it is important to set the item on the ground and clear the area. After calling 911, the authorities will assume command of the area.

College Campuses

The U.S. Department of Education (2003b) has also proposed a campus public safety program that focuses on protection from weapons of mass destruction. There are 15 million students and several million faculty, staff, and visitors on the campuses of approximately 4,000 Title IV institutions of postsecondary education in the United States. The Bureau of Justice estimates that there are 30,000 campus police officers on these campuses. Proactive steps can be integrated to deter, or respond to, terrorist attacks. While not all-inclusive, they can be modified for inclusion within the campus response plan.

While some of the recommendations for elementary and high school planning apply to college campuses, colleges must also consider how its plan fits with the larger community response plan. The unrestricted access and the variety of students pose a challenge to becoming prepared.

Prevention and Mitigation

Campuses must bring together local and regional leaders. Looking toward prevention of incidents on campus, college officials can establish a relationship with the supervisory agent in charge of the nearest FBI field office, or the regional Joint Terrorism Task Force (JTTF), so that the institution receives information about threats. Liaison

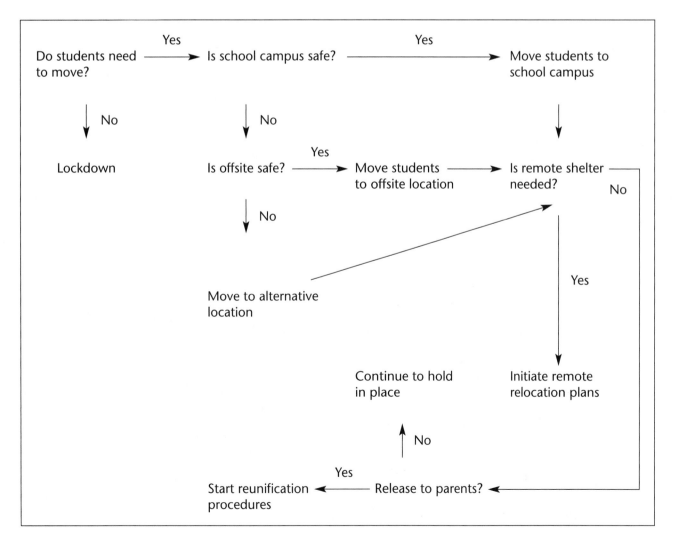

Figure 8–1. Decision tree for school crisis. *U.S. Department of Education http://wwwe.ed.gov/admins/lead/safety/emergencyplan/crisisplanning.pdf*

officers between international student groups may elicit information and build trust. These officers can also reduce fears among international students (U.S. Department of Education, 2003d).

Mitigation is defined as "any sustained action taken to reduce or eliminate long-term risk to life and property from a hazard event" (U.S. Department of Education, 2003c). In regard to a college or school, it means that they have taken all necessary actions to create a safe environment.

To deter attacks with weapons of mass destruction, a campus management team can review and direct the implementation of the emergency operations plan, as well as the terrorism incident annex, and mutual aid agreements with local partners. This review will guide the education of faculty, students, and staff. The mutual aid agreements outline potential campus assets that will be of value during and following a disaster. Increased visibility of security officers may provide additional security.

During periods of heightened alert, increasing physical checks of critical areas, establishing single point of access for critical facilities, making strict identification checks, and limiting public access may provide additional protection. Campus security should also increase inspections of persons and vehicles through video monitoring. Communication between faculty, staff, students, and parents is also vital.

Resources

Experts in terrorism believe that schools are viable targets for terrorism. Terrorism seeks to cause fear and anxiety with a hope of influencing government policies and concessions. Although innocent people were not targeted in the past, today terrorism and chaos in valued places is a goal. Is there another population more innocent than children? Assistance is available for schools through the U.S. Department of Education (2003b); Project SERV (School Emergency Response to Violence) assists schools that have experienced trauma by providing funding for mental health services and security, so that the learning environment can be resumed.

TABLE 8–2. PROACTIVE AWARENESS AND PREVENTION CHECKLIST

RECOMMENDATIONS	STEPS
Review employment and screening policies	All workers?
	Courthouse, not database searches
	Social Security traces
	Screening of subcontractor employees
Review physical security of buses, garages, and transportation security	Alarms in place?
	Storage areas locked and lighted
	Daily inspection of vehicles
	Buses with two-way radios
	Awareness of vehicles following buses
	Student rosters with contact information
Review physical security around buildings	Working alarms on all buildings
	Control of passkeys
	Changing of pass codes after terminations
	Exterior and interior lighting at night
Review access control procedures to increase awareness	Locked doors from outside
	Approach all strangers
	Visitor sign-in and badge policy
Education on reporting suspicious events	Suspicious activities and vehicles
	Routine inspections
	Suspicious activity policy
	Education
	Mandatory identification of all backpacks
Tip-line for anonymous reporting	Zero tolerance for threats
	Mandatory reporting
Collaboration with law enforcement and health officials	Enforcement of parking regulations
	Building plans with outside agencies
	Collaborative exercises
	Contact protocols
Education about potential threatening packages or letters	Posting of FBI, Postal Inspection Service advisories
	Distribute to community

Adapted from http://www.fema.gov/ofm/bc/shtm *and* http://www.ed.gov/admins/lead/safety/emergencyplan/crisisplanning.pdf

Being Proactive in Prevention

The Texas School Safety Center (2003) has made recommendations for becoming proactive in preparing schools for terrorism (Table 8–2). This checklist provides an organizational framework on which to base preparatory efforts. There are suspicious characteristics about packages or letters that should raise suspicion. These include the package being unsolicited; addressed to a title, not a name; addressed to a person no longer at the address; irregular in appearance; excessive tape or string; restrictive delivery instructions; excessive postage; and leaking powder, liquid, or strange odor.

BUSINESS ENVIRONMENTS

Preparation

It is not enough for cities and states to develop general response plans for helping their citizens to remain safe during disasters. Businesses or places where multiple people work must also prepare. Businesses of any type and any number of employees must plan for how they will respond to mass casualty events. The occupational health nurse will assume a leadership role in the development of a response plan. Participation of the occupational health nurse ensures the incorporation of any unique employee needs, such as hearing or mobility impairment with the plan. In addition, the occupational health nurse can be an effective liaison with outside responders. Some of the organizations and institutions that provide response guidelines include:

- American Red Cross
- Centers for Disease Control and Prevention
- State and local health departments
- Professional specialty organizations

To effectively plan for a disaster, businesses can follow the four-step process recommended by FEMA (2003a). (See MediaLink.) The four steps in the FEMA plan are as follows:

- Establish a planning team.
  - Form a group that will encourage participation and increase the amount of time participants are able to give, in addition to providing a broader perspective of the situation.
  - Include members from all levels of the workforce so that all employees accept responsibility for their role during a disaster.
- Analyze the capabilities and hazards of the organization.
  - Determine the current state of planning to ensure that it is regularly reviewed and updated.
  - Examine all current plans, such as fire and safety, and meet with outside groups, review existing codes and regulations, and identify critical products, services, and operations.
  - Review the internal resources and capabilities.
  - Review the external resources and insurance coverage.
  - Conduct a vulnerability analysis, listing potential emergencies of all types, such as geographic, technological, physical, and human error.
  - Assess the vulnerabilities of the business.
- Develop the plan.
  - Include an executive summary, emergency management elements, response procedures, and support documents.
  - Address the challenges and prioritize activities.
  - Write the plan and establish a training schedule.
  - Conduct training, and revise as needed.
  - Distribute the plan to all involved, and ensure that a portable copy exists for outside responders.
- Implement of the plan.
  - Integrate the plan into company operations.
  - Reevaluate and modify the plan as needed.
  (FEMA, 2003a)

Recovery

In addition to the previous development plan, FEMA (2003b) also provides a *checklist* for the creation of a recovery manual for the business. The manual is suggested as a guide for the execution of a recovery of a business following a disaster. It is appropriate for use in organizations of any size, and in manufacturing, retail, or corporate settings. The only prerequisite is that the individual has the authority to create the plan for the business and provide education and exercises so that its implementation proceeds smoothly. For the company that has previously developed a disaster response plan, the checklist may be useful to determine whether business controls are a part of the plan and to assess the readiness of the plan and the documentation associated with it. The checklist contains four sections.

- Level 1: Executive Awareness/Authority
- Level 2: Plan Development and Documentation
- Level 3: Management and Recovery Team Assessment and Evaluation for Effectiveness
- Level 4: Management and Recovery Team Assessment of Readiness and Plan Maintenance

Levels 1 and 2 contain an assessment form to establish a base level of the company's business recovery plan (BRP). This concise instrument provides an objective assessment about the awareness of those in authority about the need for or presence of a written plan. See Figure 8–2.

Standard Checklist Criteria for Business Recovery

Completed By:

Name: _____

Company: _____

Room: _____

Street: _____

City, State, Zip: _____

Phone Number: _____

Business Recovery Plan for: _____

Business Recovery Plan (BRP)—LEVEL 1 (Executive Awareness/Authority).	Y	N	N/A

1. Has a BRP been:
  a. Developed?
  b. Updated within the last 6 months?			

Business Recovery Plan (BRP)—LEVEL 2 (Plan Development and Documentation).	Y	N	N/A
1. Has a classification (critical, important, marginal) been assigned to the Business Process/Function/Component that this Facility/Function supports?			

2. Has a BRP been:
  a. Documented?
  b. Maintained?			

3. Does the BRP include the following sections:
  a. Identification?
  b. Incident Management?
    i. Responsible company officer?
    ii. Personnel responsible for updates?
  c. Response?
  d. Recovery?
  e. Restoration?
  f. Plan Exercise?
  g Plan Maintenance?
  h. Business Recovery Teams and Contact Information?			

4. Does the BRP identify hardware and software critical to recover the Business and/or Functions?			
5. Does the BRP identify necessary support equipment (forms, spare parts, office equipment, etc.) to recover the Business and/or Functions?			

Figure 8–2. FEMA checklist criteria for business recovery form for levels 1 and 2. *(http://www.fema.gov/ofm/bc1_2.shtm)*

Standard Checklist Criteria for Business Recovery (continued)

Business Recovery Plan (BRP)—LEVEL 2 (Plan Development and Documentation). (continued)	Y	N	N/A

6. Does the BRP require an alternate site for recovery?
   a. Does the BRP provide for mail service to be forwarded to the alternate facility?
   b. Does the BRP provide for other vital support functions?			

7. Are all critical or important data required to support the business being backed up? a. Are they being stored in a protected location (offsite)?			
8. Do you conduct a walk-through exercise of your plan at least annually? (This should include a full walk-through as well as "elements" of your plan (i.e. accounts payable, receivable, shipping and receiving, etc).			

9. Does the walk-through element exercises have a prepared plan which includes:
   a. Description
   b. Scope
   c. Objective			

10. Is a current copy of the BRP maintained off-site?			
11. Do all users of the BRP have ready access to a current copy at all times?			
12. Is there an audit trail of the changes made to the BRP?			
13. Do all employees responsible for the execution of the BRP received ongoing training in Disaster Recovery and Emergency Management?			

Figure 8–2. *continued.*

Levels 3 and 4 focus on the regular exercises held to familiarize employees and management with the BRP, so that its implementation during an actual disaster proceeds smoothly, each person aware of his or her role and the roles of others. Education about the response plan should be included within the new employee orientation. See Figures 8–3 and 8–4.

Responses by Threat Level

The American Red Cross (2003b) has categorized the appropriate responses for businesses according to the threat level, or risk of attack. Each level's activities are based on the assumption that the business has completed the suggested activities for the preceding lower activities. During a low risk or green alert level, the focus of ef-

forts within a business is the planning process itself. Those responsible for the preparation of the business develop written plans that outline the notification processes during a disaster, as well as the offsite location for personnel to meet if evacuation becomes necessary. The plan for communication with employees must consider that telephone communication may not be possible. Consideration should be given to alternative methods of notification, such as e-mail, radio, cell phones, or television. Each business plans for the possibility that employees will not be able to return to work in the same location for an extended period of time. Locating this alternate site contributes to a sense of continuity among employees. American Red Cross brochures and educational programs ensure that consistent information is given to all employees.

Standard Checklist Criteria for Business Recovery

Business Recovery Plan (BRP)—LEVEL 3 (Management & Recovery Team Assessment and Evaluation For Effectiveness)	Y	N	N/A
1. Has the business officer and management team approved the BRP?			
2. Does the business owner maintain: a. The master copy of the BRP? b. An audit trail of the changes made to a BRP?			
3. Do all aspects of physical and logical security at the alternate site conform with your current security procedures?			
4. Are the physical and logical security at the alternate site at least as stringent as the security at the disaster location?			
5. Have all employees and their alternates responsible for executing a manual work-around for a mechanized process been identified in the BRP and properly trained?			
6. Has an independent observer documented the simulation exercise(s) noting all results, discrepancies, exposures, action items, and individual responsible, etc.?			
7. Was a debriefing held within a reasonable period of time (typically two weeks) after the simulation exercise(s) to ensure all activities have been accurately recorded?			
8. Did the exercise coordinator publish a simulation exercise(s) report within a reasonable period of time (typically three weeks) after the completion of the simulation exercise(s)?			
9. Did the exercise report include: a. what worked properly as well as any deficiencies and recommendations for improvement? b. responsiblity and due date for the development of the Corrective Action Plan?			

Figure 8–3. FEMA checklist criteria for business recovery form for level 3. *(http://www.fema.gov/ofm/bc3.shtm)*

Blue Level (Guarded Status)

During a blue or guarded status, review and reeducate about the response plan as necessary. Communicate and document preparedness and response plans to emergency management and responders, government agencies, community organizations, and utilities. Be sure that needed equipment has been purchased and employees instructed in its operation.

Yellow Level (Elevated Risk)

During an elevated or yellow alert, consider using onsite security officers or a private security firm to conduct a risk assessment, and to determine what support or reinforce-

ment would be available in case of a disaster. Contact area volunteer organizations about a possible role for employees during a mass casualty event.

Orange Level (High Risk)

When the alert level reaches high, or orange, it is important to conduct more frequent reviews of the emergency plan, continuity plan, and media materials. If access to the business itself cannot be limited, screen and reinforce everyday security measures. Finalize the company's plans with venders to obtain supplies should an incident occur.

Standard Checklist Criteria for Business Recovery (continued)

Business Recovery Plan (BRP)—LEVEL 3 (Management & Recovery Team Assessment and Evaluation For Effectiveness)	Y	N	N/A
10. Was a Corrective Action Plan developed by the Exercise Team to address any deficiencies identified by the exercise?			
11. Is there a retention plan for the Exercise Plans and Corrective Action Plans (minimum retention 3 years)?			
12. Has a walk-through element exercise been performed at least quarterly?			
13. Did each walk-through element exercise have a prepared plan which includes: a. Description b. Scope c. Objective			
14. When there is a change in hardware, software, or a process that might impact the Business Recovery Plan, is the BRP reviewed and updated within 30 days of the changes: Sign-Off By Officer: by whom? Name: _____ When? Date: _____			
15. Based on the Joint Assessment has the Team determined that the BRP is effective?			

Figure 8–3. *continued.*

Red Level (Severe Risk)

Finally, during a red or severe level, be sure that communication between employees can be maintained via television or radio. Work with government and community organizations to determine how employees will fit with response plans. Consider working with a smaller workforce or stopping work for a period of time to protect the workforce.

FEMA *Guidelines*

FEMA (2003) also issues guidelines for emergency management that can be grouped under the following core operational considerations or functions.

- **Direction and control** defines the chain of authority during an event. The incident command system is specified as well as the emergency operations center, security, and coordination with outside responders. All those with managerial responsibility should be familiar with the authority structure during and after a disaster.
- **Communication** covers communication with outside agencies and family who should be notified.
- **Life safety** includes the examination of the evacuation plans, shelter, and family preparedness.
- **Encourage** employees to develop an emergency plan for their families.
- **The property protection function** focuses on protection systems, mitigation, and record protection so that the business can more easily return to operation following the event.
- **The community outreach function** explores involvement with the community, mutual aid agreements, and media relations.
- **The recovery and restoration function** focuses on keeping people employed and the business running, through insurance, employee support, and resumption of activities.

Standard Checklist Criteria for Business Recovery

Business Recovery Plan (BRP)—LEVEL 4 (Certification) (Management & Recovery Team Assessment Of Readiness and Plan Maintenance)	Y	N	N/A
1. Has the component BRP been approved by the owner(s) of the Business Function(s)?			
2. Has the entire BRP simulation exercise been performed at least annually?			
3. Has the Corrective Action Plan been completed and closed?			
4. Did the BRP simulation exercise have a prepared plan which includes: a. Description b. Scope c. Objectives			
5. Did the component BRP simulation exercise meet the acceptable Recovery Time Objective set by management?			
6. Based on the Joint Assessment has the Team determined that the BRP and Exercises have met all requirements to provide reasonable assurance that the plan will work in the event of a disaster?			
7. Does the BRP specify the maximum acceptable Recovery Time Objective (RTO)?			
8. Does the BRP specify the level of service (which the business owner has agreed to be acceptable) to be provided while in recovery mode?			
9. Have all changes relating to RTO in the BRP been approved by the process owner?			

Figure 8–4. FEMA checklist criteria for business recovery form for level 4. *(http://www.fema.gov/ofm/bc4.shtm)*

- **The administration and logistics function** covers authority within the business before and after an event, and the technical process of getting equipment and supplies.

Managers and supervisors must look critically at the heating, ventilation, and air-conditioning system to determine if it is secure or if it needs to be upgraded to better filter potential contaminants. Access to these systems should be protected and restricted. Multiple persons must know how to turn it off if the need arises.

Sheltering in Place

An option that may be available during an event is *sheltering in place*. The process is the same as sheltering in place at home. The windows and doors are closed and locked, air conditioning turned off, all occupants move to a pre-specified room, the windows and doors are sealed with plastic and duct tape, and the television or radio tuned for updates.

When sheltering in place at a business, some things are different from sheltering in place at home. Plans must be in place should the employees be unable to go home. Appropriate supplies must be available. The unique considerations within a business environment are that employees cannot be forced to remain in the building. There is a need to develop an accountability system to determine who is in the building, the assignment of specific duties to each employee, and the need to plan and implement practice exercises regularly, at least twice a year. Sheltering in place sample plans are available from the National Institute for Chemical Studies (2003).

HIGH-RISE BUILDINGS

A less obvious vulnerable population is those who live or work in high-rise buildings, which increase the population density of a given area. In a study by the RAND Corporation, the city of Los Angeles was analyzed for safety in its high-rise buildings following 9-11. The purpose of the study was to identify generic threats, identify exemplary practices, discuss potential actions after an event, and suggest preparations to be considered. See FEMA (2003a) for a vulnerability analysis chart sample for use in analyzing other locations.

Risk Reduction Matrix

Although business owners cannot prevent catastrophic terrorist events, such as what occurred on 9-11, they can and should manage and mitigate the consequences of such attacks. The first lines of defense are access control and perimeter security, but attention must also be given to the emergency preparedness plans and tenant education. Using a risk reduction matrix, the threats to a high rise can be grouped into categories: highly unlikely, unlikely, more likely, and preventable. This matrix can then be used to determine the need for increased or different security measures within the response plan. The horizontal axis is the severity level of consequences (negligible to catastrophic), while the vertical axis is the vulnerability (minimal to severe) (FEMA, 2003e).

Vulnerabilities

Building vulnerabilities include structural, operational, and contextual characteristics. Structural vulnerabilities include sprinklers, air ducts, and the blast resistance of the building. Structural vulnerabilities include what is intrinsic to the building that could be exploited. Consider whether the structure can withstand the blast of bombs of different sizes, placed in varying locations.

Operational vulnerabilities refer to the dynamic building-specific characteristics that motivate a terrorist, as opposed to the static structural vulnerabilities. Operational vulnerabilities may be the occupants that make it attractive to terrorists, for example, embassies, government offices, the ease of entry, and the occurrence of regular evacuation exercises.

Finally, contextual vulnerabilities include the building's proximity to other targets and the overall risk level for an attack as determined by the Department of Homeland Security. If nearby buildings are attractive targets, the building owners in close proximity should plan for the aftermath of an attack on the attractive target.

Considering the horizontal axis or consequences category, two issues are significant. In the first, the building specific consequences, or things unique to the building, are related to the effect on the population of an attack with high profile casualties. The second, or general consequences, re-

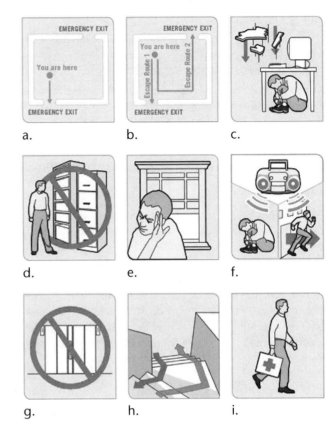

Figure 8–5. Department of Homeland Security vulnerability icons.

sult from an attack on any similar building. This reflects the general fear and vulnerability felt after the attack.

Generally, educate the tenants of a high-rise building that they must be aware of the closest emergency exit, as well as an alternate route in case the original choice is destroyed (Figure 8–5a, b). Use all information available to reach the decision on your preferred exit. If debris is falling, protect yourself by taking shelter under a desk or table (Figure 8–5c). Avoid areas near file cabinets, bookshelves, or other structures that may topple and injure them (Figure 8–5d). Also avoid facing areas with large amounts of windows or glass to prevent being cut by flying shards (Figure 8–5e). Similarly, distance yourself from exterior walls that may crumble or be destroyed. Locate a battery powered radio or television so that you can listen to news and emergency directions (Figure 8–5f). This will alert you to whether you should vacate the building or shelter in place. Once a decision has been made to leave the building, do not use the elevators (Figure 8–5g). As you descend the stairs, stay to the right side so that you do not hinder emergency workers ascending (Figure 8–5h). If it has not been contaminated, carry your emergency supply kit with you (Figure 8–5i).

The preparation or use of icons or universally understood images will ensure that all persons in the building understand the message and actions needed during a disaster. To protect high-rise buildings, the building owners and managers must work with other building managers, sharing information between themselves and with law enforcement and intelligence agencies. The underlying goal is risk reduction through reducing the vulnerabilities of each location. The government makes many of the prevention decisions, such as intelligence funding, law enforcement, and customs policies, but the building owners and managers have a responsibility to *harden the target* and increase the ability to deter and detect potential terrorists.

PERSONS WITH PHYSICAL OR MENTAL CHALLENGES

The initial step in planning for the evacuation of persons who may not be able to evacuate themselves during a disaster is the identification of those who would require additional assistance. These persons can be identified by a voluntary survey of current students or employees, or by asking specific employees with known disabilities what they would require. General accommodations may include alarms signage for the emergency exit routes, a buddy system or team approach, or designated areas of rescue assistance, such as an operating telephone, cell phone, closing door, smoke-blocking supplies, or a window with a help sign.

Those with motor impairments may require evacuation devices to be moved down stairs or over rough surfaces. Evacuation assistance devices could be a three-person wheelchair carry device, or Evac-u-Straps that permit the wheelchair to be lowered down the stairs. It is also important to remove all physical barriers on the exit route, and perhaps don heavy gloves for the manual wheelchairs and removal of debris. The person may require a one- or two-person carry technique for evacuation. Persons with sensory impairments may need visual or vibratory alarm devices and tactile signage and maps. If a guide or service dog is used, plan for the evacuation of the animal also. If you must take the dog while helping the owner, hold the leash, not the harness (FEMA, 2003c).

Persons with cognitive or psychiatric impairments may find picture signage or color coding of escapes helpful. Exercises may increase or decrease anxiety levels so this will have to be individualized for the specific person or area. Break down information into simple steps. Do not talk down to people or treat them like children.

INCARCERATED INDIVIDUALS

Those who are incarcerated are another unique vulnerable population. Security is a primary concern with this group. Prison facilities provide onsite medical care for many conditions and some facilities are supported through telemedicine. Should evacuation become necessary, officials have elaborate plans in place for the management following a terrorist event or mass casualty event. These plans are not available to the general public due to security reasons. The correctional health nurse within prisons or correctional fa-

cilities is an integral part of the planning team and an expert liaison with authorities outside the facility. This nurse appreciates the unique health care challenges as well as the security issues faced during and following a disaster (Clark, 2003; Couklin, Lincoln, & Tothill, 2000).

PARISH NURSES

Another group of community-based nurses who can be valuable members of community planning teams is parish nurses, who are located within churches and who provide health education and care for church members facing acute and chronic health challenges. Parish nurses can work with local and regional authorities in providing education about planning and responding to a mass casualty event to a variety of community citizens. They are a trusted member of the church and a valuable access to groups of community members.

Parish nurses can work with smaller subgroups of the community and provide education and reinforcement about what can be expected during and following a disaster. This permits a more personalized program of education to a smaller group, reinforcing the generalized education provided by community leaders to larger populations. Parish nurses are also valuable sources of information about specific health needs of the parish population related to medications or equipment.

SUMMARY

Different locations within each community pose unique risks and challenges when preparing for multiple casualty events. Some of the risks and challenges result from the location itself, such as the height of a building, while some result from the populations within, such as schools and prisons. Deterrence results from the visibility of effective preventive measures. On 9-11, the terrorists were convinced of their ability to succeed. To be effective, strategies should involve multiple layers focusing on preventing an attack, in addition to responses to mitigate the consequences if an attack should occur. It is necessary to plan multiple ways to achieve the objective, because this redundancy decreases the likelihood that one area or characteristic will result in catastrophe, and redundancy increases the building's resistance to various threats. Additional assistance in planning ways to protect schools, businesses, and high-rise buildings can be obtained from local authorities and other responding agencies. Fire departments, law enforcement agencies, or regional planning committees are excellent sources of information about effective planning and coordination of each business or institution's plan within the regional planning efforts.

Advance planning to protect vulnerable populations will maximize the effective use of resources. Without this planning, these groups will sustain a greater proportion of casualties during and following a disaster. As professionals, nurses are in a position to influence the planning process and become leaders during the implementation of the response plan.

CASE STUDY

Occupational Health Nurse and Plan Development

You are a new occupational health nurse at a large computer manufacturing firm. During your orientation you are told that it is your responsibility to ensure that the company is prepared for any possible terrorist event.

1. How will you begin this project?
2. Who will you need to contact?
3. How will you disseminate this information to the employees?

TEST YOUR KNOWLEDGE

1. You are the school nurse in an elementary school having 500 students. What are the significant factors to consider when planning the amount of needed supplies to have following a terrorist event?
2. What is the appropriate response when a suspicious package is found within a school setting?
3. Identify things that can be done on a college campus to prevent or mitigate a terrorist event.
4. What specific assessments and interventions are appropriate during a period of high alert?
5. What steps are recommended by FEMA to prepare businesses for possible terrorist events?
6. How would a business begin the process of analyzing capabilities and hazards within its organization?
7. Describe the process of *sheltering in*.
8. When looking at high-rise buildings as a location for possible terrorist attack, differentiate between structural, operational, and contextual characteristics of the location.
9. Identify important information to include in an educational program for tenants of a high-rise building.
10. What types of accommodations are necessary for people with handicaps?

EXPLORE MEDIALINK

Interactive resources and an audio glossary for this chapter can be found on the Companion Website at http://www.prenhall.com/langan. Click on Chapter 8 to select the activities for this chapter.

REFERENCES

American Academy of Pediatrics. (2003). *AAP Senate testimony*. Retrieved May 15, 2003, from http://www.aap.org/terrorism

American Red Cross. (2003a). *Model emergency response and crisis management plan*. Retrieved November 11, 2003, from http://www.redcross.org/disaster/masters/supplies.html

American Red Cross. (2003b). *Preparing your business for the unthinkable*. Retrieved May 8, 2003, from http://www.RedCross.org

American Red Cross. (2003c). *Emergency management guide for business and industry*. Retrieved May 8, 2003, from http://www.RedCross.org

Campus safety. (2003). Retrieved May 8, 2003, from http://www.ed.gov/offices/OSDFS/emergencyplan/campussafe.html

CDC's Division of Adolescent and School Health. (2003). Retrieved May 8, 2003, from http://www.cdc.gov/healthyouth

Clark, M. J. (2003). Care of clients in correctional settings. In M. J. Clark, Community health nursing (4th ed.) (pp. 603–621). Upper Saddle River, NJ: Pearson Education.

Conklin, T. J., Lincoln, T., & Tothill, R. W. (2000). Self-reported health & prior health behaviors of newly admitted correctional inmates. American Journal of Public Health, 90, 1939–1941.

Department of Homeland Security. Retrieved November 12, 2003, from www.ready.gov

Federal Emergency Management Agency (FEMA). (2003a). *Emergency management guide for business and industry*. Retrieved May 8, 2003, from http://www.FEMA.gov/library/biz1.shtm

Federal Emergency Management Agency (FEMA). (2003b). *Standard checklist criteria for business recovery*. Retrieved July 15, 2003, from http://www.fema.gov/ofm/bc.shtm

Federal Emergency Management Agency (FEMA). (2003c). *FEMA emergency procedures: Providing assistance*. Retrieved November 13, 2003, from http://www.ican.com/news/fullpage.cfm?articleid=OF9ED43-25E2-46B8-98787F369A

Federal Emergency Management Agency (FEMA). (2003d). *Terrorism fact sheet or federal response plan*. Retrieved May 8, 2003, from http://www.FEMA.gov

Federal Emergency Management Agency (FEMA). (2003e). *Vulnerability analysis chart*. Retrieved May 8, 2003, from http://www.FEMA.gov/graphics/library/vulanal.gif

Hale, R. W., & Zinberg, S. (2001). *Summary letter about anthrax*. American College of Obstetrics and Gynecology. Retrieved April 25, 2003, from www.acog.org/from_home/misc/anthrax.cfm

McEvoy, P., & Reineke, C. (1997). The central office role in school emergencies. *School Administrator*. http://www.aasa.org/publications/sa/1997_11/focmcelvoy.htm

National Association of School Nurses (NASN). (2002). *School nurse role in bioterrorism emergency preparedness: Position statement*. Retrieved November 13, 2003, from http://www.nasn.org/positions/bioterrorism.htm.

National Institute for Chemical Studies. (2003). *Sheltering in place at your office*. Retrieved May 15, 2003, from http://www.nicsinfo.org/SIP%20plan%20for%20offices%20NICS%20feb2003.pdf

Public Broadcasting System. (2001). *America responds: Classroom resources—9-12*. Retrieved May 15, 2003, from http://www.pbs.org/americaresponds/tamingterrorism.html

Texas School Safety Center. (2003). *Proactive guide for the threat of terrorism in schools*. San Marco, TX: Southwest Texas State University. http://www.edfacilities.org/rl/disaster.cfm

U.S. Department of Education. (2003a). *Emergency planning for America's schools*. U.S. Department of Education. Retrieved May 1, 2003, from http://www.ed.gov/news/pressreleases/2003/03/03072003.html

U.S. Department of Education. (2003b). *CDC and U.S. Department of Education collaborate to help schools prepare for possible terrorism*. PHTN satellite broadcast and webcast on May 16, 2002. Retrieved November 13, 2003, from http://www.phppo.cdc.gov/PHTN/schools/

U.S. Department of Education. (2003c). *Practical information on crisis planning*. Retrieved November 12, 2003, from http://www.ed.gov/admins/lead/safety/emergencyplan/crisisplanning.pdf

U.S. Department of Education (2003d). *Campus public safety: Weapons of mass destruction terrorism protective measures*. Retrieved 11/12/03 from http://www.ed.gov/admins/lead/safety/emergencyplan/campussafe.html

White, S. R., Henretig, F. M., & Dukes, R. G. (2002). Medical management of vulnerable populations and co-morbid conditions of victims of bioterrorism. *Emergency Medicine Clinics of North America, 20*(2), 365–392.

CHAPTER 9

Considerations for Vulnerable Populations

Joanne C. Langan and Dotti C. James

LEARNING OBJECTIVES

1. Identify the groups of people who require special consideration during a mass casualty event.
2. Explore the special needs of pregnant women and their unborn during and after a disaster.
3. Discuss the unique needs of older persons during and after a mass casualty event.
4. List key concepts to be shared with immunocompromised patients in preparing for disasters.
5. Discuss the needs of those with cognitive, mobility, or communication challenges in preparing for and responding to disasters.

MEDIALINK www.prenhall.com/langan

Resources for this chapter can be found on the Companion Website at http://www.prenhall.com/langan. Click on Chapter 9 to select the activities for this chapter.

CHAPTER OUTLINE

Know Your Terms
Audio Glossary
Web Links
    Cancer Resources
    Literacy Resources
MediaLink Applications
    Case Study: "Operation Medicate" Disaster Drill

GLOSSARY

Cancer prevalence. The number of people alive today who have been diagnosed with cancer

Disability. A limitation in functional ability resulting from impairment

Fetal vaccinia. A rare, serious infection of the fetus, that can occur following vaccination for smallpox to the mother

Generalized vaccinia. Vesicles or pustules appearing on normal skin distant from the vaccination site

Hemorrhagic smallpox. Also known as purpura variolosa, symptoms include fever, backache, diffuse, copper-red rash

Impairment. Loss of psychological, physiological, or anatomical structure or function

Literacy. An individual's ability to read, write, and speak in English and compute and solve problems at levels of proficiency necessary to function on the job and in society

New Americans. Persons in the community whose primary language is not English

Outreach workers. Persons found in neighborhood health centers, community centers, or public health departments, who hold formal positions as case workers or volunteer as interpreters in the community

Progressive vaccinia. Also known as vaccinia necrosum, a severe, potentially fatal illness characterized by the rapid and progressive necrosis in the area of the smallpox vaccination

Vaccinia Immune Globulin (VIG). A treatment for people who have serious reactions to smallpox vaccine

Vulnerable. A population or aggregate susceptible to injury, illness, or premature death

Yersinia pestis. The bacteria that causes plague

INTRODUCTION

As nurses we have multiple responsibilities in times of disaster preparation and in disaster response. This chapter focuses on the unique issues nurses must keep in mind when caring for **vulnerable** populations. A vulnerable population is described as "a population or aggregate susceptible to injury, illness, or premature death" (Smith & Maurer, 2000, p. 342). Some individuals have personal or social conditions that make them unusually susceptible, resulting in a decreased ability to deal with traumatic situations. This vulnerability causes them to be more dependent on assistance from others. Some of the vulnerable populations this chapter considers include perinatal, neonatal, older persons, disabled, learning impaired, communication impaired, and immunocompromised.

PERINATAL AND NEONATAL POPULATIONS

Special attention must be paid to women who are pregnant during a mass casualty event. These women pose distinct challenges for those planning for management of casualties. Gas-filled structures sustain the primary category of blast injuries from the overpressurization wave that is produced by high-order explosives, such as C-4, Semtex, nitroglycerin, and dynamite. Some of these structures include the lungs, GI tract, and middle ear, and pose a risk of rupture. Rupture of abdominal structures can result in abdominal hemorrhage, globe or eye rupture resulting in vision deficits, and concussions may be present without any obvious physical signs of head injury. The secondary category of injuries includes trauma resulting from flying debris and bomb fragments, while tertiary injuries result from individuals being thrown by the blast wind.

Whereas some injuries are obvious, some may not be easily seen. Careful nursing assessment is needed to ensure prompt emergency treatment that is necessary for the safety of the woman and baby. The gravid uterus must be assessed to rule out uterine rupture or abruptio placenta. Obstetricians and perinatal nurses are uniquely qualified to perform these assessments because of their understanding of the effects of altered maternal physiology and anatomy during pregnancy. Open peritoneal lavage to assess for intraperitoneal hemorrhage has been used safely during pregnancy (American Academy of Pediatrics [AAP], & American College of Obstetrics and Gynecology [ACOG], 2002).

Postdisaster Perinatal Assessment

During the initial assessment, supine hypotensive syndrome can be prevented by using a wedge or positioning the patient in the lateral decubitus position to deflect the uterus off the inferior vena cava. When pregnancy approaches viability, continuous fetal monitoring is recommended for 2 to 6 hours following the trauma (AAP & ACOG, 2002). Pregnancy does not exclude the use of traditional diagnostic, pharmacologic, or resuscitative procedures. When a laparotomy is necessary, it is not always an indication to perform a cesarean delivery. Maintenance of adequate oxygenation and perfusion may enable the fetus to tolerate surgery and anesthesia, and pregnancy to continue. The uterus should be carefully inspected for damage during the laparotomy. Rh-negative pregnant women should be given 300 mcg. of anti-D immune globulin within 72 hours to protect against Rh-isoimmunization. To evaluate for the need for additional anti-D immune globulin, perform the Kleihauer-Betke test or other quantitative assay of fetal-maternal hemorrhage to detect a fetomaternal hemorrhage of 30 ml or more (AAP & ACOG, 2002). After the woman is stabilized, perform a secondary survey to thoroughly evaluate the pregnancy. This may include ultrasonography to evaluate the placenta, fetus, amniotic fluid volume, and presence of intra-abdominal fluid (AAP & ACOG, 2002). Rupture of the uterus in women who have not had a previous cesarean birth is rare and more likely to occur with women who sustain blunt abdominal trauma. The presence of symptoms depends on the degree of rupture and may be confused with other conditions. The symptoms of uterine rupture include:

- Nonreassuring fetal heart rate (FHR) pattern
  - Impairment of fetal oxygenation
  - Late decelerations, reduced variability, tachycardia, bradycardia
- Sudden, abrupt decrease in FHR
- Uterine abdominal pain—may not be severe
  - May describe a *giving* way
- Loss of presenting part
- Increased vaginal bleeding
- Chest pain between scapulae or on inspiration
  - Due to irritation of blood below the diaphragm
- Hypovolemic shock from hemorrhage

(Cunningham, et al., 2001)

Abruptio placenta is the premature separation of a normally implanted placenta from the uterine wall. It is a complication in 40% to 50% of women who experience severe trauma (ACOG, 1998). Abruptio placenta typically presents shortly after the injury. Symptoms of abruptio placenta include:

- Dark, vaginal bleeding (may be bright or absent in concealed abruptio)
- Severe abdominal pain
- Firm, tender uterus
- Shock, more than apparent blood loss
- Contractions
- Frequent, low amplitude

Abruptio placenta is considered an obstetric emergency and should be managed as an inpatient so that delivery can be immediate if the separation is moderate (grade 2) or severe (grade 3). Perimortem cesarean birth after 5 minutes of unsuccessful maternal cardiac resuscitation can result in the survival of the fetus. Neonatal survival is unlikely when a postmortem cesarean delivery occurs more than 10-15 minutes after maternal death. Neonates surviving have an increased risk of adverse neurodevelopmental deficits (AAP & ACOG, 2002).

During pregnancy, the woman's susceptibility to infections is altered. Normally there are hormonal, cellular, and humoral changes that work together to suppress the immune response to the fetus, which is a foreign body. Typically, a humoral response, or antibody-mediated response, occurs when there are antibodies in the body fluids or humors. In addition, the high circulating levels of steroids inhibit the normal humoral response. Progesterone, the hormone that relaxes smooth muscle, also relaxes the respiratory tract, which can lead to stasis of secretions and provide an environment conducive to an increased level of local bacterial growth (White, Hen-

retig, & Dukes, 2002). Although the circulating white cell count is slightly increased, neutrophil chemotaxis and adherence, cell-mediated immunity (lymphocytes attack what is foreign or invading), and natural killer cell activity decrease. Together this lowering of defense mechanisms results in the woman being more susceptible to circulating pathogens. These normal mechanisms of pregnancy, coupled with a concern for fetal safety, pose unique challenges.

Another issue to be considered when caring for pregnant women during and following mass casualty events is vaccination. The terrorist event could include the use of biologic agents such as smallpox and anthrax. It is not generally recommended to immunize women during pregnancy. The debate occurs over whether to immunize pregnant women if a release of a biological agent is confirmed or suspected. Contracting any of these diseases results in significant morbidity and mortality to the pregnant woman, as well as unknown risks to the fetus.

Consider the possible effect of smallpox on a pregnant woman. The CDC, in collaboration with the Department of Defense and the Food and Drug Administration (FDA), is monitoring the outcomes of pregnancy in women exposed to smallpox vaccines. The data are summarized in the National Smallpox Vaccine in Pregnancy Registry (CDC, 2003a). Normally, when the virus enters the respiratory tract, it multiplies and spreads to regional lymph nodes. A 12-day incubation period begins with the prodromal phase, followed by the characteristic skin eruptions. Variola can cross the placenta and infect the fetus. Previous research has documented that during pregnancy, there is an increased susceptibility to the variola infection with greater severity of illness due to the previously discussed changes in the maternal immune system. Maternal mortality approaches 50%, compared with 30% for men and nonpregnant women (White et al., 2002). If infection occurs during the first trimester, it results in a high rate of fetal loss. During the latter half of pregnancy, infection is associated with an increased rate of prematurity.

Because the smallpox vaccine is a live virus, vaccination is not recommended unless the woman is in a high-risk area. There is a theoretical risk of teratogenicity with the smallpox vaccine.

CDC and ACIP recommend that all pre-event smallpox vaccination programs include pregnancy screening and education components with these elements: questioning about the possibility of pregnancy before vaccination and excluding those at risk, asking about the date of the last menstrual period, providing education about fetal vaccinia, counseling women to avoid becoming pregnant during the month after vaccination, recommending abstinence or highly effective contraception, and advising women who believe they might be pregnant to perform a first morning urine pregnancy test on the vaccination day. (CDC, 2003a)

In addition, if infected, pregnant women are more susceptible to **hemorrhagic smallpox,** or purpura variolosa. Symptoms include fever; backache; diffuse, copper-red rash; and a rapid decline in the health status of mother and baby. Research suggests that within 24 hours of the onset of symptoms, the woman will develop spontaneous ecchymoses, epistaxis, bleeding gums, an intense erythematous rash, and subconjunctival hemorrhages. Laboratory analysis during this period may demonstrate thrombocytopenia, increased capillary fragility, and depletion of coagulation factors and fibrinogen (White et al., 2002). Death would generally result from sepsis.

A rare, serious infection of the fetus, **fetal vaccinia,** can occur following vaccination for smallpox. Congenital variola ranges from 9% to 60% during epidemics of the disease. It is characterized by giant dermal pox and diffuse necrotic lesions of viscera and placenta. Fetal vaccinia typically results in stillbirth or death of the infant soon after delivery. In some cases, maternal immunity may protect the fetus. Smallpox vaccine is not known to cause congenital malformations (CDC, 2003a).

Vaccinia immune globulin (VIG) is a treatment for people who have serious reactions to smallpox vaccine. It is made from the blood of people who have gotten the smallpox vaccine more than once and contains antibodies that offer protection from vaccinia infection.

If the pregnant woman is accidentally exposed to smallpox, the prophylactic use of VIG is not indicated during pregnancy, due to the risk of fetal vaccinia. The few reported cases of fetal vaccinia infection usually occurred after an accidental primary vaccination of the mother in early pregnancy, or the woman becoming pregnant within 28 days of vaccination, although smallpox vaccine is not known to cause congenital malformations. Exposed pregnant women are encouraged to contact their health care providers or their state health department for assistance in enrolling in the registry (see above). Health care providers in private practice or from state health departments are encouraged to report all exposed pregnant women to the registry (CDC, 2003a, 2003b). When a woman with complications from smallpox vaccine could be treated with VIG, administration of VIG for her is acceptable while she is pregnant (CDC, 2003d).

Considering other biologic agents, there is little research available about pregnancy complicated by an anthrax infection. However, if there is documented risk, the potential for significant morbidity and mortality offsets the risk of disease. Current recommendations from ACOG and the CDC about exposure to anthrax include

- referral of pregnant women exposed to anthrax or other biologic agents to their primary obstetric or infectious disease health care provider. The Committee on Obstetric Practice recommends limiting the prophylactic treatment of pregnant and lactating women to those with known exposure to a high-risk source of contamination.
- Cipro or ciprofloxacin is the first-line drug for the initial prophylaxis of pregnant women exposed to anthrax. Although there are few clinical trials evaluating the effect of Cipro on pregnancy and lactation, it is thought that this drug is unlikely to be associated with fetal malformations. The recommended adult prophylaxis is 500mg. p.o. every 12 hours for 60 days.
- If the specific strain of anthrax is susceptible to penicillin, the initial prophylaxis therapy should be amoxicillin. This drug is generally safe during pregnancy, but not recommended to treat diagnosed anthrax.
- Caution should be used when prescribing doxycycline during pregnancy due to its effects on the fetus, the staining of primary teeth, defective dental enamel and depressed bone growth.

  (AWHONN, 2002; Center for Drug Evaluation and Research, 2001; CDC, 2003a; Hale & Zinberg, 2001; Henretig, Cieslak, & Eitzen, 2002; Morbidity and Mortality Weekly Report, 2001)

With inhalation anthrax, the early administration of antibiotics, generally ciprofloxacin, is a primary determinant of maternal-fetal outcome. Breastfeeding women should be offered prophylaxis with the same medications. All of these medications are excreted in breastmilk. The babies should be treated with an antibiotic that is safe for the prophylactic treatment of the infant.

During pregnancy, infection with **Yersinia pestis,** the bacteria causing plague, typically results in abortion or miscarriage. However, more favorable outcomes have been seen since the postantibiotic era, primarily in the treatment of bubonic plague. The recommended treatment of plague is the administration of streptomycin for 5 days, but gentamicin is the recommended treatment for breastfeeding women (CDC, 2002). Other infections resulting in fetal loss include Ebola and Lassa fever.

The Association of Women's Health, Obstetric, and Neonatal Nurses (AWHONN) (2002) has made the following recommendations to prepare pregnant women for bioterrorism or other terrorist events.

1. Keep a copy of the prenatal records on hand in case care is needed at another health care agency.
2. Prepare a list of emergency phone numbers, such as physician, midwife, family, and friends.
3. Have an additional supply of prescription medications.
4. Prepare an emergency birth kit.
5. Keep a supply of ready-to-feed infant formula. Avoid powders and concentrates because the water supply may become contaminated.
6. Prepare a disaster supply kit containing items recommended by the American Academy of Pediatrics or the American Red Cross.

OLDER PERSONS

Life expectancies have risen and older adults are not immune to terrorist attacks. When older persons become victims of disasters, they may lack the physical stamina to recover quickly. Although many older adults remain active and interested in life events and adapt well to changes brought on by chronic conditions, others may experience some type of debilitation or degree of infirmity. Nurses need to be alert and assess the level of each individual's adaptation and level of functioning and independence. The nurse will also evaluate the client's family, caregivers, socioeconomic influences, and community to assess actual or potential health care needs and resources.

One goal of many older adults is to maintain as much independence as possible for as long as possible. To achieve this goal, teaching about disaster preparedness may be needed as well as frank discussions about the feasibility of the older person being able to shelter in place during or following a disaster, or the necessity of evacuating the home and seeking shelter elsewhere in the community.

A primary factor to be considered is the level of the person's independent functioning. If the person requires no assistance in bathing, dressing, ambulation, shopping for groceries, or cooking, then no special arrangements except education may be necessary when preparing for a disaster. However, if the client requires services such as assistance with activities of daily living, administering multiple medications, in-home personal care, transportation, assistance in restructuring the home environment to facilitate mobility and wheelchair accessibility, physical therapy, or speech therapy, then special planning will be necessary. Frail, aged clients who require multiple home care services may find the process of finding these services complex and overwhelming. This process is compounded in times of disaster.

Nurses often educate clients and their families about current disease processes, management of symptoms, mobility, medications, diet, bowel and bladder function, and normal health promotion activities. In teaching disaster preparedness, the instruction is expanded to include specific preparation for evacuation should a disaster occur. It is very important for the older person to keep an accurate list of current medications, doses, and times of administration in an easily accessible and secure place. In addition, the names and phone numbers of significant persons, relatives, those with power of attorney, health care providers, or any others to be notified in case of emergency should be kept in a place that could be accessed quickly and easily. Other important documents including eyeglass prescriptions, the style and serial numbers of medical devices such as pacemakers, health care policies and numbers, identification, list of allergies, blood type, checkbook, credit cards, insurance agent's name and number, and driver's license should be kept in a routine place so that they can be grabbed quickly in case of evacuation. Additional items that should not be left behind during evacuation include a 72-hour supply of medications, dentures, eyeglasses, special dietary needs, sturdy shoes and warm clothing for cold or inclement weather, blankets, incontinence briefs, prostheses, hearing aids, hearing aid batteries, extra wheelchair batteries, oxygen, and other assistive devices (American Red Cross, 2001).

Older persons who live in assisted living or skilled care facilities pose a challenge during the evacuation of a building. Advance planning for these facilities must include alternative methods for evacuating residents, or plans to protect them within the facility itself. In some parts of the world, a core of reinforced rooms has been developed within existing facilities (Figure 9–1). These rooms have a dual purpose; some are used for recreation or exercise therapy during normal daily activities and are used as protected environments in times of danger. If this type of protected room is not possible, plans must include adequate personnel to assist in moving residents to another location.

If the older person requires a great deal of assistance during the evacuation, it is important to speak clearly, not shouting, to the person's face so that he or she may read your lips if hearing impaired. Remain calm and reassuring, yet firm in your directions. It is often important to move quickly and confidently, but not with such speed that it causes panic and further disorientation.

Persons in need of help or transportation during an evacuation are encouraged to register with their local government. The local emergency management office will provide information and suggestions about what to do during an evacuation. Evacuation of older persons from homes may also involve the evacuation of young children. It is estimated that 3.4 million children live in a grandparents' household, and many children visit their grandparents often (Federal Emergency Management Agency & American Red Cross, 2001).

An essential element of the community assessment portion of the disaster planning process is the identification of sites such as nursing homes and senior citizen complexes to develop an understanding of the status and needs of the residents. The polypharmacy of the aged may pose a significant challenge during and after a terrorist attack. Since skilled or assisted care facilities must be self-sufficient for at least 72 hours following a disaster event, medications for that time period must be readily available and portable to accompany residents should evacuation or relocation become necessary. Placing medications in a portable, secure carrier, or developing mini-backpacks complete with medical and medication history to be placed on the chairs of older residents, can accomplish the portability and accessibility of essential documents and medication. However, either method requires that a professional nurse check the medications at regular intervals to ensure that the most current medications are available.

The aged are at increased risk from many forms of terrorist attacks. Preexisting medical conditions common among older persons place them at risk in several ways. Potential drug–drug interactions and adverse effects from

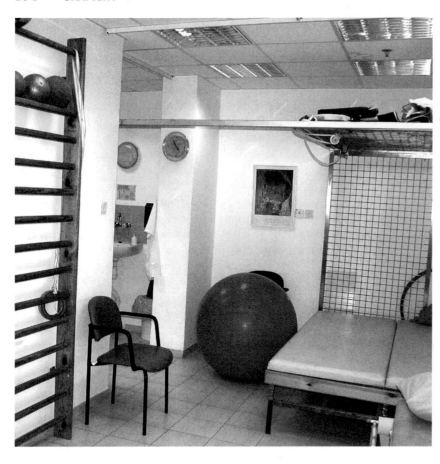

Figure 9–1. Physical therapy room in nursing home that doubles as a bomb shelter. *Photo courtesy of J. Langan.*

antibiotics used in treatment or prophylaxis would be increased in this group. Health care providers should become familiar with the more common conditions among the aged and be prepared to meet their needs. If respiratory deficits are present due to emphysema or cardiac disease, aerosolized biological or chemical agents can further damage already compromised tissue and result in severe respiratory distress. The skin of the aged is more fragile and friable than that of younger persons. This makes older persons more vulnerable to agents absorbed through the skin. Vesicants and corrosives may produce greater damage to the older person because of compromised skin integrity. Agents that produce vomiting or diarrhea place the older person at an increased risk due to the potential for fluid and electrolyte imbalance and rapid dehydration. A too-rapid infusion of intravenous fluids coupled with the biologic or chemical agent can compound the effect of either, resulting in severe complications from preexisting cardiac, respiratory, and renal disease. If preexisting dementia or confusion is present, additional vulnerabilities may surface. The older person may have diminished motor skills, making it difficult to escape from the release site of a chemical, biological, or other terrorist event. They may also lack the cognitive ability to figure out how to escape from the danger or to follow directions from those in authority.

Education must be provided for the caregivers so that they can effectively manage these potential victims. Some of the education should include:

1. Information about the more common conditions of the older person and signs and symptoms of developing complications, such as hypoglycemia or hyperglycemia, respiratory distress, or stroke.
2. Awareness that a lack of understanding or confusion about what is occurring, or the personal protective equipment of the health care providers themselves, may be frightening, causing the older person to struggle against needed treatments, safety equipment, or evacuation.
3. Information about the importance of remaining calm and using appropriate mental health techniques as needed.
4. Knowledge about the different effects of chemical and biological agents on the aged whose body systems are compromised. This group may become ill with smaller doses of the agents.

Red Cross shelters may be opened if a disaster is widespread, large numbers of persons are affected, and the emergency cannot be resolved quickly. Persons should be informed that they may be asked to go to a shelter if the

---

BOX 9–1   **Disabilities and Impairments in the U.S.**

- Over 68 million Americans have activity limitations
- Over 19 million Americans have visual impairments
- Over 34 million Americans are hearing impaired
- Almost 2.7 million Americans have speech impairments (1996)
- 7.4 million Americans use assistive technology devices (ATDs) to accommodate mobility impairments (1994)

- 4.6 million Americans use ATDs to accommodate orthopedic impairments (1994)
- 4.5 million Americans use ATDs to accommodate hearing impairments (1994)
- 500,000 Americans use ATDs to accommodate vision impairments (1994)

Sources: Vital and Health Statistics Series 10, No. 200, and 205 and Advance Data 292
Source: Vital and Health Statistics Series 10, No. 205 (1997)

---

area is without electricity, a chemical emergency is in the area, flood water is rising, or their homes have been severely damaged (American Red Cross, 2001).

However, if there should be a chemical emergency, persons may be advised to shelter in place. The American Red Cross and other emergency management services will instruct persons on the proper procedure to shelter in place; in this case persons are advised to stay indoors as the air outside is unsafe to breathe.

An important consideration when caring for older persons during and following a disaster is to meet their mental health needs by helping them to cope with fear and anxiety. Their immediate reactions will be related to their cognitive and physical level of functioning, as well as past experiences. They may experience psychological injuries, such as post-traumatic stress disorder. They may also have witnessed injuries and deaths in the past that have produced short- and long-term psychological trauma.

The vulnerability of the older person to disasters is summed up by Fernandez, Byard, Lin, Benson and Barbera (2002) as they report their research findings.

. . . their impaired physical mobility, diminished sensory awareness, chronic health conditions, and social and economic limitations that prevent adequate preparation for disasters, and hinder their adaptability during disasters. Frail elderly, those with serious physical, cognitive, economic, and psychosocial problems, are at especially high risk. (p. 67)

PERSONS WITH MOBILITY AND SENSORY DEFICITS

Before discussing the needs of this population, it is necessary to review the definitions of disability, impairment, and handicap. The International Classification of Impairments, Disabilities, and Handicaps (ICIDH) defines a **disability** as a condition that involves any restriction on, or lack of, ability to perform an activity in the usual manner or within the normal range. An **impairment** is an anatomical, mental, or psychological loss or other abnormality. A disadvantage re-

sulting from impairment or disability is a handicap (Pope and Tarlov, 1991). The World Health Organization defines impairment as the "loss of psychological, physiological, or anatomical, structure or function. Disability is a limitation in functional ability resulting from impairment" (Larson, 1998, pp. 529–530). Batavia (1993) suggests another way to consider the relationship among these terms: An impairment affects a human organ on a micro level; disability affects a person on an individual level; and a handicap involves society or an effect on a macro level.

The U.S. Department of Health and Human Services (HHS) has estimated that 13% of the U.S. population in 1998 experienced some form of activity limitation due to a chronic condition (2000).

See Box 9–1 for the number and incidence of three impairments: hearing, visual and speech, as well as numbers indicating use of assistive technology devices.

Those who are disabled require special assistance in meeting their needs. Those with physical disabilities require advance planning in order to provide necessary support during and after a disaster. If the individual is dependent on a wheelchair for mobility or has vision or hearing deficits, arrangements must be made in advance to provide adequate numbers of volunteers or staff to assist when this group must be relocated or regrouped in a safe room. Advance planning provides an opportunity to solicit input from these individuals about what services are needed. It also permits time for the creation of appropriate communication aids, such as printed cards or pictures that will facilitate rapid movement when necessary. The communication or mobility explanations also promote a collaborative effort that will maintain choice and human dignity during emergency situations. If elevators are disabled, and stairs are the only egress from the building, adequate personnel will be required to move wheelchair-bound individuals to safety. Building managers, program coordinators, and first responders should be aware of the location, number of residents, and challenges facing each person in this group so that their needs can be met and their health protected during a mass casualty event.

The hearing impaired may need to be able to look at the face of the person teaching about disaster preparedness to read lips and to use the facial expression cues. Typically, written directions will be very helpful, as will visual aids. However, it is appropriate with this group of individuals to assess literacy as well, not assuming that all members of a given group are literate.

Those who cannot speak may rely on sign language or the use of electronic phones or similar devices to obtain emergency aid. It is important to assess how individuals learn best. Some learn best visually, others are auditory learners, and still others rely on tactile information and practice the material to retain what is being taught.

Additionally, it has been recommended that emergency personnel or rescue teams learn a few basic phrases in American Sign Language. Deaf persons respond best when the rescuer's symbol of authority is clearly visible and the worker appears confident. Rescuers and those assisting in the care of deaf persons should carry notepads and pencils to use to enhance communication (University of Florida, 1998).

Those who are visually impaired will be able to hear the educator's spoken instruction but may require large print materials or recordings of disaster preparation guidelines and directives. They may appreciate cues received by the tactile sense in reviewing the items in a disaster preparedness display.

PERSONS WHO ARE COGNITIVE OR LANGUAGE-PROCESSING DELAYED

When planning for those who are cognitively or language-processing delayed, all involved in routine care and education should be consulted about the best ways to communicate with each person. The lower the level of developmental maturity, the greater the chance that the individual will focus on the present situation, rather than bringing past experiences to the current situation. During a mock disaster exercise or actual event, care must be taken to avoid the appearance of panic or frustration as these may cause fear or be interpreted as anger. Working with the daily caregivers provides an opportunity to develop plans that can be shared with those responsible for evacuation or protection. In addition, advance planning permits those close to individuals with cognitive or language-processing challenges to become involved in teaching what would happen during an event, to minimize panic. If it is not possible to reach all of the caregivers in a disaster education program, then caregivers must at least be familiar with the plans in the event of a real-time disaster. It is also important to remember that those who are mentally impaired will need training and constant reinforcement to learn steps to save themselves (University of Florida, 1998).

Meeting the needs of older persons and the disabled populations can be met through education and modest in-

vestments. It is suggested that the following questions be asked to assess readiness for disasters.

- Can the hearing and visually impaired interpret alarms?
- Are there provisions for TV crawl notices for the hearing impaired, strobe lights for the deaf, and elevator accommodations for the disabled during an evacuation?
- Will elevators be sent to the first floor automatically in a fire?
- Are special size letters being used for training and announcements to accommodate the visually impaired?
- Are emergency classes being conducted for the hearing impaired with an interpreter present?
- Does emergency training exist for the mentally impaired at rehabilitation or vocational schools?
- Is the number of special vehicle conveyances in your area adequate for a large-scale emergency?
- Are there special provisions for search and rescue of the elderly and disabled?

(University of Florida, 1998, pp. 1–2)

NON-ENGLISH SPEAKING POPULATION

Over 175 languages are used in the United States. It has been estimated that over 8 million U.S. residents live with no one 14 years or older who speaks fluent English. In other words, 38% of 7 million households are headed by immigrants or refugees (SIL International, 2003). Table 9–1 lists a sampling of languages and the approximate number of persons who speak the language.

We all must be aware of persons in the community whose primary language is not English. For these persons, sometimes called "**New Americans,**"communication is a challenge even when dealing with every day activities such as grocery shopping or getting information about bus routes. One can only imagine how frightening it would be to attempt to access emergency personnel if one did not know the English language. Persons who speak English as a Sec-

TABLE 9–1. SAMPLE OF LANGUAGES SPOKEN IN THE U.S.

LANGUAGE	LANGUAGE SPEAKERS IN U.S.
English/Hawaiian/Spanish	274,000,000
English	210,000,000
Spanish	22,400,000
French	1,000,000
German	90,000
Hawaiian	1,000
Hopi	5,264
Navajo	148,530
Sea Island Creole English	125,000
Zuni	6,413
American Sign Language	100,000-500,000 out of nearly 2,000,000 profoundly deaf

SIL International (2003)

ond Language (ESL) are often highly intelligent but have not yet grasped the complexities of the English language. Additionally, some have not had the opportunity to learn to read or write in their native languages. We cannot assume that all non-English speakers will be able to read and follow directions even if translated to their own, primary language.

A public health nurse tells the story about a group of nurses who discovered that a number of Afghan women who immigrated to the Midwest did not know how to read or understand numbers. The public health nurses obtained the assistance of a nurse who spoke Farsi. They tried to explain to the Afghan women how to dial 911 on the telephone for emergencies. The Afghan women told the Farsi interpreter that they had not learned about numbers in their primary language and, therefore, could not understand what was being taught. It was also revealed through home visiting that many new Americans who have immigrated to the United States do not listen to the local radio stations or watch the local news stations on television. Broadcast warnings, even in a number of different languages, would not benefit those who watch movies from their native countries instead of the local news stations. Some people are used to hearing air-raid sirens in their native country, especially if they have been exposed to war conditions. However, they are not used to hearing, nor do they understand, weather advisory sirens (personal communication, I. Kalnins, May 7, 2003).

Therefore, the following key suggestions or strategies may help to prepare English as a second language speakers for disasters.

1. Assess the literacy of New Americans in their primary language and in English. In its 1991 National Literacy Act, Congress defined **literacy** as "an individual's ability to read, write and speak in English, and compute and solve problems at levels of proficiency necessary to function on the job and in society, to achieve ones goals, and develop ones knowledge and potential" (National Institute for Literacy [NIFL], n.d., p. 1). In 1988, Congress directed the Department of Education to carry out an assessment of the literacy skills of American adults. The National Adult Literacy Survey (NALS) was conducted. The NALS is a monumental study that remains the most comprehensive, statistically reliable source of data on literacy in the United States. Literacy is scored along a continuum of 1 to 5. The lowest level of literacy is level I. At this level, an individual can usually sign one's name, identify a country in a short article, locate one piece of information in a sports article, locate the expiration date on a driver's license, and total a bank deposit entry (NIFL, n.d.). The nurse may use these skills as a means of assessing clients' literacy both in their primary language and in English.

2. Obtain the assistance of an interpreter, preferably a community outreach worker, with whom the learners are familiar. The outreach workers or caseworkers often have a telephone tree or call list to assist in getting information to the community. Word of mouth can help the spread of important information, especially if there is no phone in the home. Community **outreach workers** can be found in neighborhood health centers, community centers or in public health departments. They may hold formal positions as caseworkers or simply volunteer as interpreters throughout the community. The local community church may be able to recommend someone who knows many of the neighborhood residents and is acknowledged as an advocate for the residents.

3. Obtain the information and guidelines in the learners' primary language. Prepare communication aids for use during an emergency. These may include key phrase translations (Table 9–2).

4. Practice the steps given in the emergency literature. For example, bring a toy telephone to the instructional meeting and have participants practice dialing 911 and giving specific information to the dispatcher so that the appropriate rescue personnel and equipment will be deployed.

5. The use of visual aids can be most helpful. Bring the actual items that are suggested as emergency items. For example, have a display set up on a table with gallon jugs of water, a flashlight, batteries, blankets, emergency telephone numbers, medicines, lists of medicines, eyeglass prescriptions, physician telephone numbers, etc.

6. Do not use children as interpreters if adults are available. At times, the stress of the added responsibilities of interpretation can be overwhelming to the children and this practice places unnecessary burden on these young persons.

TABLE 9–2. KEY PHRASES DURING AN EMERGENCY

PHRASE	SPANISH	FRENCH	GERMAN	PORTUGUESE
Are you hurt?	¿Es lastimado usted?	Vous êtes endommagé?	Sind Sie hurt?	São você hurt?
Call 911 for help	Llame 911 para la ayuda	Appeler 911 pour aider	Rufen 911 um Hilfe	Chamada 911 para a ajuda
You must leave this building	Usted debe salir esta construcción	Vous devez ceci partir construire	Sie müssen dieses Gebäude lassen	Você deve deixar este edifício

Developed by D. James

PERSONS WHO ARE IMMUNOCOMPROMISED

Cancer prevalence is the number of people who have been diagnosed with cancer and are alive today. Considering the incidence of cancer in the United Sates, it is likely that many of the patients in your community will have a compromised immune system. According to the National Cancer Institute, there are 9.6 million cancer survivors. This represents approximately 3% of the population. The statistics are as follows:

- 61% of survivors are currently over the age of 65.
- Breast, prostate and colon/rectum are the three most prevalent cancer sites.
- Approximately 14% (N = 1,368,674) of the 9.6 million estimated cancer survivors were diagnosed over 20 years ago.
- The current average age of male and female cancer survivors is 69 and 64, respectively.

(National Cancer Institute, 2003).

A compromised immune system may be due to treatments such as chemotherapy, those who have had organ or bone marrow transplants and are on immunosuppressive drugs, or from an underlying disease process such as HIV. If a bioterrorist attack should occur within this population, the rate of complications and death would be greater than in the general population. The antibiotics recommended for treatment in the general population are also recommended for those who are immunocompromised.

A potential complication following smallpox vaccination is generalized vaccinia. In the past, it was estimated to occur in 242 million primary persons who are vaccinated. It is believed to result from a vaccinia viremia with skin manifestations. In the noncompromised population, **generalized vaccinia** consists of vesicles or pustules appearing on normal skin distant from the vaccination site. The rash is generally self-limited and usually requires only supportive therapy. However, patients with underlying immunosuppressed illnesses may have a toxic course and require vaccinia immune globulin (VIG), available only from the CDC (CDC, 2003c; Cono, Casey & Bell, 2003).

Another, more serious complication of smallpox vaccination is progressive vaccinia. **Progressive vaccinia,** also known as vaccinia necrosum, is a severe, potentially fatal illness characterized by the rapid and progressive necrosis in the area of vaccination, often with lesions at places other than the vaccination site. It is painless and without apparent healing after 15 days. The virus continues to spread locally through viremia, or spread of lesions, through the lesion to skin, viscera, and bone. Initially, there is little inflammation at the site and little if any pain. Bacteria may result in a superinfection. In the past, it was estimated that progressive vaccinia occurred in approximately one to two per million primary vaccinations, and was almost always fatal before the introduction of VIG and antiviral agents. Rare in the past, it may be a greater threat today, given the larger proportion of susceptible persons in the population and the greater number with immunocompromise. Nearly all instances of progressive vaccinia occur in people with defined cell-mediated immune defect or T-cell deficiency (Cono, Casey & Bell, 2003).

Treatment involves prompt hospitalization and aggressive use of VIG. Massive doses of VIG are necessary to control the viremia, up to 10ml. per kilogram of intramuscular VIG has been used. There is no proven antiviral therapy effective in the treatment of progressive vaccinia. Preliminary studies with cidofovir show some antiviral effect in vitro, although the results of studies in animals are pending. An immediate consultation with the CDC is recommended to determine if any experimental antiviral drugs are available.

The development of progressive vaccinia should be an index of suspicion for possible immunocompromised or immunodeficient conditions. Fear of not receiving what is perceived as a lifesaving treatment, the vaccine may cause some persons to omit significant parts of their medical history. Health care providers should ask questions about needle sticks, sexual history, IV drug use, and transfusions to determine whether HIV infection is possible. To assess for a cancer-related immunocompromised condition, ask questions about recurrent infections, constitutional symptoms, easy bruising, headache, or nonspecific coughs. Because progressive vaccinia occurs almost exclusively among persons with cellular immunodeficiency, this assessment is critical. It can also occur in persons with humoral immunodeficiency or those revaccinated after they have become immune suppressed.

The best prognosis is with those whose immune suppression results from systemic steroids, and is, therefore, reversible. Once the diagnosis is made, the recommended treatment is aggressive therapy with VIG. There are newer antiviral drugs in development but these have not been tested in humans. The second-line treatment agent is cidofovir. Surgical debridement has met with variable success. It is important to differentiate progressive vaccinia from a *severe take,* which resolves in 1 to 2 weeks without therapy. The prophylactic use of VIG or cidofovir is not indicated, but administering it should not be delayed should inadvertent vaccination of individuals with contraindications occur.

Nurses working with patients who are immunocompromised should have additional precautions defined for these patients in case of disaster or emergency. For example, do the patients know of an alternative site to visit for chemotherapy if their usual office is inaccessible? Do they know not to eat raw seafood or drink water that is possibly contaminated?

Among the many issues to be discussed pertaining to cancer patients and their preparation for disaster events is infection control. It is important that health care providers know exactly where these patients are in their treatment program and also in their disease process at any

Patient Information

Name_____

Address_____

_____

Home Phone_____ Cell phone _____

Emergency Contact _____

Relationship_____ Phone _____

Medical History

Problem	Treatment	Date

Surgeries	Date

Doctors:

Name_____
Phone_____ Fax #_____
Address_____
_____
_____

Name_____
Phone_____ Fax #_____
Address_____
_____
_____

Figure 9–2. Patient information record. *Reprinted with permission: Saint Louis University Cancer Center Patient Record T. Dunleavy, RN, BSN, OCN*

point in time. Patients are given treatment calendars to carry with them at all times (personal communication, T. Dunleavy, May 15, 2003). The advantages of carrying the treatment calendars with them at all times is that the patients have information available concerning their treatment protocols and medicines and any health care provider can review these treatments and medicines at a glance to save valuable time, should an emergency arise. See Figures 9–2 through 9–4.

There is also a need for a mechanism for bone marrow transplant patients in need of red blood cell and platelet transfusions, including irradiated platelets. This mechanism may be set up through the American Red Cross or

through the individual's treatment center. Patients are counseled to have an alternative site for treatment in mind if they are unable to travel to their cancer center. They are instructed to go to the nearest emergency room if they are in trouble and to take their treatment information with them so that they can give the health professionals a starting place in which to assess and treat them.

Many immunocompromised patients must travel long distances to get to their cancer center. The bone marrow transplant patients have specific, and often complicated instructions. They are given specific criteria for seeking medical assistance as well as specific orders before they are discharged to their homes in the community.

Name _____

Diagnosis _____

Stage _____T_____N_____M_____

Allergies _____

Treatment

Surgery	Date	Date
_____		
_____		

Chemotherapy	Date	Date	Date	Date	Date	Date
Course	1	2	3	4	5	6
_____						
_____						
_____						
_____						
_____						
_____						
_____						
_____						

Radiation	Date	Start	Finish

Figure 9–3. Treatment record. *Reprinted with permission: Saint Louis University Cancer Center Patient Record T. Dunleavy, RN, BSN, OCN*

Distance becomes a dangerous issue, especially if the patient is neutropenic and has a fever. They should be seen in a medical facility within 1 to 2 hours of spiking a fever. The health care team would prefer that these patients receive medical care within 1 hour of spiking the fever and certainly would not want them to wait any longer than 2 hours to reach a health care facility, as this is a life and death situation. Patients are taught to recognize symptoms and what to expect. If patients were to experience a disaster in their area, they are advised to go to the nearest emergency room that they can safely reach (personal communication, T. Dunleavy, May 19, 2003).

Immunocompromised patients need to be taught to consider a number of alternative routes to emergency care, as their usual routes may not be accessible. For example, if a tornado has gone through an area, one would expect fallen trees and downed power lines. Major streets and thoroughfares may be impassable due to flooding. Accidents may tie up traffic for extended periods of time. Large volumes of traffic will clog major arteries and will be at a standstill if large-scale evacuations take place. If patients are doing central line dressing changes they need to have supplies readily available to accomplish that task. In the event of flash flooding, they would need

Sunday	Monday	Tuesday	Wednesday	Thursday	Friday	Saturday

Treatment of nausea and vomiting: _____

Treatment of
diarrhea: _____

Treatment of constipation: _____

If symptoms persist more than 24 hours please call _____ , Monday thru
Friday until 5pm. Nights, weekends and holidays please call 314-577-8000 and ask for
the Oncologist on call

Pharmacy _____

Lab work to be drawn at: _____

Figure 9–4. Symptom Log. *Reprinted with permission: Saint Louis University Cancer Center Patient Record T. Dunleavy, RN, BSN, OCN*

to carry their supplies with them. The supplies need to be double bagged to keep them dry, especially if they must wade through waist-deep water and transfer into rescue boats.

As we have already mentioned, infection control is a major issue for immunocompromised patients. Considering this, teach patients to have bottled water ready and not to risk drinking water of questionable purity. Bone marrow transplant patients are instructed *not* to eat fresh fruits and vegetables due to the risk of contamination and subsequent infection. As communities lose power due to disasters, residents need to be careful about consuming foods from their freezers and refrigerators. If there is a propane gas supply, it may be safe to cook the foods over a barbecue if the temperatures can get hot enough. This is only recommended

for foods still cold or frozen. It is safest for this population of patients to leave this type of food alone and to consume processed or canned foods if they can be heated to the proper temperatures.

Another danger associated with disasters is the cleanup efforts of those persons anxious to return to some kind of "normalcy." Many will go outdoors and try to work with heavy equipment such as chainsaws, even if they have never operated this type of equipment prior to the disaster. The aftermath of the disaster causes many persons to experience minor injuries and more serious insults such as cardiac arrest and the loss of body extremities. This is a major concern for those having bleeding problems. With low platelets, they are more susceptible to bleeding, in addition to the high risk of infection. Due to nervous system changes, patients are cautioned to avoid exposing fingers and toes to very hot or very cold temperatures. They are to wear sturdy shoes that fit well at all times. These suggestions may become huge challenges especially in times of unexpected disasters. For example, if there is a severe fire in the patient's building, evacuation becomes a priority. Without time to collect the appropriate clothing, exposure to extreme cold in the winter months and stepping through broken glass and debris could threaten the patient's well-being. Emotional issues are also important to address. Persons diagnosed with cancer and their families go through the entire gamut of emotions including anxiety and depression. A disaster situation only compounds such emotions. Cancer treatment and the possible loss of work and time in school can greatly impact a family's finances too. If the family's home is destroyed by a tornado or any kind of disaster, they would have that additional burden. Probably all of the emotions would be magnified (personal communication, T. Dunleavy, May 19, 2003). See Chapter 4 for promotion of mental health.

In summary, it is helpful to develop a patient record/treatment book for immunocompromised patients. Items to include are as follows:

- medication log
- medication list (with side effects)
- health insurance information
- cancer treatment
- allergies
- blood type
- home care instructions
- calendars that include appointments
- tips on what to do in specific situations
- list of who to contact

(personal communication, T. Dunleavy, May 19, 2003)
See Figures 9–5 and 9–6.

SUMMARY

During the planning and implementation of a disaster response plan special attention must be paid to those populations who, because of physical conditions, psychosocial conditions, environment, or cultural situations, are more at risk during manmade or natural disasters. To provide an adequate response, additional preparations must be made to meet their unique needs, to elicit their cooperation, and to protect those responding to a mass casualty event. Preparations to address the needs of vulnerable populations requires the participation of those with expertise in working with these groups. These vulnerable groups may not be in a position to advocate for themselves. Their vulnerability becomes a mandate for the professional nurse involved in disaster

response planning, a mandate challenging all involved in preparing a response for mass casualty events.

CASE STUDY

Chemotherapy Patient and Potential Flood

The home health nurse is visiting a 59-year-old married, male client who was discharged from the hospital yesterday. The purpose of the visit today is to review the care and dressing change instructions for his new central line catheter through which he will receive chemotherapy. While driving to the home, the nurse notices the couple's close proximity to the town's main river. They have a dock at the back of their home. It has been raining off and on for the past 3 days and the forecast calls for several more days of heavy rainstorms.

1. What types of questions will the nurse ask this client and his wife regarding their proximity to the water?
2. What will the nurse assess regarding their preparations for emergencies?
3. What types of items should the couple keep with them at all times, especially if swift evacuation is required?
4. What will the nurse teach about foods and water if they should lose power to their home?
5. What other types of information will the nurse be sharing to prepare them for emergencies?

TEST YOUR KNOWLEDGE

1. An effective communication technique to use with the older person is to shout as loudly as you can in an emergency because the person probably cannot hear you otherwise.
   A. True
   B. False
2. Immunocompromised patients may eat raw fruits and vegetables as long as they are rinsed for at least 1 minute under running water.
   A. True
   B. False
3. During pregnancy, the woman's susceptibility to infections is increased.
   A. True
   B. False
4. The community health nurse can safely assume that at least one person in a household of New Americans can speak English and dial 911.
   A. True
   B. False

Health Insurance Telephone Log

Health Insurance Provider _____
Insurance Numbers _____
Casemanager _____
Phone Number _____

Date/Time	Who you talked to	Authorization or Referral Numbers	Date and service covered by number	Notes

Figure 9–5. Health insurance telephone log. *Reprinted with permission: Saint Louis University Cancer Center Patient Record*
T. Dunleavy, RN, BSN, OCN

173

Medication Log

Day/Date	Drug _____ Dose _____	Drug _____ Dose _____	Drug _____ Dose _____	Drug _____ Dose _____	Drug _____ Dose _____
Sunday	Time ____ Time ____ Time ____ Time ____	Time ____ Time ____ Time ____ Time ____	Time ____ Time ____ Time ____ Time ____	Time ____ Time ____ Time ____ Time ____	Time ____ Time ____ Time ____ Time ____
Monday	Time ____ Time ____ Time ____ Time ____	Time ____ Time ____ Time ____ Time ____	Time ____ Time ____ Time ____ Time ____	Time ____ Time ____ Time ____ Time ____	Time ____ Time ____ Time ____ Time ____
Tuesday	Time ____ Time ____ Time ____ Time ____	Time ____ Time ____ Time ____ Time ____	Time ____ Time ____ Time ____ Time ____	Time ____ Time ____ Time ____ Time ____	Time ____ Time ____ Time ____ Time ____
Wednesday	Time ____ Time ____ Time ____ Time ____	Time ____ Time ____ Time ____ Time ____	Time ____ Time ____ Time ____ Time ____	Time ____ Time ____ Time ____ Time ____	Time ____ Time ____ Time ____ Time ____
Thursday	Time ____ Time ____ Time ____ Time ____	Time ____ Time ____ Time ____ Time ____	Time ____ Time ____ Time ____ Time ____	Time ____ Time ____ Time ____ Time ____	Time ____ Time ____ Time ____ Time ____
Friday	Time ____ Time ____ Time ____ Time ____	Time ____ Time ____ Time ____ Time ____	Time ____ Time ____ Time ____ Time ____	Time ____ Time ____ Time ____ Time ____	Time ____ Time ____ Time ____ Time ____
Saturday	Time ____ Time ____ Time ____ Time ____	Time ____ Time ____ Time ____ Time ____	Time ____ Time ____ Time ____ Time ____	Time ____ Time ____ Time ____ Time ____	Time ____ Time ____ Time ____ Time ____

Figure 9-6. Medication log. *Reprinted with permission: Saint Louis University Cancer Center Patient Record*
T. Dunleavy, RN, BSN, OCN

5. It is a good idea to bring visual aids or actual items for learners to see and touch as a reinforcement of instructions given when teaching about emergency preparedness.

   A. True
   B. False

6. It is not generally recommended to immunize pregnant women.

   A. True
   B. False

7. A rare, serious infection of the fetus, fetal vaccinia, can occur following vaccination for smallpox.

   A. True
   B. False

8. During pregnancy, infection with Yersinia pestis, the bacteria causing plague, will be of little or no consequence.

   A. True
   B. False

9. During a fire, it is only acceptable to transport patients in wheelchairs in the elevators to facilitate rapid evacuation of residents.

   A. True
   B. False

10. Involving patients with varying cognitive, physical and sensory abilities in the disaster planning at a facility will assist health care personnel with maintaining the dignity of the residents even in disaster situations.

    A. True
    B. False

See Test Your Knowledge Answers in Appendix B.

EXPLORE MEDIALINK

Interactive resources and an audio glossary for this chapter can be found on the Companion Website at http://www.prenhall.com/langan. Click on Chapter 9 to select the activities for this chapter.

REFERENCES

American Academy of Pediatrics (AAP) & American College of Obstetrics and Gynecology (ACOG). (2002). *Guidelines for perinatal care* 5th ed. Chicago: American Academy of Pediatrics.

American College of Obstetrics and Gynecology. (1998). *Obstetric aspects of trauma management* (ACOG Educational Bulletin No. 251). Washington DC: ACOG

American Red Cross. (2001). *Disaster Preparedness for seniors by seniors*, Retrieved June 19, 2003, from http://www.redcross.org/services/disaster/beprepared/seniors.html

Association of Women's Health, Obstetric, and Neonatal Nurses (AWHONN). (2002). *How can nurses advise pregnant women to prepare for bioterrorism events?* Retrieved December 3, 2002, from http://www.awhonn.org/awhonn?pg873-8010-3350-6890

Batavia, A. I. (1993). Relating disability policy to broader public policy: Understanding the concept of "handicap." *Policy Studies Journal 21*(4), 735–739.

Center for Drug Evaluation and Research. (2001). *Cipro (Ciprofloxacin Hydrochloride) for inhalation anthrax*. Retrieved February 10, 2004, from http://www.fda.gov/cder/drug/infopage/cipro/cipro_message.htm

Centers for Disease Control and Prevention (CDC). (2002). CDC plague home page. Retrieved December 15, 2002, from http://www.cdc.gov/ncidod/dvbid/plague/index.htm

Centers for Disease Control and Prevention (CDC). (2003a). Women with smallpox vaccine exposure during pregnancy reported to the National Smallpox Vaccine in Pregnancy Registry–United States, 2003. *MMWR, 52*(17), 386–388.

Centers for Disease Control and Prevention (CDC). (2003b). National smallpox vaccine in pregnancy registry–United States, 2003. *MMWR, 52*(12), 256.

Centers for Disease Control and Prevention (CDC). (2003c). Recommendations for using smallpox vaccine in a pre-event vaccination program. *MMWR, 52*(RR07), 1–16.

Centers for Disease Control and Prevention (CDC). (2003d). *Smallpox vaccination information for women who are pregnant or breastfeeding*. Retrieved May 9, 2003, from www.cdc.gov

Cono, J., Casey, C. G., & Bell, D. M. (2003). Smallpox vaccination & adverse reactions. MMWR, 52(RR04), 1–28.

Cunningham, F. G., MacDonald, P. C., Gant, N. F., Leveno, K. J., Gilstrap, L. C., Hankins, G. D., & Clark, S. L. (2001). Williams Obstetrics (21st ed.). Stamford, CT: Appleton & Lange.

Department of Health and Human Services, & Collins, J. D. (1997). *Prevalence of selected chronic conditions: United States, 1990–92*. Vital and Health Statistics, Series 10(194). Publication No. (PHS) 97-1522. Washington, DC: U. S. Department of Health and Human Services.

Federal Emergency Management Agency & American Red Cross. (2001). *Family disaster plan*. Retrieved June 18, 2003, from http://www.redcross.org/services/disaster/beprepared/familyplan.html

Fernandez, L. S., Byard, D., Lin, C. C., Benson, S., & Barbera, J. A. (2002). Frail elderly as disaster victims: Emergency management strategies. *Prehospital and Disaster Medicine*, 67–74. Retrieved June 18, 2003, from http://www.seas.gwu.edu/~icdm/67-74%20Fernandez.pdf

Hale, R. W., & Zinberg, S. (2001). *Summary letter about anthrax*. American College of Obstetrics and Gynecology. Retrieved April 25, 2003, from www.acog.org/from_home/misc/anthrax.cfm

Henretig, F. M., Cieslak, T. J., & Eitzen, E. M. (2002). Biological and chemical terrorism. *The Journal of Pediatrics, 141*(3), 311–326.

Larson, P. D. (1998). Rehabilitation. In I. M. Lubkin & P. D. Larson (Eds.), *Chronic illness: Impact and interventions* (4th ed.) (pp. 528–547). Boston: Jones and Bartlett.

McReynolds, J. (2003, July). M&Ms used to "treat" Anthrax exposure. *Missouri Department of Health and Senior Services, Public Health Preparedness and Response UPDATE,* 1–2.

Missouri Department of Health and Senior Services. (2004). *Public health preparedness and response update*. Retrieved April 16, 2004, from http://www.dhss.state.mo.us/BT_Response/DHSSPrep/RespUpdate.March_2004.pdf

Morbidity and Mortality Weekly Report (MMWR). (2001). Updated recommendations for antimicrobial prophylaxis among asymptomatic pregnant women after exposure to bacillus anthracis. *MMWR, 50,* 960.

National Cancer Institute, Cancer Control & Population Sciences. (2003). *Estimated US cancer prevalence counts*. Retrieved October 28, 2003, from http://cancercontrol.cancer.gov/ocs/prevalence/

National Center for Health Statistics (NCHS). (1990). *Current estimates from the National Health Interview Survey, United States, 1990*. Hyattsville, MD: Author

National Center for Health Statistics (NCHS). (1996). *Current statistics from the National Health Interview Survey, United States, 1996*. Retrieved June 19, 2003, from http://www.cdc.gov/nchs/fastats/disable.htm

National Center for Health Statistics (NCHS). (1997). *Vital statistics of the Centers for Disease Control and Prevention/National Center for Health Statistics, 1997*. Retrieved June 19, 2003, from http://www.cdc.gov/nchs/fastats/disable.htm

National Center for Health Statistics (NCHS). (2003). Disabilities/limitations. Retrieved April 30, 2004, from http://www.cdc.gov/nchs/fastats/disable.htm

National Commission of Correctional Health Care Standards. (2002). *Emergency Plan (essential)*. J-06, 7.

National Institute for Literacy (NIFL) (n.d.). *Search literacy information*. Retrieved October 27, 2003, from http://www.nifl.gov/reders/!intro.htm

Pope, A. M., & Tarlov, A. R. (Eds.). (1991). *Disability in America: Toward a national agenda for prevention*. Washington, DC: IOM, National Academy Press.

SIL International. (2003). *Ethnologue: Languages of the world* (14th ed.). Dallas: Author. Retrieved October 26, 2003, from http://www.ethnologue.com

Smith, C. M., & Maurer, F. A. (2000). *Community health nursing: Theory and practice,* (2nd ed.). Philadelphia: W. B. Saunders.

United States Bureau of the Census. (1997, August). *Current population reports: Americans with disabilities: 1994–95*. Washington, DC: Author www.census.gov/prod/3/97pubs/p70-61.pdf.

United States Department of Health and Human Services. (2000). *Health United States, 2000*. Washington, DC: Author.

University of Florida, Cooperative Extension Service, Institute of Food and Agricultural Sciences. (1998). Disaster planning for elderly and disabled populations. In *IFAS Disaster Handbook for Extension Agents* (Document DH-031).

White, S. R., Henretig, F. M., & Dukes, R. G. (2002). Medical management of vulnerable populations and co-morbid conditions of victims of bioterrorism. *Emergency medical clinics of North America, 20*(2), 365–392.

CHAPTER 10

Preparing Nurses to Plan and Care for Children During Disaster Situations

Nina K. Westhus, Diana Fendya, and Vered Kater

LEARNING OBJECTIVES

1. Review physiological, psychological, and psychosocial differences of children that influence their response to disaster.
2. Identify specific physiological vulnerabilities that increase children's response to chemical, biological, and nuclear weapons of mass disaster.
3. Discuss the impact of disaster on the psychological and psychosocial well-being of children.
4. Increase the knowledge of health care providers in preparing and caring for children during mass causality disaster situations.
5. Discuss interventions and action steps that health care providers can employ to decrease the impact of mass casualty disasters upon children and their families.

MEDIALINK www.prenhall.com/langan

Resources for this chapter can be found on the Companion Website at http://www.prenhall.com/langan Click on Chapter 10 to select the activities for this chapter.

CHAPTER OUTLINE

Know Your Terms
Audio Glossary
Web Links
    Pediatric Resources
MediaLink Applications

GLOSSARY

Family readiness kit. Holds specific items believed to be essential to help children and families cope with the effects of a disaster. It gives not only general information necessary for all disasters but also specific instructions related to various types of disaster and how to respond to each of these

Go box. A box that can be taken by the school nurse (health care worker) when a crisis occurs

The contents of the box should include:

    List of students and staff

    List of students and staff with significant health problems

Medication list

Blueprint of school property

Evacuation plan

Walkie-talkies

Cell phone or beeper

Current yearbook

Phone numbers

For young children, the box may contain safety items, as well as a favorite object such as a stuffed animal

Mock disaster drill. Practice essential safety routines for various types of natural and man-made disasters

Pediatric specialty resource centers. Pediatric facilities with expertise in a particular area, such as critical care, trauma, etc., designated at regional and state level

Family disaster plan. Plan developed at a family meeting, practiced regularly, about every six months. It should include several escape routes from the home and places to meet in case family members get separated

Rally points. Preselected meeting places at locations where members of the family spend a significant amount of time (e.g., schools, neighborhood, and workplaces)

INTRODUCTION

Millions of people are affected by natural and man-made disasters, violence, and acts of terrorism each year. Terrorism, or threatened acts of violence directed against property or individuals, strives to induce fear and coerce governments or others for political, ideological, or religious purposes (Institute of Medicine [IOM], 2003). While the lives of adults are seriously affected by these situations, the lives of children are affected to an even greater degree (Cieslak & Henritig, 2003). Such purposeful acts place children at risk and threaten safe worlds that foster growth and development, previously developed coping skills, and trust, the most basic of developmental milestones.

This chapter will explore the impact of disaster on children and their caregivers from a physiological, psychological, and developmental perspective. Children are not merely little adults; their response to illness, injury, and to all happenings in life is a response influenced by physiological differences and life experiences contributing to personality development.

and transmission, is immature in the young child. This immaturity makes full assessment and prediction of recovery following traumatic insult difficult. Acetylcholine, and its role in neural transmission, can be interrupted when certain toxic agents interfere with the less resistant esterase enzymes of children including acetylcholinesterase. As acetylcholine accumulates, heightened excitability occurs at nerve junctions resulting in seizure activity (Rotenberg, 2003).

PEDIATRIC PHYSIOLOGICAL DIFFERENCES CONTRIBUTING TO ILLNESS AND INJURY RESPONSE

Cranial and Neurological System

The child's head is proportionately larger in relation to body size than the adult's head. The size and weight of the child's head predispose the child to head trauma. A lack of neck muscle strength, combined with a large heavy head, focus stress upon the child's cervical (C) spine region. Significant stress is often responsible for cervical spine fractures in the C1 and C2 vertebrae. Approximately 70% of cervical fractures in children occur in this area, whereas cervical fractures in the adult occur in these vertebrae only 15% of the time (Eichelberger, 1993).

The cranial bones are thinner, providing less protection to underlying brain structures. Vital vascular structures and fragile neural tissues are more vulnerable. Blood vessels are thinner and more fragile, succumbing to shearing and tearing forces more easily than in the adult. Nerve conduction also differs in children. Myelinzation, critical to nerve synapses

Airway and Respiratory System

The child's tongue, the first anatomical structure of the airway, is larger in proportion to the child's oral pharynx than the adult's tongue is in relation to the adult oral pharynx. The tongue's large size often leads to airway obstruction. The large tongue and contrasting small intraoral airway make securing the child's airway difficult. Young children first explore their environment by putting much of it into their mouths. Foreign bodies are often found when assessing the airway that can also lead to airway obstruction.

The trachea, small and narrow, is flexible. Unless positioned with the head in a neutral or sniffing position, it can be kinked easily and obstructed. When in a supine position, the child's large occiput produces a natural flexion of the neck causing airway obstruction. Because of the small size of the internal lumen of airway structures, secretions and edema can quickly occlude the child's airway. Even small amounts of edema or secretions contribute greatly to increased airway resistance, increasing the work of breathing. The child's larynx is funnel shaped and lies higher and more anteriorly. Its position makes visualization of the glottis and subsequent endotracheal intubation difficult. The epiglottic structure is longer, floppier, and narrower, decreasing protection of the lower airway structures and increasing the risk of esophageal intubation as well as aspiration of secretions or foreign bodies (American Heart Association, [AHA], 2002).

The pediatric chest wall or rib cage does not extend as far down the child's torso as the adults. As a result, the child's liver and spleen, already disproportionately large, are exposed and vulnerable to injury. The child's rib cage is not comprised of true bone, but rather cartilage that provides minimal protection to underlying structures. The cartilage is estimated to be twice as compliant as the rib cage of the adult. Upon impact, the child's rib cage, being flexible, often bends, resulting in rare rib fractures. Without the protection of the ribs, the energy forces of trauma are often transmitted to underlying structures within the chest, resulting in pulmonary and/or cardiac contusion(s).

Ventilation also differs in the child. Younger children breathe through their nares as opposed to nares and mouth. They depend upon the diaphragm to assist with pulmonary expansion and exhalation. Any abdominal trauma can impede the diaphragm's movements, leading to respiratory compromise. Intercostal muscles that assist adults in ventilation are poorly developed in the child, contributing to the stridorous appearance of children struggling to breathe. Alveoli within the lungs are fewer, with 24 million in the infant as opposed to approximately 300 million in the adult. This results in smaller tidal volumes. Increased respiratory rates are necessary (increased minute ventilations) to ensure adequate oxygenation (Hazinski, 1992). Meanwhile, the oxygen demand of the child is twice as great as that of the adult (6 to 8 mL/kg compared to 4 mL/kg in the adult). Consequently, hypoxemia occurs more rapidly in the child with inadequate alveolar ventilation or apnea (AHA, 2002).

Circulatory System

Adults have a total circulating blood flow (TCBF) of 65 mL/kg. The child has 80 mL of TCBF per kg/wt. Although the TCBF is greater in mL/kg, the lesser weight of children reduces the TCBF greatly. Hypovolemia is a frequent complication of injured children or children experiencing significant gastroenteritis accompanied by diarrhea and/or vomiting. Children generally have strong hearts that compensate for a reduction in CO or TCBF. Constriction of peripheral vasculature causes a prolonged capillary refill (15% to 40% blood loss). Real heart rate increases occur prior to falling blood pressures (loss of 31% to 40% of CO). Caregivers need to be aware of this phenomenon. The compensatory mechanisms of the child are effective in masking impending shock, especially if injuries are not obvious, hidden, or internal, causing hemorrhage and reduction in cardiac output. See Table 10–1.

Integumentary System

The skin is the largest organ of the body. In a child, the skin measures approximately 4 to 5 square feet. In proportion to the child's weight, the integumentary system covers a much larger body surface area than in an adult. As a result, children succumb to cold stress more quickly and easily. Caregivers must provide normothermic conditions or implement special measures to conserve heat when caring for the child. As in the adult, the child's skin consists of three layers—the epidermis, which is thinner in the child, the dermis, and subcutaneous layers. It should be noted that the thickness of the skin layers also varies significantly as

TABLE 10–1. PEDIATRIC SYSTEMIC RESPONSE TO BLOOD LOSS

SYSTEM EVALUATION	MILD HEMORRHAGE, SIMPLE HYPOVOLEMIA - COMPENSATED SHOCK (<30% BLOOD VOL. LOSS)	MODERATE HEMORRAGE, MARKED HYPOVOLEMIA (30%–40% BLOOD VOL. LOSS)	SEVERE HEMORRHAGE, PROFOUND HYPOVOLEMIA (>45% BLOOD VOL. LOSS)
Cardiac	Mild increase in heart rate (+)	Increased heart rate (++)	Heart rate elevated (+++)
	Peripheral pulses weak (−)	Peripheral pulses thready (−−)	Peripheral pulse absent (−−−)
	Central pulse present	Central pulse weak (−)	Central pulse thready (−−)
	Blood pressure low—normal (systolic blood pressure greater than 70 mm Hg = 2 X age in years)	Hypotensive (systolic blood pressure less than 70 mm Hg + 2 X age in years)	Hypotension profound (systolic blood pressure less than 50 mm Hg)
Respiratory	Respiratory rate increased (+)	Increased respiratory rate (++)	Respiratory rate increased greatly (+++)
Neuro	Anxious, irritable, confused	Agitated, confused — progressing to lethargy (pain response decreased)	Obtunded, nonresponsive, comatose
Skin	Capillary refill greater than 2 seconds	Capillary refill greater than 3 seconds	Capillary refill greater than 5 seconds
	Skin cool/clammy and mottling may be evident	Skin cool to touch and pallor in appearance	Extremities cold
			Cyanotic in appearance
Renal	Urine output greatly decreased	Urine output decreased	Anuric
	Specific gravity increased	BUN (blood urea nitrogen) increased	

Adapted with permission from Advanced Trauma Life Support Course, Chicago, Illinois, American College of Surgeons, Student Manual, 1997, p. 297, Chapter 10.

to the body region or area of location. The skin serves multiple functions, all of which are critical in the maintenance of physiological stability in the child. Beyond thermoregulation, the skin also serves as a protective barrier and aids in maintaining fluid and electrolyte balance.

FACTORS INFLUENCING THE CHILD'S RESPONSE TO ILLNESS AND DISASTER

Psychosocial and Cognitive Development of the Child

Foundations for healthy development proceed by achieving defined tasks and developmental milestones. Interruptions in the achievement of these milestones may contribute to the development of unhealthy adults. Assisting children to reach these milestones, even in turbulent times, assists the child to build a healthy mind and become a healthy adult.

Infants (0 to 1 year)

Infants understand their world through sensory awareness and motor activity. They find gratification in consistently having their basic needs of food, warmth, and comfort met by their primary caretakers (Figure 10–1). Their primary developmental task is establishment of a sense of trust. Parents are the usual primary caregivers and through them the infant forms basic attitudes toward life from experiences with parents perceived as reliable, consistent, available, and caring—or the negative counterpart. Ongoing nurturing relationships are essential; disruption can cause regression (Betz & Sowden, 2004; Brazelton & Greenspan, 2000; DeHart, Sroufe, & Cooper, 2004).

Toddlers (1 to 3 years)

Toddlers not only find gratification in having their daily care and feeding needs met, but also in learning to assert themselves in the expression of these needs. They are learning to be autonomous. Parents continue to be the primary caregivers, but also help children learn socialization for management of acceptable behavior (Figure 10–2). Toddlers must learn to delay immediate gratification, despite an immature conception of time. External disruption can be critically damaging to toddlers (Betz & Sowden, 2004; Brazelton & Greenspan, 2000; DeHart et al., 2004).

Preschoolers (3 to 6 years)

Preschoolers develop a sense of initiative (Figure 10–3). They have the ability to form mental images of objects and people never perceived, which leads to fantasies and possible fear. They are developing a beginning concept of time.

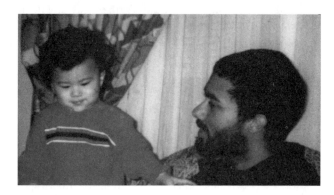

Figure 10–2. Toddler.

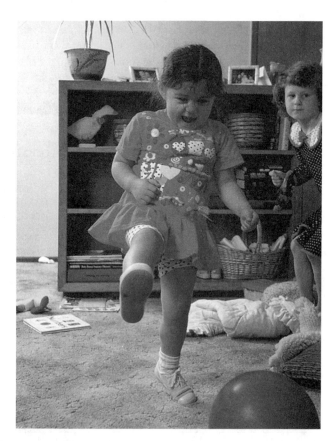

Figure 10–3. Pre-schooler.

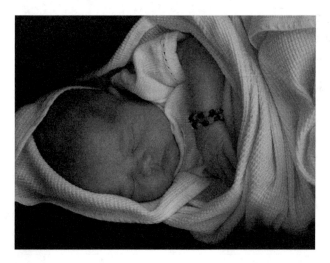

Figure 10–1. Infant.

Preschoolers are egocentric. They are bound by centration, a focusing on one aspect of a situation. The family continues to be their primary base and frame of reference. They are beginning the process of becoming aware of other people and children. Through dramatic play, preschoolers enact roles of parents. Preschoolers do not understand that reality and fantasy are two distinct realms. They believe powerful beings cause events and find it hard to grasp the finality of death (Betz & Sowden, 2004; Brazelton & Greenspan, 2000; DeHart et al., 2004).

School-Age Child (6 to 12 years)

School-age children's thinking becomes abstract and symbolic. These children are able to form mental images that are assisted by their perceptual abilities. They can tell time and understand the concepts of past, present, and future. Language is their way of interacting with the world. School-age children are developing a sense of industry (Figure 10–4). Home and family continue to be important, but their significance diminishes, while the peer group takes on an added significance. School-age children have a sense of right and wrong.

These children have a background of experience that helps them appraise situations more realistically. They understand verbal explanations and have within themselves a degree of self-mastery that younger children have not yet acquired (Betz & Sowden, 2004; Brazelton & Greenspan, 2000; DeHart et al., 2004).

Adolescent (12 to 18 years)

Adolescent thinking approaches the level of an adult. Adolescents are able to take on the perspective of another and think of solutions to problems. They are searching for their identity, coming to know who they are, what they believe in and value, and what they want to accomplish (Figure 10–5). Fairness and justice are important to them. Adolescents use language to convey ideas, opinions, and values (Betz & Sowden, 2004; Brazelton & Greenspan, 2000; DeHart et al., 2004).

CARING FOR CHILDREN DURING DISASTER SITUATIONS

Man-Made Disasters and Their Impact on Children

The impact of disasters, whether natural or man made, is epitomized in the changing characters of communities, human death, and suffering. Man-made disasters, such as deliberate use of or accidents involving chemical and biological agents, bombings, and nuclear radiation exposures, are becoming more common and raising concerns of the general public, government officials, and health care workers. When such disasters occur, children will be victimized more than adults. "Children are more vulnerable to the effects of such disasters than the general population. Besides their proportionately greater level of exposure, children will also be affected by loss of parents, displacement from their homes, and post traumatic stress" (American Academy of Pediatrics [AAP], 2003a, p. 1). Their unique physical and cognitive aspects put them at enhanced risk. Agents that may not be lethal to the general population put well children at risk, and may be lethal, if their victim is a child with special health care needs or a child with chronic illness.

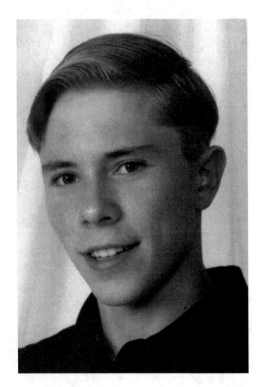

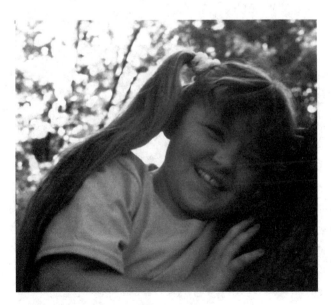

Figure 10–4. School-age child.

Figure 10–5. Adolescent.

The Centers for Disease Control and Prevention (CDC) has identified that the release of chemical or biological agents is one of the imminent terrorist threats (AAP, 2000). Chemical and biological weapons though easy to develop, are often difficult to detect. These weapons are often disseminated through the air without odor or taste.

Chemical Agents and Their Impact on Children

Children are at increased risk to chemical agents that are absorbed through the skin or inhaled. Inhalation agents can be classified as type I, acting on the proximal, tracheobronchial portion of the respiratory tract. Type II agents act primarily on the gas exchange region in the respiratory bronchioles and alveoli. Agents that affect the body systemically are referred to as type III (Burklow, Yu, & Madsen, 2003). Mucosal irritation and coughing, sneezing, hoarseness, and strider and/or wheezing are noted with type I inhalant agents. Children exposed to type II agents frequently are short of breath and have nonradiographic depicted pulmonary edema. Disseminated in high doses, most inhalant chemical agents can cause both type I and type II injuries.

Chlorine, phosgene, ammonia, nerve agents, and mustard gas are corrosive chemical agents. They can injure skin, eyes, and nasal mucosa. Inhaled they can cause life-threatening pneumonitis. Chlorine and phosgene are vaporized easily and are pulmonary, inhalational, or choking agents. Chlorine, as a gas, is heavier than air. When released, it settles close to the ground, the breathing space of most small children, putting them at greater risk of exposure to greater concentrations of the gas than adults. Increased concentrations and the increased respiratory rates of children lead to increased inhalation of this toxic substance.

After the child has been moved from the source of the chlorine gas, it is important to irrigate skin, eyes, and mucosal membranes with water to prevent continued irritation and injury. With type I injuries, warm moist air with supplemental oxygen should be provided. Bronchospasm is common with these injuries and treatment with bronchodilators may be necessary. Type II injuries require oxygenation, and positive end expiratory pressure (PEEP) may assist inflation of damaged alveoli. Fluid resuscitation will be required if the child has progressed into pulmonary edema (Burklow, et al., 2003).

Phosgene is used in the making of dyes, pesticides, and plastics. This chemical gas is also heavier than air, putting a child at greater risk. This agent does not have a readily detected odor, making it more difficult to detect prior to reaching toxic levels. It penetrates airways poorly due to its poor water solubility (Burklow, et al, 2003). Once the agent reaches the airways, it attacks the surface of the alveolar capillaries causing leakage of serum from the capillaries in the lung into alveolar septi. As the fluid leaks into the alveoli, massive amounts of fluid pour out of the circulation causing volume depletion. Due to the limited circulating blood flow, pulmonary edema caused by both

chlorine and phosgene gases put children at risk of hypovolemic shock as fluid shifts occur from vascular spaces to the pulmonary interstitial spaces.

Nerve agents include tabun, sarin, and soman, which are toxic and volatile. They are colorless liquids at room temperature, but form into easily dispersed toxic vapors that are inhaled by victims. Sarin gas is dense and more concentrated closer to the ground, increasing the likelihood that children will inhale it. Organophosphorus nerve agents are well absorbed through intact skin. Children have a unique susceptibility to organophosphorus compounds. The compounds inhibit esterase enzymes causing acetylcholine to accumulate at neuromuscular junctions. The accumulation of acetylcholine heightens the convulsive effect of the nerve agents, which cause a cholinergic syndrome. It should be noted, though, that children respond differently to organophosphorus compounds. They do not commonly demonstrate autonomic signs of excessive glandular secretion, nor is miosis seen in all children as it is with adults (Rotenberg, 2003).

Severe nerve agent exposure will necessitate the use of an antidote. Atropine is the antidote of choice. Muscle weakness and respiratory failure may persist even after administration of the atropine. Atropine should be repeated until airway resistance and secretions have been reduced. The Mark I kit is a combination of atropine and pralidoxime chloride (2-Pam, Protopam Chloride) utilized by the military (Quinn-Doggett, Stewart-Craig, & Doak, 1998). This drug combination is available in an auto-injector for use. The auto-injector enhances the rapid absorption of the medication (Figure 10–6). Unfortunately, medication dosages in the auto-injector have been calculated for adults and are inappropriate for children. It should be noted that the needle of the Mark I auto-injector may also cause injury if used to treat a child. A child-size auto-injector has been developed but is awaiting the approval of the FDA. However, because of the greater impact of nerve agents on children, the Center for Pediatric Disaster Pre-

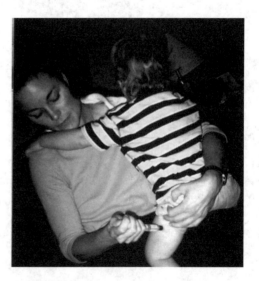

Figure 10–6. Auto-injector.

paredness is recommending use of the adult auto-injectors until appropriate child size devices are available (Markenson, 2003). Diffuse muscle twitching and seizure activity indicates progression of the nerve agent insult. Diazepam is the drug of choice for treatment of seizures. Intramuscular diazapam results in erratic absorption; thus, intravenous administration is recommended (Rotenberg, 2003).

Because nerve agents are absorbed through the skin, decontamination and the preservation of body warmth are essential when caring for a child exposed to these agents. After decontamination, care should focus on providing adequate respiratory support—nerve agents induce both apnea and muscle weakness. Apnea and muscle weakness, accompanied by an increase in secretions, bronchospasm, and airway resistance, may necessitate the use of ventilator support. Vomiting, associated with nerve agent exposure, increases the risk of aspiration. Fluid intake and output should be monitored to ensure that hypovolemia from vomiting does not occur. Intravenous fluids should be administered and essential electrolytes monitored and replaced if necessary.

Cyanide forms, including hydrogen cyanide and cyanogen chloride, are potent poisons that interfere with the cell mitochondria's ability to use oxygen. Organs requiring high-energy and high-oxygen utilization, such as the brain and the heart, are affected first. Cyanide acts as a neurotoxin. Cell membranes are disrupted and an increase in excitatory injury in the central nervous system occurs. Cyanides, type III agents, are distributed to all tissues and organs of the body. Initial symptoms include upper airway and mucous membrane irritation. Significant exposure causes rapid progression of symptoms. Hyperpnea, anxiety, and restlessness quickly lead to loss of consciousness, seizures, apnea, and death. Cyanide poisoning can impact the autonomic system causing salivation, emesis, urination, and defecation. The higher respiratory rate of children puts them at greater risk for cyanide poisoning. The thinner layer of their stratum corneum allows greater and more rapid systemic absorption of liquid forms of cyanide (Rotenberg, 2003).

Treatment for cyanide poisoning is primarily supportive. After initial decontamination with warm water, 100% O^2 should be administered and intravenous access established. If symptoms persist, providers should consider use of a multistage antidote kit. These kits use two drug agents to neutralize the cyanide—nitrites and thiosulfates. Nitrite aids in shifting the cyanide from the mitochondrial enzyme. Unfortunately, nitrate treatment in children has been associated with methemoglobinemia and hypotension. If hypotension is identified, fluid resuscitation or vasopressors are needed to reestablish perfusion. Special care is required with infants when adjusting cyanide antidotes due to the risk of methemoglobinemia. The second drug in the kit, thiosulfate, acts as a detoxifier of cyanide, enabling the kidney excretion of cyanide (Rotenberg, 2003).

Vesicant agents, such as mustard-sulfur and nitrogen and lewisite, can cause significant prolonged morbidity (Yu, Burklow, & Madsen, 2003). Mustards can be both a vapor inhalation and liquid contact hazard capable of penetrating clothing. Clinical effects of mustard agents can be delayed typically for 2–48 hours even though chemical cellular damage occurs within minutes of exposure. Mustard causes local damage to skin, airways, and eyes, as well as systemic effects involving the hematopoietic and gastrointestinal systems (Quinn-Doggett, et al., 1998).

The effects of mustard on children are more severe than on adults. The thin, delicate skin of the child quickly begins to show erythema and blisters resulting from the vesicant agent. Blister occurrence in children is more severe. Vaporized, these agents have a greater density than that of air, resulting in enhanced vapor concentration in the child's environment, increasing the incidence of ocular damage, inhalation, and gastrointestinal injuries. Airway inflammation and necrosis can lead quickly to increased resistance and obstruction in the child's small airways, contributing to respiratory arrest unless caregivers facilitate airway protection. Caregivers should be aware that these injuries are quite painful and management of pain is essential for these victims.

Lewisite, a military vesicant, is extremely irritating. Initial exposure produces visible lesions quickly. It is also absorbed by the eyes, skin, and lungs. The nose and sinuses are affected immediately; trauma to upper airway structures prevents injury extension to the lower airways and lungs. Lewisite also causes an enhanced capillary permeability leading to volume depletion and hepatic and renal injury. Lewisite does not damage the bone marrow (Quinn-Doggett, et al., 1998).

Vesicant or blister agent exposure should be treated with prompt decontamination as these agents cause irreversible effects within 3 to 10 minutes. A binding agent, e.g., powder, flour, charcoal, or earth, should be applied to exposed areas first. Then these areas should be washed with water. Thinner skin layers put children at risk of greater skin lesions. Damage from these agents occurs in a shorter exposure period than the adult. Antibiotics should be avoided initially to prevent the development of resistant organisms. The occurrence of pulmonary symptoms warrants early intubation and mechanical ventilation, and the use of PEEP may be helpful. Damaged skin, allowing for fluid loss, and vomiting often accompany these exposures. Children will be at risk for hypovolemic shock, and intravenous fluid resuscitation should be initiated. Ocular injury is common with vesicant exposure. The eyes of victims should be irrigated with copious amounts of water. Injury from exposure to these agents is very painful. Comfort and pain medications should be offered for both eye and skin trauma (Yu, Burklow, Selanikio, 2003).

Biological Weapons and Their Impact on Children

Whereas decontamination is the primary and initial treatment for many of the chemical agents, treatment of exposure to biological agents will be determined by the agent and method of exposure. The use of microorganisms (bacteria, viruses, fungi) or toxins from living organisms to infect humans, animals, and plants or to cause death is referred to as biological warfare. Biological weapons are considered the oldest and most lethal of warfare weapons. Due to their ease of manufacture and deployment, they are often referred to as the poor man's bombs.

The CDC has focused attention on those biological weapons that pose the greatest threats to public health and safety. These agents have been divided by threat severity, with A posing the greatest threat and C posing a lesser threat. Because they are nonvolatile or do not evaporate, these agents are usually dispersed in an aerosolized form. Because of their size, molecules may stay suspended in the air for hours. Inhaled organisms are often deposited into the terminal air sacs of the lungs. Because symptoms do not occur readily, illnesses from these agents may go unrecognized in their initial stages. Time delay to detection, until large numbers of individuals present with similar symptoms, can result in widespread secondary exposure. New real-time surveillance systems still under development may assist in quicker identification of infectious processes.

Depending on the infectious agent, injuries from biological weapons range from incapacitation to death (CDC, 2003). One of the best defenses for these weapons will be the development and dissemination of effective vaccines for both adults and children. Commonly identified biological weapons include bacteria, viruses, and toxins. Bacteria, such as anthrax, plague, and tularemia, cause diseases in animals and humans by invading tissues, causing an inflammatory reaction, or manufacturing toxins that are poisonous to cells.

Anthrax is a spore-forming bacillus organism. Its lethality is related to its ability to form resilient spores that can be aerosolized. Spores are able to survive without nutrients or moisture for long periods. Anthrax occurs in three forms—cutaneous, gastrointestinal, and inhalational. If aerosolized, anthrax spores act like a gas. Upon entering a host, anthrax spores are incompletely cleared by macrophages. Spores migrate to the mediastinum via the lymphatics, and germinate into a vegetative bacterium. The inhaled form is the rarest, and has the highest associated mortality. This mortality rate may be even greater for the young child due to increased respiratory rate and inhaled aerosol concentration. Children older than 2 years of age frequently demonstrate symptoms similar to adults (Cieslak & Henretig, 2003).

Early diagnosis of anthrax is difficult due to the nonspecific, flulike symptoms. The most accurate diagnoses are made with blood or fluid cultures. Cutaneous anthrax, the most common, presents with mild, constitutional symptoms, progressing to a systemic disease with lymphangitis and lymphadenopathy. The characteristic sign of cutaneous anthrax is a black eschar over the skin ulcer. Administration of intravenous antibiotics and a course of postexposure chemoprophylaxis is the present treatment plan for children (Cieslak & Henretig, 2003).

Plague, frequently found in infected rodents, is usually carried by fleas, and can be spread to humans. If inhaled, the organism causes a pneumonic infection, and if the organism escapes from lungs or lymph nodes, septicemia can occur. Because of their higher minute ventilation rates and greater concentrations of these agents within their breathing zones, children would inhale a larger number of these pathogens and experience more extreme symptoms. Circulating blood transports the organisms to secondary sites—liver, spleen, lungs, and the brain (Cieslak & Henretig, 2003). Pneumonic plague symptoms are nonspecific and include sudden flulike fever and chills. These quickly develop into pneumonia with liver cellular damage causing coagulation abnormalities and septicemia. Coagulation abnormalities can lead to disseminated intravascular coagulation, hypovolemia, and shock. Primary oropharangeal infections rapidly lead to airway compromise in the young child (Quinn-Doggett, et al., 1998). Isolation precautions and intravenous administration of antibiotics will be necessary (Cieslak & Henretig, 2003).

Tularemia causes an infection characterized by inflammation and necrosis of the pulmonary, oropharynx, eye, skin, and lymph node tissues. Alveolar septa and regional node necrosis often accompany inhalational tularemia. Chills, headache, generalized muscle pain, nonproductive cough, pneumonia, and regional lymphadenopathy are symptoms occurring within 2 to 10 days of inhalation. A combination of higher minute respiratory rates and greater concentrations of the aerosolized agent put children at greater risk. Once diagnosed, treatment consists of antibiotic therapy for 10 days. Prophylaxis treatment, in anticipation of biological attack during wartime, may be of value (Quinn-Doggett, et al, 1998).

Smallpox is caused by an orthopoxvirus declared eradicated in 1980 (Figure 10–7). Stockpiles of the agent still exist, raising concern that it might be utilized as a weapon. Once infected, the virus replicates in the upper respiratory tract. The infection spreads to the spleen and liver where a second viremic phase begins. Present recommendations discourage pre-outbreak vaccinations of children younger than 18 years. Infants under 1 year of age should not be vaccinated. They are at particular risk for postvaccinal encephalitis or encephalomyelitis, a severe complication (Waecker & Hale, 2003). Another concern is the shedding of the virus postvaccination from day 3 or 4, until the scab falls from inoculation sites. Recently vaccinated individuals should not be around children until their scab falls off or approximately 21 days postvaccination.

Viral hemorrhagic fever (VHF) is characterized by high fevers and generalized vascular damage (Cieslak & Henretig, 2003). The most familiar filovirus, Ebola, is of grave concern especially for children. Its mortality rate is extremely high at 50% to 80%. Lower TCBF put children at major risk for shock. Clinicians should be vigilant for early indicators of shock. Measures should be available to treat volume deficiencies and ensure sufficient blood oxygenation transport capabilities.

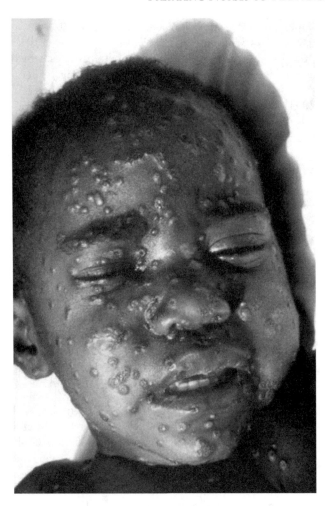

Figure 10–7. Smallpox. *Source: CDC.*

Botulinum, a neurotoxin, is produced by bacteria C botulinium and is considered one of the most lethal compounds. Inhaled or ingested, symptomology is the same. Symptom onset varies depending on agent entry route. Botulinum has the capability of irreversibly binding the presynaptic neuromuscular junction and preventing the release of acetylcholine, resulting in bulbar palsies and skeletal muscle weakness (Cieslak & Henretig, 2003). Symptoms include blurred vision, mydriasis, diplopia, ptosis, photophobia, dysphagia, and dysarthria. A descending paralysis occurs soon after bulbar palsy symptoms are noted. Symptoms progress quickly to respiratory failure that ultimately leads to death. The disease progresses rapidly with death often occurring within 24 hours (Quinn-Doggett, et al., 1998). Children, because of their smaller size, experience quick progression of the disease. Their inability to discuss or describe the bulbar symptoms places them at greater risk to these toxins.

Ricin, a by-product of castor oil production, is a powerful cytotoxin. It blocks protein synthesis within cells. Pulmonary tissue exposed to ricin becomes edematous with severe hemorrhagic and necrotic areas. Signs and symptoms occur within 4 to 8 hours of exposure and include fever, chest tightness, cough, shortness of breath, nausea, and joint pain (Quinn-Doggett, et al., 1998). Children usually succumb to cardiac arrest if respiratory compromise persists or progresses. If ingested, victims exhibit nausea, vomiting, severe diarrhea, and gastrointestinal (GI) hemorrhage. Because of lower TCBF and associated fluid deficits resultant from diarrhea and GI hemorrhage, children will be at risk of shock. Associated shock and necrosis of the liver, spleen, and kidneys will lead to death within 3 days.

Staphylococcal enterotoxin B (SEB) is a common food poisoning bacterium. Symptoms vary with the route of entry, either inhaled or ingestion. The toxin stimulates the proliferation of T-cell lymphocytes and production and secretion of cytokines. Victims will experience fever, headache, myalgias, chills and a nonproductive cough approximately 3 to 12 hours after inhalation (Quinn-Doggett, et al., 1998). Greater concentrations and amounts of the bacteria are likely to be inhaled by children, leading to severe shortness of breath and chest pain, thereby impeding respiratory function. Even though patients experience significant respiratory symptoms with the inhaled form, they tend to stabilize quickly. Close monitoring and the utilization of respiratory support devices may be necessary. Ingested, SEB can cause severe nausea, vomiting, and diarrhea resulting in significant fluid deficits as well. When ingested by a child, close monitoring of fluid status and assessing for signs and symptoms of shock is essential.

Biological agents causing dehydration and shock will have a greater impact on a small child than on an adult. Antibiotic dosages and antidotes for many of these agents will differ significantly for children. Vaccines have been developed for both anthrax and plague, but neither has been perfected and none have been recognized as effective and safe for children.

Unfortunately there is little evidence-based information on the appropriate management and antidote dosing for the pediatric patient for these kinds of weapons. Auto-injector antidotes need to be developed in appropriate doses.

Explosive Bombing and Its Impact on Children

Bombings create the potential for multisystem life-threatening trauma to many. Risk of death is increased when explosions occur in confined spaces such as large vehicles (e.g., the suicide bombing incidents of passenger buses in Israel), mines, and buildings such as the Murrrah Federal Building, site of the Oklahoma City bombing on April 19, 1995.

Explosive incidents will put children at major risk of head trauma resulting from falling or being thrown, acceleration/deceleration trauma (i.e., the shearing and tearing of vessels and neural axons within the brain), environmental structures falling, and potential bomb or environmental debris penetrating the skull. Children are uniquely at risk for tympanic membrane rupture, resulting from overpressurized bomb blast shock waves.

Environmental and bomb debris increase the likelihood that children will experience significant penetrating injuries. Thinner layers of skin and major organs lying closer to the child's body surface, without protective adipose tissue, increase their risk to these injuries. Major penetrating vessel and organ injury is to be expected.

Impact trauma from being thrown will put children at risk for extremity fractures and internal blunt injuries. The liver and spleen are particularly vulnerable. Blunt trauma puts children at a higher risk of death. Sustained injuries are difficult to assess in the young child. Because the cardiopulmonary system initially compensates for internal bleeding, children quickly develop shock, making fluid resuscitation difficult and death common.

Quaternary traumatic injuries include burns, asthma, inhalation, and crush injuries. Burns may result from a bomb flash, hot gases, steam, or combustion of the surrounding environment. Thin layers of the child's skin increase the likelihood of deeper burn trauma. When a child is in a closed space or close to the combustion agent, breathing and airway assessment are essential. Upper airway structures coated with soot should alert the caregiver to the potential of airway compromise. Small airway structures readily close with subsequent secretions and edema. Appropriate preparations are necessary for airway management.

In the Oklahoma bombing, 19 children died and six were transported to care facilities as survivors. These children experienced significant head trauma, crush injuries from collapsing environmental structures, blunt trauma, extremity fractures, penetrating trauma (glass/concrete/plastic bomb fragments), and burns from the explosive flame, steam, and/or heat. Common injuries resulting from mass bombings include ocular trauma resulting from particles entering the ocular space, sprains, strains, minor wounds, and ear trauma. Sprains and strains are often the result of trying to escape from the blast scene or being pushed by the bomb blast.

Flying debris, brushing against sharp jagged objects or dismantled environmental rubble, and falling while trying to leave the scene will account for many of the superficial wounds experienced by victims. Caring for the child who has been involved in a blast explosion will be much like caring for a major pediatric trauma patient. Resuscitation should focus on airway and cardiopulmonary resuscitation and stabilization with cervical spine precautions. Unique physical differences of the child, as previously discussed, should be kept in mind during both initial assessment and resuscitation. Assessment should be systematic beginning with the head and moving down the body. Vigilance should be taken on examination when looking for embedded debris and penetrating injuries. Open wounds should be cleansed with dressings and topical antibiotic ointments applied.

Nuclear Bombs

Nuclear disasters lead to devastation as a result of the emitted radiation. Ionizing radiation can consist of alpha particles, beta particles, gamma rays or photons, or neutrons.

Alpha particles can be inhaled, ingested, or enter via an open wound. Children can be shielded from these particles by a thin layer of paper or clothing. Beta particles, which are smaller and faster, are moderately penetrating. If left on the skin, beta radiation can cause skin injury or burns (Yu, 2003). Photons or gamma rays, able to travel and penetrate most materials, are more destructive. Neutrons can be the most damaging. Their ability to penetrate tissue and cause tissue damage is estimated to be 20 times more powerful than gamma radiation (Quinn-Doggett, et al., 1998).

Radioactive materials are readily available in radioactive isotopes for medical use and in nuclear power plants. Severity of injury and impact of nuclear radiation exposure is a reflection of dispersal mode, radiation dose, and length of time of exposure (Quinn-Doggett, et al., 1998). Radiation injury can result from external irradiation where the body or a part of the body is exposed to radiation, and the radiation is absorbed (e.g. during X rays). Injury also occurs during contamination when radioactive materials (solid, liquid, or gas states) are dispersed and victims are exposed externally or internally via the lungs or open wounds. Target organs for absorption of radioactive materials include bone, liver, thyroid, and kidney.

Children have an enhanced susceptibility to the effect of radiation exposure. Experiences at Chernobyl and Three Mile Island identified unique vulnerabilities and consequences of children being exposed to radiation. Children have relatively greater minute ventilation compared with adults, increasing their exposure to radioactive gases. Nuclear particles quickly settle to the ground. A higher concentration of radioactive material will exist in the spaces where children live and breathe.

Care of the child who has had significant exposure to radiation will be dependent on the type of radiation, degree of exposure, and associated injuries. Studies have shown that children exposed to radiation have a greater risk of developing cancers later in life. Decontamination is an essential first step of care. Removal of clothing is directly related to the effectiveness of decontamination and reduction of exposure to radiation. Once clothing is removed and stored appropriately, the child should be examined carefully for embedded radioactive debris. Skin should be washed with warm water while trying to maintain the child's warmth. Once decontamination has been completed, but within two hours of exposure, preventive treatment should be begun with the administration of potassium iodine (KI). Potassium iodine reduces thyroid uptake of radiation and subsequently decreases the effect of radiation on thyroid tissue. The protective aspect of KI lasts approximately 24 hours, necessitating administration of subsequent doses if radioiodines persist.

The thyroid of children seems to be particularly sensitive as a target organ for the radiation uptake. This increases their (children 5 years and under) risk of thyroid cancer. Postradiation-induced thyroid cancer is well documented in studies of children who were exposed to radiation in the Chernobyl disaster of 1991. Within 5 years of exposure, 577 children and adolescents developed thyroid cancer. Prior to the disaster only 59 children in the area had been diagnosed with thyroid cancer within a 5-year period. The cancer of these children was much more aggressive than typically seen. Children 5 years of age and younger were at the greatest risk (Balk & Miller, 2002).

Exposure to large doses of radiation can also lead to nausea and vomiting, requiring children to be treated with emetics and fluid resuscitation. Radiation burns and subsequent infections are also seen with large doses of radiation exposure or prolonged exposure to radioactive materials necessitating burn wound management. Bone marrow suppression also occurs with significant exposure, thus increasing risk of infections. The National Consensus Conference on Pediatric Preparedness for Disasters and Terrorism recommends the administration of marrow stimulative agents when children are victims of radiological terrorism or exposed to radiation through a nonterrorism event such as Chernobyl (Markenson & Redlener, 2003).

INFLUENCES ON THE CHILD'S RESPONSE TO DISASTER

Just as there are unique physiological vulnerabilities in children because of their developing bodies, there are also specific psychological and psychosocial challenges to children's developing minds (AAP, 2003c). These characteristics need to be taken into consideration when planning for children's needs during a disaster.

Children's Response to Disasters

Children's response to disaster or an act of terrorism depends upon the previously discussed physical and psychological maturity, as well as the emotional well-being of their parents or caretakers, the children's level of experience, coping skills, and supportive resources within their family and community (AAP, 2003d; Schonfeld, 2003).

Children's chronologic age, cognitive level, developmental stage, past experiences, and ego strength influence their adjustment to a new situation. Age is an important factor in the child's adjustment. As children grow and develop, they have experiences that help them develop the ego strength necessary to master difficult situations.

Assess Impact of Disaster

When children are exposed to a stressful event, they may react in a variety of ways including disinterest, shock and numbness, sadness, anger, guilt, or transient unhappiness. They may be dazed, disoriented, or bewildered. They may keep their concerns hidden or inside. Hurt et al (2001) found that neither caregivers nor teachers recognized the symptoms of psychological trauma or distress expressed by children. It is essential that caretakers (parents, teachers, and others who are in contact with children) be informed about, understand, and be able to evaluate children's reactions to disaster (Table 10–2). (AAP, 2003d; Milgram, 2002). The health care professional can obtain information by interviewing parents and children and observing for normal and unusual responses. The initial reaction is often

TABLE 10–2. CHILDREN'S REACTIONS TO DISASTER EVENTS

*CHANGES IN BEHAVIOR	*CHANGES IN MOOD	*CHANGES IN RELATIONSHIP PATTERNS
Sleep disturbances	Easily upset	Clinging or wanting to be alone
	Anxious	Fear of separation
Difficulty falling asleep	Crying	Social isolation
Sleeping too little or sleeping too much	Fearful	Increased or decreased arousal
Night terrors—may last up to two years	Depressed or irritable mood	Lack of responsiveness
Trauma-specific dreams	Sad	Hypersensitivity
Nighttime waking	Upset	Hyperactivity (new onset)
Afraid to sleep alone or with the light off	Argumentative	Repetitive or obsessive play concerning the
Regression—regress developmentally and adopt	Angry	traumatic event so that it interferes with
behavior more typical of a younger child,		normal activities
Regression in service of the ego, e.g.,		
thumbsucking or bedwetting		
	Apathetic	
	Depersonalization	
	Loss of interest in normal activities	
	Feeling overwhelmed	
	Guilt	
	Withdrawal	
Difficulty concentrating in school	Occurrence of stress-related physical symptoms, e.g., headaches, stomachaches, nausea, vomiting, diarrhea, shaking, anxiety, feelings of guilt, being secretive	Loss of appetite
Confusion	Energy loss	
Drop in school performance		
Absenteeism		

Note. From AAP, 2003d; Davidhizar & Shearer, 2002; Hanze, 2002; Milgram, 2002.

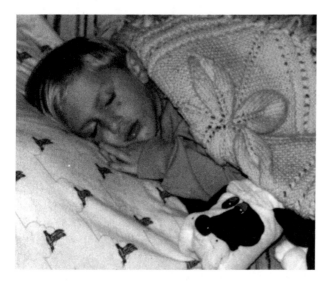

Figure 10–8. Sleeping child.

one of shock, disbelief, and numbness. These reactions may occur from the first hours after the event for up to 2 weeks. However, some children may act as though nothing has happened. They may seem disinterested and unconcerned about the event. The concern in this instance is that children are repressing their emotions (Milgram, 2002).

The AAP points out that adolescents may be especially vulnerable to these events and that parents should "watch for signs such as: sleep disturbances, fatigue, lack of pleasure in activities enjoyed previously, and initiation of illicit substance abuse" (AAP, 2003b, p. 1). Disaster events have such an impact on people that these events immediately affect our brain, which can result in traumatic stress and grief reactions (Milgram, 2002). Normal reactions are a concern when they become severe or persistent.

While there is no particular way to respond and no set time in which to respond, the AAP suggests that parents or caretakers should be concerned and seek help if a child (Figure 10–8):

- Becomes withdrawn and refuses to talk with parents
- Expresses thoughts of self-harm or harm to others
- Has severe, persistent problems sleeping and/or eating
- Displays intense irritability and extreme behavior outbursts

(AAP, 2003e)

Post-Traumatic Stress Disorder

When caretakers have concerns about children's behaviors, referrals to mental health services are appropriate. All children are at risk for post-traumatic stress disorder from experiencing devastating events, grave or catastrophic injuries, and deaths of strangers, parents or loved ones, and significant others such as teachers or caretakers (AAP, 2003d; Schonfeld, 2003) (See Chapter 4).

CARING FOR CHILDREN DURING DISASTER SITUATIONS

Psychological and Psychosocial Considerations and Support for Children

The most significant, character-forming interactions occur in childhood, largely within the context of the family. Families are a source of physical and emotional care that ideally results in healthy growth and development. Families have a crucial influence on the formation of the individual's identity and feelings of self-esteem. The family not only serves as the mediator between the individual and society, but also functions to meet the individual needs of its members. Parents are the primary teachers, because they interpret the world and society to their children. Parents are the ones who translate to their children the major meanings these outside forces have. It is beneficial to children's health when health care providers support children indirectly by educating their parents and guardians after a disaster (Davidhizar & Shearer, 2002; Milgram, 2002). See Nursing Vignette 10–1.

Preparation

Parents need to be prepared to meet the unique needs of children and adolescents in a disaster. An important step in preparing for a natural or man-made disaster is to have a plan of action in place. This plan is crucial to ensure optimal management, provide a sense of security, and enable the safety of children and their families. The plan must be updated regularly and practiced routinely. When parents become familiar with disaster-related materials, they will indirectly prepare for questions from their children. Preparation for a new experience supports the child's ego. It gives the child the opportunity to become adjusted to the situation. This reduces anxiety and makes energy available for mastering the situation and combating fear. Many groups, e.g., National Association of School Nurses, are in the process of developing emergency care plans for children and adolescence when disaster strikes. With the help of 250 families, Mulligan-Smith (2003, AAP, 2003d) developed a family readiness kit to help families prepare for these situations. The kit includes a list of specific items believed to be essential to help children and families cope with the effects of a disaster. It gives general information necessary for all disasters, but also it gives specific instructions related to various types of disaster and how to respond to each of these. See "Before a Disaster" below for more information on planning.

When disaster strikes, children may not be at home or in the presence of family members. Children spend a large proportion of their day in child care, school, and a variety of afterschool programs, or in transit to these locations. Caretakers in these settings must define the

Nursing Vignette 10-1   Ways to Decrease the Impact of Disaster Traumas in Children

A mobile therapy center manned by Arabic-speaking psychologists has been touring the West Bank since March 2003. Many living there cannot travel to established clinics, so this clinic is a realistic answer to a need.

In Israel, social workers receive ongoing training to help families when a disaster occurs. Teachers at all schools (including preschools) are taught how to communicate with their pupils when tragedy strikes. Regular school programs are then discontinued, and teachers, sometimes with help of a nurse or social worker, discuss what happened and suggest ways of coping.

Nurses working in the community and in schools help parents familiarize children with protective equipment, which may be needed in the event of an attack. In school, children are encouraged to draw on the box containing their gas mask. In Israel, all citizens possess a gas mask and everyone knows where the nearest bomb shelter is located.

Frequent drills occur in which the teachers guide their pupils into the bomb shelters where they continue their teaching sessions. Many houses have their own shelter since a law was passed in 1992 that requires all buildings to include a bomb shelter (IDF, 2003). Parents are advised to store favorite toys, games, and books in the shelter.

Several non-government organizations have begun to visit the families of victims. They answer an unmet need. Frequently, the helpers and those being helped become close, which can decrease tension. Teenagers can participate in a free program where they learn therapeutic leadership activities for their age mates (Kidsforkids, 2003).

Hospitals in Israel have a "walking wounded" area manned by social workers and nurses. All children and adults can receive care without payment. Frequently, the "patients" arrive only one or two days after the incident. During a disaster, all hospitals open a "family room," a room where nurses and social workers help families to identify their wounded family members. In cases in which a family member has been killed or severely wounded due to terrorism, a team, including a physician, makes a home visit to inform the family. Transportation to the hospital is arranged for the family. Out of respect, no victims are filmed for television or other purposes.

The psychological needs of children are addressed relative to television programming. In times of unrest, such as a war, a clinical psychologist advises the program presenter of the children's television in "real time" when and how to interrupt the program. Children have a need to know, and it is important to inform them in a language they understand. In times of increased tension, parents often allow the child to watch many hours of television. This helps the parent to cope. To interrupt the childrens' television program with "adult" announcements may cause unnecessary tension.

In the hospital, art therapists work with the children. Drawings and other creations help clarify what the child is experiencing. This is also a means that can identify the child who is in need of more intensive therapy. Nurses are often among the first to convince the child to participate.

Finding a balance between permissiveness and safety is very hard for parents. Keeping one's children completely safe is almost impossible in our world. The question remains, "How do you give a child the freedom they need to grow and mature, yet impose enough boundaries to keep the child safe?" There is no clear answer to this question. As nurses, we should avoid any hint of blame towards the parent of an injured child. Our task is different in each case.

The nurse is often the liaison between the parents and the child. It is a nurse's responsibility to help understand the specific needs of each child. The nurse encourages parents to create an open and supportive environment. A very important task of the nurse is to guide the parents in understanding that by permitting their child to go to the city, they are not responsible for the injury that occurred. Parents have to be taught how to avoid making unrealistic promises and becoming overly protective.

Nurses have to be aware of the specific needs of the child and the parents.

needs of children and plan for their care. These workers must be prepared to "evacuate children, take them to a safe place, notify parents, reunite children with their families, care for or arrange care for children whose parents are incapacitated or cannot reach them, and render first-aid" (AAP, 2003f, p. 7).

These practice sessions should include evacuation techniques and donning of protective gear such as gas masks, protective suits, and portable sealed rooms. When these activities are first done with the supportive care of significant others, it is less frightening. Education is most beneficial when it is done in small groups, in comfortable settings, includes preparatory materials that are similar to those used in actual situations, and allows time for discussion and counseling (Markenson & Redlener, 2003).

Further, pediatric health care professionals need to be prepared to meet the unique needs of children and adolescents in a disaster. Children with special health care needs are particularly vulnerable especially if their survival depends on technological means. From a physiological perspective these professionals need knowledge of specific types of natural (earthquakes, tornadoes, and hurricanes) and man-made (bioterrorism, radiological events, and bombings) disasters, and the knowledge and skill to recognize and treat those affected by them.

Communication

One of the consequences of a disaster is that caretakers, who are distressed or psychologically harmed, may care for children. Children are influenced by the emotional state of their caregivers. Thus, it is important for parents or caretakers to be aware of their own feelings. If parents feel stressed, anxious, and insecure, then they may be irritable, impatient, or intolerant of the behavior of their children and inadvertently handle them roughly or respond harshly. Parents must take care of themselves first in order that they will have the physical energy and emotional resources necessary to care for others. Children are careful observers of their parents' reaction to situations. When parents are a source of anxiety or fear as opposed to comfort, support, and reassurance, children may experience added stress. "Little ears" listen to what those around them have to say, and "little eyes" diligently observe the behavior of others. Children are more likely to deal successfully with problems if the adults around them are able to do so. Children of all ages can sense when a serious event takes place. They often imagine something worse than the actual event. Thus, parents and caretakers should inform children about the event as soon as possible (AAP, 2003d; Milgram, 2002; Schonfeld, 2003).

It is best to position oneself at children's eye level when speaking with them (Figure 10–9). Encourage children to tell what they know about the situation to ascertain their level of understanding. They should be allowed to express their feelings that may include anxiety, fear, and anger. The feelings of children should be respected. If pos-

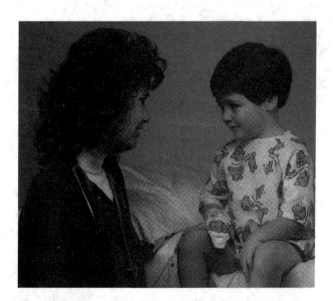

Figure 10–9. Maintain eye contact.

sible, provide them with an emotionally warm, comfortable, and peaceful environment. Children need to know that it is okay to cry. They should be encouraged to ask questions. Asking questions before giving answers is often the best way to help children reveal just what their fears or misconceptions may be (AAP, 2003d). This helps them share their concerns, fears, and feelings. It is important to listen carefully to what children have to say. To encourage verbalization, judgment should be reserved. Children may be asking something quite different from what their actual words seem to be expressing.

Discussion of the situation is an essential component of alleviating stress. Simple terms should be used when talking with children and explaining the events that have occurred. Honesty should always be a hallmark of the discussion. In a terrorism event, remind children that there are people who do "bad" things. Children need to understand that not all people of like origin or beliefs do bad things. Age-appropriate explanations are essential. Discuss the event to decrease the anxiety associated with the event. Silence may suggest the event is too dreadful to discuss (AAP, 2003g; Milgram, 2002). Children have difficulty differentiating between fantasy and reality. Some violence they see on television is real and some is pretend. Young children have vivid imaginations, and what they imagine may be much worse than reality. Children need someone they can trust. They need adults who can help them master both anxiety and reality. Caretakers should correct children's interpretation and misconceptions of what happened when necessary. Children need simple, truthful explanations of the situation, explained in a way that they can understand. This will help them accept the situation in a realistic way. Children need information pertaining to the experiences they will encounter. It is helpful when parents can let children know that the nurse or health care worker will help the parent to help the children (Cieslak & Henretig, 2003; Rogers, 2003; Schonfeld, 2003).

If the parent or caretaker can honestly do so, reassure children that they are safe. When parents reassure fearful children and explain what they have done to help ensure children's safety and protection, children are better able to cope with disaster (AAP, 2003d; Schonfeld, 2003). Reassuring comments when spoken calmly decrease anxiety (Figure 10–10). Such comments might include:

"I will be there to take care of you."

"I am going to take care of you."

"You don't need to be afraid."

"Everyone's doing the best they can to help us."

"I have done everything that I can to keep you safe."(AAP, 2003d, p. 1)

When the disaster is in an isolated area, inform children of that fact, and assure them that they are safe and will not be harmed. Children need time to process information and adults need to be physically available for further discussion.

Family-Centered Care During Disaster Situations

Children and adolescents are particularly vulnerable to the stresses of disaster because they experience a change from their usual routine, and because they have limited or immature coping skills. Separation from family, familiar objects, and routines, especially at young ages and in difficult situations, causes significant anxiety. Children need time to learn to trust others and form new attachments. The nature of the disaster situation is such that this is extremely difficult at best. Therefore, it is essential to have a communication plan that includes family contact information and a method to reunite families as quickly as possible. Directing families to have identification tags for all family members and to have designated "rallying points" enables this process. Having a "go box," a box that can be taken when a crisis occurs, that contains safety items as well as a favorite object, such as a stuffed animal, will lessen the stress of the situation. Feelings of loss of control are caused by unfamiliar environmental stimuli, physical restriction, altered routine, and dependency. Resuming usual routines and normal activities benefits the entire family and helps children feel stronger and less insecure. Pediatric health care professionals should foster parent-child relations and promote self-mastery of children. An important goal of predisaster counseling is to make the situation less strange and frightening to parents, children, and adolescents. This means that professionals must anticipate possible disaster scenarios and prepare a mock disaster drill that includes practice of essential safety routines.

Developmental Considerations

While children develop at their own pace, stages of development correspond to specific age ranges. "Children's developmental ability and cognitive levels may impede their ability to escape danger" (Markenson & Redlener, 2003, p. 2). Children need care based on their level of physical and psychosocial development.

0 to 3 Years of Age

Infants and toddlers are fully dependent on adults because of their developmental vulnerabilities. This age cannot appreciate the significance and danger of the event, but they can sense that something is wrong, Figure 10–11. They will cry and be afraid and may cling to available adults and display regressive behaviors. They have neither the motor skills, nor cognitive ability to evaluate and flee the situation. Until age two years children do not have a cognitive understanding of death. Children from two to five years view death as reversible and temporary. If they are mad at a friend and the friend dies; guilt is pervasive. "What infants and toddlers need from parents after a disaster is their usual loving care" (Leavitt, 2001, p. 7). If they have been separated from their parents or guardians, children need to be reunited with them as promptly as possible. These children need to have their basic needs of food, warmth, and shelter (a quiet, private area) met. They need to be held and comforted, and spoken to quietly and softly. They are used to a particular style of interaction and benefit from usual activities. Such games as the "Itsy, Bitsy Spider," "Pat-a-Cake," "So Big," and the usual stories read prior to the disaster will be comforting to them (Henderson, 2003; Leavitt, 2001, p. 7).

3 to 6 Years of Age

Because very young children in this age group are incapable of verbal expression of their anxieties and fears, these are usually expressed in play. Young children need opportunities for nondirected play with restrictions only in so far as safety is concerned. Children are able to tolerate anxiety

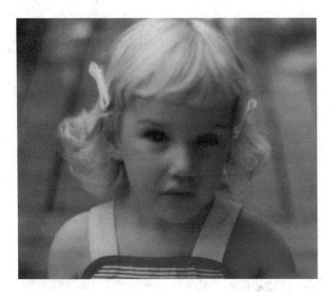

Figure 10–10. Reassurance.

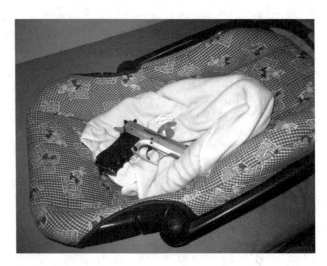

Figure 10–11. Gun in child safety seat.

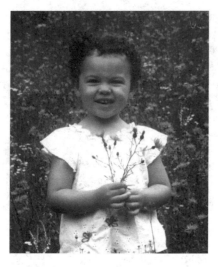

Figure 10–12. Developmental stage.

through the use of fantasy and play, which allows them to break events down into manageable parts (Figure 10–12). It helps children master the reality of the world. Older children in this age group are incapable of mature verbal expression and moral reasoning of right and wrong. They may believe that something they did caused the event. Adults can reassure these children that they did not cause the event. These children often experience nightmares, so a nightlight may be helpful for them. Children need adults who can empathize or feel with them. They need the loving care of adults and family and a return to familiar surroundings, toys, and their normal daily routine. Parents and health care workers who can observe and listen to children's play will gain understanding of the meaning of the event to the child. Only then will the parent or health care provider be able to support and guide the child. Leavitt (2001) believes these children ask questions because they are insecure and suggests reassuring children with comments such as, "Mommy loves you and is here to take care of you" (Henderson, 2003; Seideman et al., 1998).

6 to 12 Years of Age

School-age children have the cognitive ability to comprehend what has happened during a disaster situation. They may become alarmed, frightened, and fearful for their safety. These children may have nightmares and problems eating. Because they understand the difference between right and wrong, they may be bewildered about the circumstances surrounding the event. They may be angry. These children are aware of the irreversibility and inevitability of death. In the latter years of this age group, children have abstract reasoning about death and begin to understand death much as an adult understands death. They know all people die and that they could die (AAP, 2003d; Henderson, 2003; Seideman et al., 1998).

These children need adults who are available to listen to them, available for questions, and able to discuss the

events that have transpired (see "Communication" earlier in the chapter). Leavitt (2001) suggests that significant adults express feelings of sadness, but add reassurance for children. For example, "I am sad about what happened, but I am happy that we are together" (p. 11). These children need step-by-step general information of events as they are unfolding. Their involvement in recovery activities can be elicited to help them cope with the situation. They need familiar surroundings and a return to the structure of their daily routines. They should return to school as soon as possible. Peers are essential for this age group and a return to activities with their friends will help them cope with the event (Henderson, 2003; Seideman et al., 1998).

12 to 18 Years of Age

At times of crises, adolescents may seem self-centered. Adults need to be aware that this is a normal initial reaction and should not find fault or berate teens for these egocentric feelings (Schonfeld, 2003). Adolescents are developing a sense of identity and are "trying on" values and beliefs in an attempt to discern which ones are important to them, which ones "fit." They still need assistance when these values and beliefs are "put to the test." Adolescents may experience a variety of emotions. They may feel sad and/or angry. Initially, they may want to strike out at those responsible for the event. They will need help directing their feelings of anger. They may experience difficulty sleeping (AAP, 2003d; Henderson, 2003; Leavitt, 2001; Seideman et al., 1998).

Adolescents will communicate with their peers about the situation, but will be interested in parents' thoughts and feelings (see "Communication" earlier in the chapter). They need to know that parents will listen to them, discuss events, and "are still available to help and protect them" (Leavitt, 2001, p. 13). Adolescents can be included in advance planning and be encouraged to help during the time surrounding the event. These young adults need familiar surroundings and a return to normal routines as soon as possible. Returning to normal routines helps them feel secure (AAP, 2003d; Henderson, 2003; Seideman et al., 1998).

Before a Disaster

Pediatric health care professionals can ascertain and evaluate resources available in the local area that contain timely and accurate information. They can make this information available to parents or caretakers of children. Issues related to children are underrepresented at local, state, and regional planning meetings for preparation for disasters. Pediatric specialty care experts can be advocates for children and families by working with federal, state, and local legislatures to develop a disaster plan or response plan and protocols that are inclusive of children. Decontamination systems should be designed "so that they can be used for decontamination of children for all ages (including infants), of the parentless child, of the non-ambulatory child, and of the child with special health care needs" (Markenson & Redlener, 2003, p. 12). Pediatric health care facilities are best suited to care for children. It is essential that pediatric equipment be available at all locations at which children may be treated. Pediatric specialty resource centers (facilities with particular expertise in a particular area, such as critical care or trauma) can be designated at the regional and state level. Pediatric health care professionals can influence policy by volunteering their services (Markenson & Redlinger, 2003; Schwarz & Kennedy, 2003).

To further correct the pediatric underrepresentation discrepancy, involvement of professional and advocacy organizations with significant membership may be the most effective way to bring about necessary legislative changes. Some pediatric health care professionals often site lack of knowledge of disasters as a reason for nonparticipation, but their presence has been found to be helpful because they have expertise in caring for children. Using a team approach involving members of the disciplines of pediatric health care, psychology, education, parenting, and social work enhances understanding of the unique issues of child victims. "Collaborative leadership skills consolidate expertise and strengthen response to prevention, preparation, and recovery on behalf of children in regard to . . . disasters" (Blaschke, Palfrey, & Lynch, 2003, p. 273).

It is suggested that the family have a meeting and develop a disaster plan. The plan should be practiced regularly, about every six months. It should include several escape routes from the home and places to meet in case family members get separated. These meeting places are called "rally points." It is helpful to establish rally points at each location where members of the family spend a significant amount of time e.g., schools, neighborhood, and workplaces. It is suggested that families have an out-of-state family or friend as a single contact for all the members of the family. Each family member should have some form of identification. Child identification cards are paramount, as is a list of emergency contact phone numbers or e-mail addresses. The AAP suggests that children be warned, but not overly alarmed about disasters. Children should be reminded that there are people who can help them, and be taught how to call for help. Supplies that should be included in a disaster kit are listed in Mulligan-Smith's family readiness kit (2003) and the AAP's "Four Steps to Safety Readiness." Note that it is important that children have protective clothing, rain gear, and sturdy shoes (AAP, 2003h, 2003i, 2003j).

Once a disaster plan has been developed, it must be practiced on a routine basis. Preschool through adolescent children benefit from active participation in disaster drills. These drills provide an opportunity to detect problems and make appropriate changes prior to their implementation in an actual event. They should take place in a variety of settings. Encouraging parents to participate in disaster drills and to try to take the perspective of their child can be helpful in calling attention to problematic areas.

Pediatric health care professionals can act as advisors to caretakers and personnel in schools, day care facilities, after-school programs, and health and social welfare agencies in the area. They can work with community resources on the local level such as the health department and poison control center. Pediatric health care professionals can conduct formal and informal sessions with those who work directly with children, at the local school, church, or community center. These locations help to reach the largest number of people (Davidhizar & Shearer, 2002).

During a Disaster

Triage, decontamination, and treatment are initiated during this phase of the disaster. Each of these processes must be child and age specific. An important consideration during a disaster is communication and consultation among facilities as well as between facilities, children, and their families. Pediatric health care professionals care for children and their families in both the physical and psychosocial realms during a disaster. Injured children will need to have caregivers who are knowledgeable in the signs, symptoms, and treatment of specific types of disaster-related illnesses discussed earlier in the chapter. Further, many families will benefit from counseling for mental health issues (AAP, 2003d).

Children may be frightened by the activity during a disaster. Reactions may include running, yelling or screaming, or looking anxious or even terrified. People may be wearing protective gear including suits, gas masks or goggles. Children may be confused and frightened by the appearance of those around them and they may try to flee from the situation.

After a Disaster

All those who work with children will need to be aware not only of the range of normal reactions to a disaster, but also of the unusual or prolonged and persistent reactions. See Box 10–1. Knowledgeable health care workers can instruct those who work with children about these reactions. Further, they can evaluate children and refer them when appropriate. Community and religious organizations will need to be included in the recovery plan (AAP, 1999).

Media

Media coverage of these events is immediate and continuous in bringing images of the events into the homes of millions of families. Parents and children are able to watch

BOX 10–1   Lessons Learned: Disasters and Children

(All names are fictitious, but the events are true)

Newborn

Anna's first words after the delivery were, "It is a boy, he will have to go to the Army." These words express the thoughts of many pregnant women in Israel. As a nurse, there is no solution one can give, only hope that when Anna's child reaches the age of 18 there will be no need for him to serve in the army.

Toddler

Rimais, 37 years old, is married and the mother of four children. The youngest, Mona, was five months old when Rima was seriously injured in a city bus explosion on her way to work. Rima was hospitalized seven months, undergoing surgery several times, as well as spending time in rehabilitation. Today, 13 months after the incident, she is able to work part time. However, several metal splinters remain in her neck and she is unable to lift anything heavy. Mona is still unable to relate to her mother as a normal 18-month-old toddler. She is angry at her mother, does not want to be comforted or held by her, and cries often. Rima is extremely upset and has great difficulty understanding her daughter. The family is receiving psychotherapy to help them return to a normal family life. This is but one example of how a disaster affects the life of a young infant; the long-term influences are as yet unknown.

School Age

The Chen family had two children, a nine-year-old son, Mano, and a 14-year-old daughter. The girl was killed instantly by a suicide bomber while eating a snack with friends. Since the incident two years ago, Mano has developed learning and behavioral problems. He does not

want to listen to his parents, is abusive to age mates and his grades are barely passing. While talking with Mano, it became clear that he was angry at his parents for allowing his sister to go that afternoon. He also expressed jealousy and felt that nobody was paying any attention to his achievements and problems. The family is receiving family therapy after a long period of individual counseling.

Some of the problems in the Chen family may have been prevented if someone had prepared the parents for these expected changes in Mano's behavior. Early intervention may have resulted in a shorter period of therapy. Today, the family continues to need help and it is unclear what the long-term effects will be for Mano.

Preadolescence

On her way home from school Sara, age 14, witnessed a stabbing in which the victim was killed. She hardly talked about the incident and continued her regular activities. Two months later, she was in town when a bomb exploded. She only heard the blast but learned later that one of her schoolmates was killed. Since the second event, she started waking up frequently with nightmares, expressed fear when having to leave the house and did not want to stay home alone. After she began to fail exams at school, Sara stopped showing interest in her studies. Her sister, serving in the army at the time of the incident, tried to talk to her but all discussions ended in unpleasant arguments.

Today, almost two years later, after receiving therapy, Sara is trying to catch up at school. Her parents and sister have learned a difficult lesson; one does not have to be physically hurt in order to need help. In this case, the treatment should have started much earlier. Nurses have the ability and should take the opportunity to increase the awareness of teachers, parents and siblings regarding the influence that these events can have on a teenager.

---

the unfolding story on television, listen to the radio announcer, read widely publicized newspaper and magazine articles, and log on to the Internet at any time of the day or night. Media often present unnecessarily graphic details. Stories in the media bring the event closer to home by identifying people from the area, making the experience a personal one. Young children are not able to differentiate between actual events and replays of the events. It is important to limit media exposure, as repeated viewing of the event may continue to traumatize children and adolescents. School-age children may become alarmed and fearful because they are able to comprehend what has happened. Responsible adults should participate (listen, watch, and discuss with children) and supervise media exposure. They should discourage classroom viewing of live

coverage of the events (Leavitt, 2001; Milgram, 2003; Schonfeld, 2003; Seideman et al., 1998).

OPTIMIZING ENVIRONMENTS FOR HEALTHY CHILDREN

The school nurse has a critical role in developing and implementing strategies to assist children during a disaster situation. As mentioned, adults must take care of themselves so they have the physical energy and emotional resources to be able to assist children. The initial reaction to the disaster will depend upon the physical surroundings, including property damage, and the number and type of injuries and fatalities that occur. The first concern is restoring the safety and security of those affected by the event. Once these concerns are being met, affective reactions can be considered (Milgram, 2002).

The school should establish a policy that describes procedures to follow before, during, and after a disaster. A comprehensive plan will consider the needs of students, parents, faculty and staff. It is important to create a crises management team to establish this policy. The team should consist of the school nurse, school administrator, psychologist, guidance counselors, social workers, a security representative, and a custodian. Further, it is helpful to include members from the community such as law enforcement, the fire department, and public health agencies. The inclusion of these members increases the knowledge and resources available to the school community. It is essential that the team train periodically and establish a formal chain of command (Milgram, 2002).

An important element of this plan is the system of communication. The effectiveness of the plan depends on the group's ability to reach key personnel. There must be a way for the school community to access information to report safety and related concerns. Suggested means of communication consist of published hotline numbers, school district call-in lines, websites, television, and radio. Including community members on the planning committee expands resources to increase response capacity and lessen the burden on school resources (Milgram, 2002).

The school nurse can develop and maintain a "go box," a box that the nurse can take when a crisis occurs. The contents of the box should include the following:

- List of students and staff
- List of students and staff with significant health problems
- Medication list
- Blueprint of school property
- Evacuation plan
- Walkie-talkies
- Cell phone or beeper
- Current yearbook
- Phone numbers

It is helpful to have a second box available as a backup (Milgram, 2002).

There are several points to be considered that are specific to the school situation. It is important to maintain structure within the school. Classes should not be canceled and students should not be sent home early. When school is dismissed early, parents have additional concerns about the welfare of their children (Milgram, 2002).

After a disaster, children who previously have been eager to go to school may have mixed feelings or concerns about their own safety or the safety of family members. Children may need a personal belonging to comfort them. They may need the freedom to contact a parent(s) to ascertain that the parents are safe. Parents can reassure children that teachers are there to help them. Knowing that teachers were once children themselves and understand children's fears may help children return to school. Remind children that the reason these adults wanted to be teachers was that they like children and want to help them (Milgram, 2002).

Summary

Children have special needs. They are more vulnerable to the effects of a disaster, physiologically and psychologically. These needs often go unrecognized by health care professionals. In a time of crisis, it is essential that health care professionals consider these unique vulnerabilities in both planning and caring for children during disaster situations (Markenson & Redlener, 2003).

Case Study

School Explosion

It is 10 A.M. on a cool April morning at Dublin Elementary School. Dublin is a small, rural seven-classroom building where 160 kindergarteners and elementary students through grade 6 attend school. The school nurse has been busy seeing youngsters with minor complaints of headache, runny noses, and swollen, tearing eyes all morning—allergies run high in the small community of Dublin this time of year. Suddenly a hissing sound is heard, followed by a loud explosion. The explosion shatters windows, and belches smoke and steam. The roof collapses in the east wing, where a classroom of kindergarteners and first graders are in class.

- What should the teachers in the west wing of the building immediately do?
- What should the administrators, including the school nurse, who are centered in offices between the east and west wings do?

As the school nurse, you realize you have been unhurt and place an immediate call to 911. You then go to the classroom and see children and teachers down. The steam has decreased, but smoke persists.

- What should you do?

EMS responds and declares the scene safe for entry and asks you, the school nurse, to aid them in assessing and triaging children for transport.

- What types of injuries would you anticipate from the blast?

It is determined that the blast is a result of a faulty boiler that provides steam for the school furnace system.

- Describe critical first steps in assessment and resuscitation stabilization of the victims.
- Describe differences in airway assessment and management of the children versus the adult teachers and aide who were also involved in the blast.

TEST YOUR KNOWLEDGE

1. Which of the following specific measures can parents and professionals take to minimize the disaster's traumatic effects on children?

   A. Distract children with TV viewing of the event
   B. Let children express their feelings and name their fears
   C. Separate children from their parents, treatment for children is different from treatment for adults
   D. All of the above

2. Children are particularly vulnerable to terrorist attacks or disasters because of

   A. Past experiences
   B. Social class
   C. Unique physical and cognitive aspects of development
   D. All of the above

3. When children are exposed to a stressful event such as a disaster, they may react with

   1. Regression
   2. Disinterest
   3. Sleep disturbances (sleep too little or too much)
   4. Introversion
      A. 1 and 2
      B. 1 and 3
      C. 2 and 3
      D. All of the above

4. The school nurse has a critical role in developing and implementing strategies to assist children during a disaster. The plan should

   A. Include preparation of a "go box"
   B. Include cancellation of classes and sending children home immediately
   C. Exclude disaster drills as these create anxiety
   D. Limit communication with those outside the school except parents

5. Pediatric health care providers lessen the impact of mass casualty disasters upon children and their families by which of the following?

   1. Have a plan of action in place and update it regularly
   2. Be knowledgeable and instruct the public in comfortable, small group sessions
   3. Practice evacuation techniques including donning protective gear such as gas masks, protective suits, and use of sealed rooms
   4. Inform children about the event as soon as possible
   5. Be a member of a disaster preparation committee
      A. 1, 2, and 3
      B. 2, 3, and 4
      C. 1, 3, and 5
      D. All of the above

6. Two factors that would increase the child's inhalation of chemical or biological agents are

   1. Greater concentration of molecules dispersed within the child's breathing space
   2. Greater number of alveoli in the pediatric pulmonary system
   3. Greater minute ventilation rate
   4. Younger children are mouth breathers allowing for more molecules to enter the respiratory system
      A. 1 and 2
      B. 1 and 3
      C. 2 and 3
      D. 2 and 4
      E. 3 and 4

7. Children are at greater risk of dehydration and shock when ricin or SEB are ingested due to lower total circulating blood flow. Identify any early symptoms of impending shock and the need for circulatory support.

   1. Rosy skin color and temperature warm to the touch
   2. Decreased blood pressure
   3. Decrease in tissue perfusion due to increased vascular resistance resulting in a prolonged capillary refill, in the normothermic child
   4. Increase in heart rate
      A. 1 and 2
      B. 1 and 3
      C. 2 and 3
      D. 2 and 4
      E. 3 and 1

8. Children are at greater risk to absorption of biological, chemical, and radiation disasters because

   A. They have a thinner integumentary system
   B. They have larger body surface areas in proportion to their weight
   C. They may not cognitively comprehend risks of exposure and be exposed for greater lengths of time before leaving environments of risk
   D. All of above are correct

9. Blast injuries increase the likelihood that children will experience blunt internal trauma. The major organs at risk are

   A. Kidneys
   B. Lungs
   C. Spleen and liver
   D. Colon

10. Caretakers of children exposed to radiation should take which of the following steps?

    A. Immediate removal of contaminated clothing and discarding such in an appropriate receptacle

    B. Skin washed with cold water to decrease the occurrence of topical radiation burning
    C. Administration of potassium iodine for significant exposure
    D. A and C
    E. A and B

See Test Yourself Answers in Appendix B.

EXPLORE MEDIALINK

Interactive resources and an audio glossary for this chapter can be found on the Companion Website at http://www.prenhall.com/langan. Click on Chapter 10 to select the activities for this chapter.

REFERENCES

Along, G. (2003). *Terror leaves 42% of children with PTSD.* Retrieved June 6, 2003, from http://www.haaretz.com/hasen/pages/ShArt.jhtml?itemNo=300638

American Academy of Pediatrics (AAP). (1999). How pediatricians can respond to the psychosocial implications of disasters (RE9813). *Pediatrics, 103,* 521–523.

American Academy of Pediatrics (AAP). (2000). Policy statement: Chemical-biological terrorism and its impact on children: A subject review (RE 9959). *Pediatrics, 105,* 662–670.

American Academy of Pediatrics (AAP). (2003a). *Radiation disasters and children policy statement.* Retrieved June 23, 2003, from http://www.aap.org

American Academy of Pediatrics (AAP). (2003b). *Radiation disasters and children.* Retrieved June 23, 2003, from http://www.aap.org/policy/radiation.html

American Academy of Pediatrics (AAP). (2003c). *Children, terrorism and disasters.* Retrieved June 23, 2003, from http://www.aap.org/advocacy/releases/disasterpreparedness.html

American Academy of Pediatrics (AAP). (2003d). *Meeting children's needs in a disaster.* Retrieved May 21, 2003, from http://www.aap.org/advocacy/releases/disaster.html

American Academy of Pediatrics (AAP). (2003e). *Advice for parents.* Retrieved June 23, 2003, from http://www.aap.org/advocacy/archives.cochapter

American Academy of Pediatrics (AAP). (2003f). *Testimony before the Senate Committee on Health Education, Labor and Pensions Subcommittee on Children and Families.* Retrieved June 23, 2003, from http://www.aap.org/advocacy/washington/dr%5fwright.html

American Academy of Pediatrics (AAP). (2003g). *Meeting children's needs in a disaster.* Retrieved June 23, 2003, from http://www.aap.org/advocacy/releases/disaster.html

American Academy of Pediatrics (AAP). (2003h). *Four steps to safety readiness.* Retrieved June 23, 2003, from http://www.aap.org/family/tipp4steps.html

American Academy of Pediatrics (AAP). (2003i). *Family readiness kit.* Retrieved June 23, 2003, from http://www.aap.org/family/frk/frkit29.html

American Academy of Pediatrics (AAP). (2003j). *Family readiness kit.* Retrieved June 23, 2003, from http://www.aap.org/family/frk/frkit.html

Balk, S., & Miller, R. (2002). FDA issues KI recommendations. *AAP News, 20,* 99–103.

Betz, C. L., & Sowden, L. A. (2004). *Mosby's pediatric nursing reference.* St. Louis: Mosby.

Blaschke, G. S., Palfrey, J. S., & Lynch, J. (2003). Advocating for children during uncertain times. *Pediatric Annals, 32,* 271–274.

Brazelton, T. B., & Greenspan, S. I. (2000). *The irreducible needs of children: What every child must have to grow, learn, and flourish.* Cambridge: Perseus.

Burklow, T. R., Yu, C. E., & Madsen, J. M. (2003). Industrial chemicals: Terrorist weapons of opportunity. *Pediatric Annals, 32,* 230–234.

Center for Disease Control and Prevention (CDC). (2003). Mass trauma preparedness and response: Explosions and blast injuries, a primer for clinicians. Retrieved June 23, 2003, from www.cdc.gov

Cieslak, E. Y., & Henretig, F. M. (2003). Bioterrorism. *Pediatric Annals, 32,* 154–164.

Davidhizar, R., & Shearer, R. (2002). Helping children cope with public disasters: Support given immediately after a traumatic event can counteract or even negate long-term adverse effects. *American Journal of Nursing, 102,* 26–33.

DeHart, G. B., Sroufe, L. A., & Cooper, R. G. (2004). *Child development: Its nature and course* (5th ed.). St. Louis: McGraw-Hill.

Eichelberger, M. (1993). *Pediatric trauma, prevention, acute care, rehabilitation*. St. Louis: Mosby.

Hanze, D. (2002). How to help children and adolescents deal with the threat of terrorism. *Journal for Specialists in Pediatric Nursing, 7,* 42–44.

Hazinski, M. F. (1992). *Nursing care of the critically ill child.* St. Louis: Mosby.

Hazinski, M. F., Zaritsky, A., Nakarni, V., Hickey, R., Schexnayder, S., & Berg, R. (2002). *PALS provider manual.* Dallas, TX: American Heart Association.

Henderson, D. P. (2003, June 26). Meeting the needs of children in disasters. Speech presented at Pacific Emergency Medical Services for Children Regional Symposium, Corvallis, OR.

Hurt, H., Malmud, E., Brobsky, N. L., & Gianetta, J. (2001). Exposure to violence: Psychological and academic correlates in child witnesses. *Archives of Pediatrics and Adolescent Medicine 155,* 1351–1356.

Institute of Medicine (IOM). (2003, June). *Preparing for the psychological consequences of terrorism: A public health strategy.* Washington, DC: National Academy of Sciences.

Israel Defense Force (IDF). (2003). *Spokesperson's unit home front command. Protected space/shelters –guidelines.* Retrieved June 12, 2003, from http://www.idf.il

Kidsforkids. (2003). Retrieved June 12, 2003, from www.kidsforkids.net/where-heading.html

Leavitt, L. A. (2001). When terrible things happen: A parent's guide to talking with their children (Brochure HE3017 AB01-B318). International Pediatric Association, American Academy of Pediatrics, Johnson & Johnson Pediatric Institute, Johnson & Johnson Consumer Companies, Inc.

Markenson, D., & Redlener, I. (2003). *Pediatric preparedness for disaster and terrorism.* A National Consensus Conference, Executive Summary, Mailman School of Public Health. New York: Columbia University.

Mesa City Fire Department. (2003). *Mark I kits.* Retrieved June 24, 2003, from http://www.heds.org/Mark%201%20Kit%20'02Conf.pdf

Milgram, G. G. (Developer). (2002). Impact of disaster on children in our schools: A program for school nurses. (Available from The Education and Training Division, Center of Alcohol Studies, Rutgers, The State University of New Jersey, 607 Allison Road, Piscataway, NJ 08854-8001).

Mulligan-Smith, D. (2003). *Family Readiness Kit: Preparing to handle disasters.* Retrieved April 28, 2003, from http://www.aap.org/family/frk/frkit/html

Quinn-Doggett, K., Stewart-Craig, E., & Doak, M. (1998). *Domestic preparedness training program.* Bethesda, MD: Booz-Allen and Hamilton Inc. & Science Applications International Corporation.

Rogers, A. P. (2003). *Bioterrorism reader.* New York: Nova Science.

Rotenberg, J. S. (2003). Diagnosis and management of nerve agent exposure. *Pediatric Annals, 32,* 242–250.

Schonfeld, D. (2003). Supporting children after terrorist events: Potential roles for pediatricians. *Pediatric Annnals, 32,* 182–187.

Schwarz, T., & Kennedy, M. (2003). Disaster volunteer teams: Where to go when you want to help. *American Journal of Nursing AJN, 103,* 64AA–64DD.

Seideman, R. Y., Hutchison, B., Buckner, S. K., Myers, S. T., Miller-Boyle, D., Macrobert, M., & Heath, S. (1998). The responses of children to disaster: Do children have a greater depth of response to tragedy than we realize. *The American Journal of Maternal/Child Nursing, 23,* 37–44.

Waecker, N. J., & Hale, B. R. (2003). Smallpox vaccination: What the pediatrician needs to know. *Pediatric Annals, 32,* 178–181.

Yu, C. E. (2003). Medical response to radiation-related terrorism. *Pediatric Annals, 32,* 169–176.

Yu, C. E., Burklow, T. R., & Madsen, J. M. (2003). Vesicant agents and children. *Pediatric Annals, 32,* 254–257.

CHAPTER 11

The Role of the Infection Control Nurse in Disaster Preparedness

Terri Rebmann

LEARNING OBJECTIVES

1. Describe the phases of the emergency management model.
2. Define the role of the infection control nurse in disaster preparedness, response, recovery, and mitigation.
3. List resources that can help infection control nurses become better prepared to respond to natural and man-made disasters, as well as chemical and biological terrorism.

MEDIALINK **www.prenhall.com/langan**

Resources for this chapter can be found on the Companion Website at http://www.prenhall.com/langan. Click on Chapter 11 to select the activities for this chapter.

CHAPTER OUTLINE

Know Your Terms
Audio Glossary
Web Links
    Bioterrorism Resources
    Infection Control Resources
MediaLink Applications

GLOSSARY

Active surveillance. Direct solicitation of data from others participating in the active surveillance program that is used to detect a change or trend in the health of a population

Consequence management. The second phase of a disaster, during which FEMA is the lead federal agency. The ultimate goal of consequence management is to manage and minimize the impact of the event on the community and return to normal functioning

Crisis management. The first phase of a disaster, during which the FBI is the lead federal agency. Crisis management involves either identifying perpetrators before an attack occurs or taking steps to identify the perpetrators after an attack has occurred with the ultimate goal of capturing the perpetrators and preventing additional attacks

Decontamination. The process of removing pathogenic microorganisms from objects or people

Epidemiology. The scientific study of disease frequency, determinants of disease, and the distribution of disease in a population

Epidemiological investigation. The use of epidemiology tools to establish person, place, and time associated with an outbreak

Hospital emergency incident command system. A hospital-based incident command system used as a framework for reporting and communication, which entails assignment of specific roles to individuals in an effort to create a distinct chain of command that temporarily enacts in response to a disaster situation

Incident command system. A framework for reporting and communication, which entails assignment of specific roles to individuals in an effort to create a distinct chain of command that temporarily enacts in response to a disaster situation

Mitigation. The last phase of the emergency management model, during which sustained activities are undertaken to prevent or minimize the negative impact of an event. Mitigation also describes interventions to either prevent or reduce morbidity and mortality, and ease the economic and social impact of the event on the affected community

Passive surveillance. Data collected solely from unsolicited source reports, and are used to detect a change or trend in the health of a population

Performance measurement. A formal process for evaluating the level of disaster preparedness for a facility or community

Preparedness. The first phase of the emergency management model, during which all of the measures taken in preparing to handle an emergency, such as developing a plan and educating the workforce, are accomplished

Prophylaxis. Medication or vaccination provided to exposed or potentially exposed individuals in an attempt to decrease morbidity and mortality associated with the exposure

Recovery. The third phase of the emergency management model, during which all of the measures taken to effectively recover from an emergency and return a facility or community to baseline are accomplished

Response. The second phase of the emergency management model, during which all of the measures taken to effectively respond to an emergency, such as implementation of the disaster response plan and patient management, are accomplished

Risk communication. The science of communicating effectively in situations that are of high concern, sensitive, or controversial. Risk communication principles serve to create an appropriate level of outrage that is in direct proportion to the level of risk or hazard

Surveillance. The process of collecting and analyzing data to detect a change or trend in the health of the population

Syndromic surveillance. Collecting and analyzing nontraditional data to detect a change or trend in the health of a population. Traditionally, syndromic surveillance referred to the collection and analysis of syndrome-related data, but has expanded to include almost any nontraditional data that may indicate a potential bioterrorism event has occurred

INTRODUCTION

Infection control professionals have a vital role in maintaining the health of patients, visitors, and employees in their facilities and the community. Most infection control professionals began their careers as nurses or laboratory microbiologists. Their varied experience in both nursing and infection control provides them with a unique skill set that helps them prepare for and respond to different types of disasters.

As experts in the fields of surveillance and epidemiology, infection control nurses (ICNs) are responsible for investigating outbreaks and initiating interventions to prevent the transmission of infections that occur within health care. These epidemiological skills are well matched with the infection control professional's nursing background. During a disaster response, the infection control nurse must utilize both epidemiological and nursing skills. It will be crucial for the infection control nurse to work with all nursing departments before, during, and after a crisis to ensure an effective disaster response.

Because the infection control impact of a disaster will vary depending on the nature of the emergency, infection control nurses must be familiar with the different types of disasters and the potential consequences of each. However, while interventions will vary with different types of disaster, the general principles of surveillance and epidemiology remain the same.

Historically, the role of ICNs in emergency management has centered more on disaster response than disaster planning. Following the terrorist events of September 11, 2001, and the subsequent bioterrorism attacks using anthrax-laden letters, the role of ICNs has broadened to include preparedness responsibilities in addition to response duties.

EMERGENCY MANAGEMENT MODEL

To better understand the role of infection control and disaster management, many organizations and facilities apply the emergency management model created by the Federal Emergency Management Agency (FEMA) as the basis for their disaster planning (FEMA, 1998). The emergency management model, designed to visually display the process of facility or community preparation for emergencies, consists of four activity phases in a continuous process: preparation, response, recovery, and mitigation. Rather than displaying a simple numbered sequence starting with preparedness and ending with mitigation, this model presents a continuous cycle in which the phases can overlap or occur simultaneously (Figure 11–1). Moreover, the emergency management model emphasizes evaluation and applying lessons learned to future events. A brief, sequential description of each phase follows with an in-depth discussion of interventions for the preparedness and response phases.

The preparedness phase involves all of the measures taken in preparing to handle an emergency, such as developing a plan and educating the workforce. This is followed by the response phase, when the plan developed in the first phase is implemented. The two central components of the response phase are patient management and communication. The recovery phase of the emergency management model consists of the interventions needed to return a facility and/or community to its predisaster baseline as soon as possible. Another important component of the recovery phase is responding to the mental health impact on the community, including dealing with patients suffering from post traumatic stress disorder (PTSD). During the final phase, mitigation, sustained activities are undertaken to prevent or minimize the negative impact of an event. These include interventions to either prevent or reduce

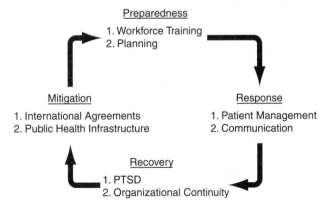

Figure 11–1. Emergency management model. *Source: Adapted from Principles of Emergency Management Student Manual (DHHS Publication No. 1998-622-686/93421) by Federal Emergency Management Agency, 1998, Washington, DC: U.S. Government Printing Office.*

morbidity and mortality, and ease the economic and social impact of the event on the affected community.

Preparedness

What is the role of the infection control nurse in preparing for a disaster? The ICN has the following seven duties:

- Assessment
- Education/training
- Surveillance
- Epidemiology
- Plan development
- Communication
- Performance measurement

Assessments During Preparedness Phase

There are four types of assessments that should be performed to prepare for an emergency. As we do not know which type of emergency is going to occur, an all-hazards approach is preferable. In this way, facilities are prepared for almost any emergency that may arise, from a flood to a terrorist attack.

The first type of assessment that should be performed is a risk assessment of the facility and community. In some cases this will be easy: Most communities are acutely aware if they are in a flood- or earthquake-prone area. Some risks are impossible to calculate, however. There is no easy way to determine the risk of a chemical or biological attack in a community. One option may be for a facility to assess its use, storage methods, and security system for chemicals and biological agents that could be used in a chemical or biological attack. Does the facility have large, unsecured containers of dangerous chemicals, such as ammonia or chlorine, that could cause morbidity and mortality if used as weapons? It would not be the ICN's role to assess the amount and type of chemicals stored at a facility, but the ICN should realize the risk and effectively communicate the need to assess for this threat.

Terrorism is on the rise, and there are more terrorist groups than ever before. Since 1996, the FBI has tracked 37 incidents of weapons of mass destruction (WMD) threats. In 2000, this number increased sevenfold to 257 threats (U.S. Department of Justice, Federal Bureau of Investigations, 1999). See Figure 11–2.

In addition to the increase in number of WMD threats, the threatened method of attack has shifted. According to the FBI, the number of nuclear, chemical, and biological WMD threats was approximately the same in 1997, but just a year later, biological agents had become the most frequently threatened method of attack (U.S. Department of Justice, Federal Bureau of Investigations, 1999). Bioterrorism accounted for more than half of the WMD threats in 1998. See Figure 11–3. In the fall of 2001, those threats became reality in the United States

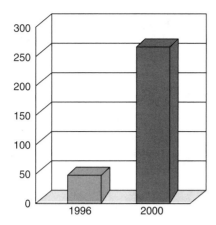

Figure 11–2. Number of weapons of mass destruction threats. *(Source: From* Terrorism in the United States, 1999 *by U.S. Department of Justice, Federal Bureau of Investigations, Counterterrorism Threat Assessment and Warning Unit Counterterrorism Division, 1999,* available from Federal Bureau of Investigations website, *http://www.fbi.org)*

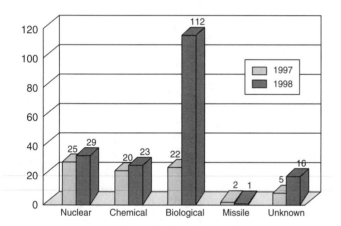

Figure 11–3. Weapons of mass destruction FBI investigations. Opened 1997–1999. *(Source: From* Terrorism in the United States, 1999. *U.S. Department of Justice, Federal Bureau of Investigations, Counterterrorism Threat Assessment and Warning Unit Counterterrorism Division, 1999,* available from Federal Bureau of Investigations website, *http://www.fbi.org)*

when anthrax was used as a bioterrorism agent in the form of letters mailed to various media organizations and politicians. More recently, the 2003 war in Iraq raised fear of a possible dirty bomb or chemical terrorism attack. Though the probability of such attacks is low, their potentially devastating consequences require preparation and vigilance.

Self-assessment is also crucial for infection control nurses, and includes knowledge and personal risk assessment. ICNs must assess their current knowledge base of disasters and take advantage of educational opportunities to increase their level of knowledge. Although it is not necessary to memorize all of the information, such as the clinical description of all potential bioterrorism agents, it is critical to have a basic understanding of how

to prepare for and respond to a bioterrorism attack and identify reliable sources of information that can be accessed during a time of crisis.

A personal risk assessment that addresses both you and your family should be performed as well. Do you or a member of your family have any underlying disease that puts you at increased risk for illness, such as a contraindication to the smallpox vaccine? Does your work or home environment contain hazards that predispose you to injury or illness? Do you have a family emergency plan, such as backup child care in case you get called to work in an emergency?

Facility assessment, a necessary but complicated task, should be performed as part of emergency preparedness. Thorough assessment should be part of the development of the facility emergency response plan, accomplished through communication and coordination with every department in the facility.

The primary goals of facility assessment include determining on-hand and back-up resources, evaluating current communication networks, and establishing a baseline of available resources and gaps that must be filled before an emergency situation arises. In the process of assessment, facilities may examine backup resources and develop memorandums of understanding between facilities or groups to enable rapid access to needed supplies during a crisis.

Quantifying available resources entails knowing how much functional medical equipment is available onsite, and how much backup equipment can be obtained from which sources. Other information to gather would include current staffing levels, sources and number of backup staff available in an emergency, the number of licensed and available beds, and the number of beds that could be filled in the time of crisis. Having this information will prevent delays that could lead to higher mortality rates in the event of a disaster.

The second goal of facility assessment is to evaluate current communication networks. This includes both physical communication systems, such as phones, radios, and other communication devices, and intangible communication networks, such as reporting structures and media spokespeople. Among the questions to address are the following:

- Are the current communication systems effective?
- Can departments communicate among themselves and with outside agencies?
- Do you have a backup plan in case of an emergency?
- Have you established auxiliary power and secondary sites?
- Is staff trained to use the systems?

Key groups that should work together to perform the facility assessment include infection control, hospital epidemiologist, infectious diseases, administration, laboratory, security, facilities engineering, nursing, pharmacy, occupational health, mortuary, respiratory therapy, central supply, housekeeping, and food and nutrition. Other departments or groups may need to be involved. Each facility should evaluate its organizational structure and determine key groups that need to participate in the assessment process.

In some facilities, the ICN will be designated as the person responsible for coordinating this assessment. The exact role of the ICN in this process may vary depending upon the needs of the facility. Regardless of whether the ICN is the designated coordinator for facility assessment, this person should play an active role in the process.

Assessment of a facility should be accomplished in an organized manner using a standardized tool such as the *Facility Mass Casualty Disaster Plan Checklist: A Template for Healthcare Facilities* (Association for Professionals in Infection Control and Epidemiology [APIC] and the Institute for Bio-Security at Saint Louis University School of Public Health, 2001). The checklist is a template designed to assess a facility in preparation for an intentional or natural incident that results in mass casualties. It incorporates elements of emergency management such as mitigation, preparedness, response, and recovery, and serves as a foundation for the development of a preparedness plan for any emergency. The checklist is an 18-page comprehensive document containing a series of questions about whether an objective has been met. It identifies action plans to fill gaps and designates the person responsible for carrying out the plan.

Many of the sections in the checklist overlap and affect departments within the facility as well as outside agencies that should be working with the facility to develop a response plan. The checklist is designed to spark communication and development of partnerships throughout the facility and between the entity and outside agen-

cies. Questions and sections can be added or amended to meet the needs of the assessing facility. This checklist is available from APIC & Institute for Bio-Security at Saint Louis University School of Public Health (2001; 2003). See MediaLink resources.

Education and Training During Preparedness Phase

Education and training, the second duty of infection control nurses in emergency preparedness, involves both education for the ICN and educational initiatives created or provided by the ICN. Educational opportunities are widely available, some specific to different types of disasters and others offering an all-hazards approach. Each ICN should decide which training topics are necessary. In addition, there are several delivery methods available for this training, including in-services, presentations at national meetings, videos, journal articles, and online resources. The ICN need not memorize all patient management information for every type of disaster; however, a basic understanding of how different disaster-related diseases typically present allows ICNs to maintain a high index of suspicion and awareness of any changes in the medical community. It is also crucial to identify reliable sources of information, which can be accessed in a time of crisis. During emergency situations, such 9-11, telephone and cell phone lines can easily become clogged or unavailable, resulting in loss of phone, fax, and Internet service. When in need of expert advice, ICNs should be able to turn to appropriate informational CD-ROMs or written versions of them, and they should keep copies on facility computer hard drives so that access to these materials is maintained in the event of loss of telephone service. See Box 11–1 for examples of appropriate materials.

BOX 11–1   **Examples of Educational Programs on Disaster Management**

- Disaster Preparedness for Nurses Certificate Program (Saint Louis University, 2003)
- Assessing Facility Bioterrorism Preparedness: A Guide for Infection Control Professionals (Rebmann, 2002)
- Anthrax: Protecting and Preparing Your Family (Franck, 2002)
- Role of the Infection Control Professional in Bioterrorism Preparedness (Rebmann, 2003)
- Clinical Description and Epidemiology of Bioterrorism Agents: Anthrax, Smallpox, and Plague (Rebmann, 2001)
- Smallpox: Clinical Description & Recommendations for a Vaccination Program (Institute for Bio-Security at Saint Louis University School of Public Health, 2003)

- Bioterrorism Toolkit II: Key Resources for Infection Control Professional and Health Care Workers (Institute for Bio-Security at Saint Louis University School of Public Health, 2002)
- Bioterrorism Toolkit: Key Resources for Infection Control Professionals and Health Care Workers (Institute for Bio-Security at Saint Louis University School of Public Health, 2003)
- Providing Health Care in Disaster (American Red Cross, 1998)
- Family Disaster Plan and Personal Survival Guide (American Red Cross, 1992)

The ICN must also generate educational materials about the epidemiological risks associated with disasters, and distribute them. Some possible topics include:

- Waterborne illnesses that may occur after floods
- Immunizations, such as tetanus and smallpox
- Biological terrorism, especially communicable diseases such as smallpox and pneumonic plague
- Proper food handling to prevent foodborne illness

Education must be created for and provided to all groups involved in implementation of the emergency response plan. This includes medical staff, such as physicians and nurses, and non-medical staff such as security, food and nutrition, and housekeeping. The education should be occupation-specific because medical worker groups, such as nurses, will require different information than nonmedical staff. Training should include an overall description of the plan, participants' roles in the plan, where and how to obtain resources, explanation of the communication system, and description of the reporting chain of command. Providing such education is a continual process, rather than a one-time event. Regular education updates are required to ensure staff comfort with emergency management processes and to alert staff to changes in the plan.

Surveillance During Preparedness Phase

Depending on the type of emergency, surveillance by ICNs for disaster preparedness may be critical. Because surveillance is already part of the day-to-day duties of the ICN, implementation during a disaster is easier. ICNs may be the first to detect a bioterrorist attack, and early detection decreases morbidity and mortality.

Indeed, in all disasters, the sooner the incident and at-risk patients are identified, the higher the likelihood of decreasing morbidity, mortality, and cost associated with the incident. The difference between bioterrorism and other disasters is that bioterrorism is more difficult to detect. With natural disasters and even traditional or chemical terrorism, you have an obvious sign that something unusual has happened. This can range from damaged buildings in an earthquake to a huge influx of patients immediately after a chemical attack.

In a bioterrorism event, however, an explosion is unlikely, and we may not know that there has been an attack unless the perpetrators announce it, because aerosolized biological particles are odorless, colorless, and tasteless. In the case of a covert bioterrorism attack, a few days or weeks after the release, patients will begin to show symptoms and will access the medical system at that point. These patients will probably go to an emergency department (ED) or some other primary care facility. Detection will be difficult because it is unlikely that all of the patients will go to the same facility or primary care provider. In this scenario, surveillance is essential to early detection of the event.

Surveillance entails collecting and analyzing data to establish a baseline and determine a point at which there is a change or trend in the health of the population. Information in a surveillance program is gathered through either active or passive data collection.

In passive surveillance, data are collected solely from unsolicited source reports when someone calls to report a change in the medical community. Passive surveillance is sufficient for most communities prior to the onset of a disaster (such as in the preparedness stage). It would be overwhelming to actively collect data on all types of potential infectious diseases that could result from a disaster.

An effective passive surveillance system requires the facility and community to maintain a high index of suspicion. If primary care providers are not considering bioterrorism agents as potential causative agents, then it is unlikely that a bioterrorism attack will be identified unless there is a sudden, huge influx of patients with the same symptom presentation. Primary care providers like the emergency department staff should be familiar with the clinical presentation, mode of transmission, and patient treatment and management of the agents most likely to be used in a bioterrorism attack.

There are potentially thousands of agents that could be used in a bioterrorism attack. However, CDC narrows the list to three categories: A, B and C, with category A agents being the most likely to be used in a bioterrorism attack (CDC, 2003). The FBI has developed its own list of agents, which are likely to be used in a bioterrorism attack (FBI, 2002). Ideally, infection control nurses should be familiar with all of the CDC category A agents as well as the FBI's list of most likely bioterrorism agents. ICNs should try to become familiar with the CDC's category B and C agents as well, and take an active role in educating staff about bioterrorism agents and how an attack may present. This will increase the level of awareness and maintain a high index of suspicion in the primary care providers.

ICNs should also know the facility or medical community's baseline of disease so that they can be alert to subtle changes or trends and respond quickly to disasters, thus mitigating potential consequences. Similar to the development of a case definition, determining the baseline as it relates to a bioterrorism attack is difficult to accomplish. Infection control issues often have standardized definitions and easily accessible lab tests, making it relatively easy to establish a baseline. However, because there are potentially thousands of biological agents that could be used in a bioterrorism attack, active surveillance is impossible for all of them. Establishing a baseline for syndromic surveillance is even more overwhelming. How difficult would it be for your facility to track the number of patients presenting with respiratory illnesses, especially during influenza season?

There are no hard and fast rules for determining a baseline in relation to bioterrorism. Every facility needs to decide how best to accomplish this, and the ICN will play a vital role in the decision. The key is to be able to quickly identify a subtle change or trend in the population. Even if a proven increased rate in some predetermined collection criteria cannot be established, it is important to notify the health department immediately of any suspected change or trend in the population. It is better to have a low threshold for alarm than to miss what may be the beginning wave of patients presenting from a bioterrorism attack or other disaster. This initiated notification process illustrates how passive surveillance works.

In contrast, active surveillance involves direct solicitation of data from others participating in the active surveillance program. Thus, for example, the data collector would contact specified people and/or groups in the community and ask for predetermined information. Most ICNs utilize active surveillance to track indicators in their facilities, such as the rate of bloodstream infections or surgical site infections.

Examples of data that could be collected and analyzed as part of an active surveillance program for bioterrorism are as follows:

- Number of patients seen in an emergency room (ER)
- Number of patients admitted to a hospital
- Number of emergency medical services (EMS) or ambulance runs performed each day, week, month, or other time period
- Other data available from the facility that may indicate a change or trend in the community

Although tracking and analyzing the number of patients seen in an ER or hospital admissions may not seem like an effective way to perform bioterrorism surveillance, keep in mind that bioterrorism surveillance is, in some ways, unlike traditional surveillance. It is much more difficult because we have no standardized definitions or collection criteria, and because most potential bioterrorism agents cause uncommon diseases such as inhalation anthrax, tularemia, and pneumonic plague. There also are no easily accessed laboratory tests for confirmatory diagnosis. In addition, most of the potential bioterrorism agents cause disease, which usually begins with nonspecific flulike symptoms. Case finding, especially during the preparedness phase, would be difficult. Therefore, most bioterrorism active surveillance programs are designed to examine the population's health status broadly and detect any sudden change.

Another form of active surveillance for bioterrorism uses syndromic surveillance, which consists of collecting and analyzing nontraditional data. Traditionally, syndromic surveillance referred to the collection and analysis of syndrome-related data.

Examples of traditional syndromic surveillance data include the following:

- Severe flulike illness indicating the release of inhalation anthrax, pneumonic plague, smallpox, or other diseases
- Flaccid muscle paralysis indicating that a neurotoxin, such as botulism toxin, may have been released
- Bleeding disorders indicating the use of a viral hemorrhagic fever agent

- Rash indicating the release of smallpox
- Apparent foodborne illnesses possibly indicating an intentional release on a food source or vendor

Newer attempts at collecting syndromic surveillance data indicate a broader definition for the term (Osterholm, 2002). Almost any nontraditional data that may indicate a potential bioterrorism event has occurred may now be classified as syndromic surveillance. Examples of newer syndromic surveillance data include the following:

- Number of patients presenting to the emergency department with flulike illness as their chief complaint
- Number of purchases of over-the-counter flu remedies
- Number of purchases of over-the-counter diarrhea medications

Surveillance of grocery sales is perhaps one of the most interesting ways to conduct syndromic surveillance. Data are gathered on the number of grocery items purchased that could indicate that patients are experiencing flulike symptoms, such as orange juice, chicken noodle soup, and facial tissues (Thompson, 2002). The rate of grocery purchases are compared to the rate of physician visits or phone calls with nursing consultation lines. Studies have been conducted in the New York area to determine if these sales correlate with an increase in the number of physician visits and health care professional phone consultations. Whether this data collection would correlate with a bioterrorism attack has yet to be determined, but it is certainly an innovative method of conducting syndromic surveillance.

Epidemiology During Preparedness Phase

Regardless of which indicators are collected as part of disaster preparedness surveillance, the data are handled and analyzed in a similar manner using epidemiological tools. Rates and means for the data are determined and tracked, and when a change in the data indicates an upward trend or spike over a predetermined threshold, an epidemiological investigation would be undertaken. This is similar to other surveillance, such as monitoring the rates of bloodstream infections or surgical site infections, conducted daily by ICNs. In this regard, there is no difference between surveillance for disasters and "regular" surveillance.

When possible, it is best to initiate the epidemiological investigation at the first suspicion of an increase, even if it means beginning a few unnecessary investigations; this is preferable to missing an actual event because the threshold for alarm was set too high. Syndromic surveillance for bioterrorism is more likely to produce false alarms since you are not tracking a specific indicator of disease. In other words, an increase in ER visits may be related to inclement weather that resulted in numerous car accidents rather than a bioterrorism attack. You will need to begin the investigation to determine the relevance of the data.

An active surveillance program can be set up and run by the ICN within the facility or in conjunction with the local health department. Alternatively, facilities may choose to participate in a passive surveillance system in cooperation with the local health department.

Regardless of which type of surveillance is chosen by a facility or community, the ICN plays a vital role in setting up and coordinating the surveillance system as well as taking part in the epidemiological investigation by analyzing the data and reporting suspected incidents to the local health department. The surveillance process and the necessary corresponding communication network will be essential to prevent morbidity and mortality associated with disasters.

Plan Development During Preparedness Phase

Another duty of the infection control nurse in disaster preparedness involves the development of the emergency response plan. It is best to use an all-hazards approach to disaster plan development that is broad enough to allow an effective response to any type of disaster, from a flood to a chemical terrorism attack.

Each facility should appoint a multidisciplinary and multiagency disaster planning committee. The committee should appoint an individual responsible for coordinating the writing of the disaster response plan. In some facilities this may be the ICN, but it could also be the hospital epidemiologist, an infectious disease physician, emergency management leader, environmental health care professional, or other knowledgeable individual.

Disaster plan development should not be the responsibility of a single person, although one person may be assigned the responsibility of coordinating the writing of the plan. The ICN plays a critical role as a member of the planning committee, but the exact role may vary. In some facilities, the ICN may be the leader, coordinator, or facilitator for the team. Each facility must assess the strengths of their own committee members and assign responsibilities accordingly.

The following is a partial list of groups the ICN needs to partner with when developing a disaster plan and before an emergency occurs:

- Public health
- Hospital epidemiologist
- Infectious diseases
- Environmental health
- Emergency department
- Security
- Facilities engineering
- Your hospital/facility administrator
- Emergency medical service personnel
- Law enforcement
- Local FBI

The development of a facility emergency response plan should occur either before or in conjunction with staff training. A facility's disaster response plan should always be considered a work in progress. Additions and updates are made as gaps are identified and policy changes emerge. Furthermore, these changes to the plan must be communicated to the staff, as response plans are only as effective as the staff implementing them.

To mount an effective response, all facility employees should be familiar with the response plan and their role in it. During a crisis, it is likely that the facility will implement a new temporary reporting and communications structure, such as the incident command system. If this occurs, staff may be assigned a job action sheet that contains duties different from day-to-day operations. Staff will most likely report to someone other than the usual supervisor. To maximize the effectiveness of your facility's disaster plan, it is best if all participants know their roles and responsibilities in advance.

Development of a disaster response plan should be initiated either after or in conjunction with the facility assessment. Facilities will need to know their baseline of readiness in order to develop an effective response plan.

One of the most important aspects of emergency response plan development is the delineation of available resources and how to access these resources. In addition to on-hand resources and backup supplies available from a facility's community, resources will be made available through state and federal agencies. These supplies will be imperative in reducing loss of life during an emergency. However, state or federal resources are of no use to a facility or community unless these resources are made available at the local level. To access these resources, facilities and communities must know what resources are available and how to access them. See Figure 11–3.

One resource that can and should be accessed during a disaster is the CDC's Strategic National Stockpile (CDC, 2003). The stockpile's primary goal is to provide necessary antibiotics, medications, vaccines, and medical supplies to the affected community in a short period of time. The exact contents of the stockpile are kept secret for security purposes, but will include medications and vaccines needed to treat and/or prophylax various diseases, including those resulting from a chemical or biological terrorism attack. Further information on the Strategic National Stockpile may be found at the CDC's website; see MediaLink.

Release of the Strategic National Stockpile, however, is only the first step in utilizing these resources. The CDC delivers the supplies to the affected area, but does not sort or distribute the equipment and medications. Each facility and community must have a distribution plan for handling and disseminating the supplies to the community members. This may involve mass prophylaxis or vaccination of thousands or millions of affected individuals in a community within a period of hours to days. Because of the short response time needed to prevent morbidity and mortality and the urgent nature of the situation, this distribution plan should be in place before an event occurs. This requires the facility to have developed the distribution plan as part of the facility or community response plan.

Communication During Preparedness Phase

Many aspects of communication that must be addressed as part of disaster planning have been discussed within the other ICNs responsibilities, such as the need to assess communication networks as part of facility assessment. Another component of communication that must be developed and implemented as part of the planning process is the reporting and communication structure, which will be used during an emergency. This usually involves the incorporation of an incident command system.

The incident command system is a framework for reporting and communication, which entails assignment of specific roles to individuals in an effort to create a distinct chain of command (K. Keith, personal communication, May 28, 2000). Individuals may be responsible for areas and personnel new to them. Specific role responsibilities are listed on job action sheets, which are provided in the incident command manual. All are expected to perform their job within the defined parameters of the job action sheets and within specific command structures. For instance, an ICN may be assigned the position of public information officer, requiring new job responsibilities and a new reporting structure to replace surveillance and epidemiology work. In such a case, the ICN would report to the incident commander rather than his or her usual supervisor. Most ICNs and other health care employees are not familiar with incident command or the terminology and structure upon which it is based. ICNs should learn the system before a crisis occurs.

The incident command system (ICS) consists of basic operating principles that ensure rapid and appropriate resource management while aiming to continue routine operating procedures of the organization (FEMA, 2003). A hospital would thus continue to evaluate and treat patients for heart attacks while responding to and treating victims of an earthquake.

An excellent model for the incident command system has been developed by the San Mateo County Health Services Agency in California. This comprehensive incident command system called the Hospital Emergency Incident Command System or HEICS (San Mateo County Emergency Medical System, 1998). HEICS is based on the incident command system (ICS), but is geared toward health care facilities, most notably hospitals. It functions as a framework for communication and delineation of the lines of authority during a disaster.

HEICS provides an organizational chart with positions that have specific missions to address during the emergency situation. Each position has a job action sheet describing responsibilities assigned to the person holding the position. Free access to a HEICS manual or additional information concerning HEICS is available from the San Mateo County website; see MediaLink. HEICS continues to change its systems and positions in response to new information or when gaps are identified during exercises (Starling & Stangy, 2003). If a facility chooses to use HEICS, the personnel in charge should check with the website regularly for updates.

How does a facility decide whether to incorporate a traditional incident command system or HEICS into its disaster plan? The community-chosen standard system should be used. If other hospitals in the area are using HEICS, all facilities in the area should try to use the same. This will allow for common terminology and position designations at different hospitals and will cut down on miscommunication, which could result in a delayed or ineffective response.

The media provide an important outlet for sharing treatment and prophylaxis information, and updates on progression of events, thus having a significant impact on response. Preparedness plans must be made for interaction with the media. In the event of a disaster involving an infectious disease, the ICN may be consulted to provide information or be the designated spokesperson.

The facility's communication plan should designate only one spokesperson, or one spokesperson for each shift. In emergency situations, media requests for information are often relentless. There may be interview requests around the clock until the disaster subsides. In the absence of an expert, the media will reach out to anyone willing to answer their questions. This can mean misleading information, confusion, and panic in the community. It is best to avoid this situation by assigning spokespeople in advance.

The spokesperson or people need to be informed, educated, articulate, and calm. In very large disasters, it is best to have a designated spokesperson that does only media communication. This allows the person to thoroughly investigate the situation for timely and accurate information and to concentrate on public relations rather than trying to juggle interviews while completing other tasks.

In the event of a large disaster, false information may be widespread, causing panic and fear in the community. Infection control nurses would need to dispel myths by providing accurate information to the public and to health care professionals who often have very little education about the transmission of infectious diseases. The need for an accurate, consistent message is especially true in a disaster that involves a communicable disease. An example is an outbreak of pneumonic plague, which is infectious and spreads from person to person via respiratory droplets. In such a case, the ICN communicates the risk to the public and explains how people can protect themselves. The information would include a definition and description of who is at risk (i.e., people who came within six feet of an infected patient since the onset of symptoms, especially those with close contact such as household members or health care providers caring for the patient before the patient was isolated and started on appropriate antibiotic therapy). ICNs would also need to communicate prophylaxis options available and where and how to obtain prophylaxis and follow-up care.

Facilities should try to prevent anyone other than the designated spokesperson or people from speaking to the media in order to avoid mixed messages that may result in further confusion and panic in the community. Messages should be planned in advance and, if possible, written answers or fact sheets should be readily available. This will make the spokesperson more comfortable and provide the media an accurate reference to which they may refer in future reports.

To provide short newsbytes and prevent misquotations, spokespersons should be instructed to avoid speculation. They should provide to the media only verified facts in short, easy-to-understand terminology. In addition, the spokesperson or people must rehearse. Mock interviews should be incorporated as part of the facility's response plan exercise program. One option is to videotape the mock interviews so that participants can critique their own performance and identify opportunities for improvement. If the ICN is to be a designated spokesperson, he or she should participate in these mock interviews and in the development of written messages.

Performance Measurement During Preparedness Phase
Once the disaster response plan is developed, staff should be taught about the plan and their role in it. Finally, a formal process for evaluating the response plan must be developed, as it is an integral component of effective planning. Health care and regulatory agencies require performance-based evaluation. Performance measurement of disaster preparedness must, therefore, be integrated into emergency management plans.

Currently there are no standardized, validated performance measurement tools to assess bioterrorism preparedness (Rebmann, Shadel, Clements, & Evans, 2002). Most facilities and communities use subjective evaluations of the outcomes of exercises and drills to determine disaster preparedness. Disaster response plan exercises and drills provide the following benefits to a facility.

- Identify and correct gaps in resources
- Clarify participants' roles and responsibilities
- Enhance coordination between internal and external agencies
- Demonstrate plan implementation
- Provide introduction to the new reporting and communication structure

Exercise programs can make the difference between a poor and an effective response, which will translate into lives and resources saved. In addition, some regulatory agencies, including the Joint Commission on Accreditation of Healthcare Organizations (JCAHO), require annual execution of plans in the form of natural events or planned drills. One such exercise program created by FEMA is entitled *An Orientation to Community Disaster Exercisers* (FEMA, 1995). FEMA's exercise program consists of a five-stage process of exercises, which increase intensity and realism as you progress through the program.

Infection control nurses should participate in a facility's disaster plan drill and help organize the exercise. Responses to all types of disasters require practice, whether they are mass casualty disasters such as a bombing, response to victims of chemical terrorism, or mass vaccination programs in the face of a bioterrorism attack. By exercising different aspects of the disaster plan, ICNs ensure that staff members are comfortable responding to any type of disaster.

In Israel, hospitals hold approximately 20 drills each year (K. Keith, personal communication, May 28, 2000). Each drill focuses on a different type of emergency and the scenarios are rotated so that staff members are exposed to drills for floods, bombings, chemical terrorism and bioterrorism attacks. The United States can learn a great deal about responding to disasters from Israel.

While the ICN's responsibilities are the same, regardless of the phase of the emergency, the implementation of the duties changes. Assessments must be performed before, during, and after an event, but the nature of the assessments will be different. For example, assessments performed before an emergency are generally broader and should have an all-hazards approach. During an emergency, assessments are situation specific and are usually quick and dirty.

Response

Organization of the Response
To discuss the ICN's role in disaster response, we must first describe the organization of the response. The response will depend on a number of factors, including the type and scope of the disaster, and how rapidly the event is identified. Even the role of responding agencies will be different.

Once the response plan is initiated, who will be in charge? It depends on whether the organization or community is in the crisis or consequence management component of the response. The terms crisis and consequence management were first used in the Presidential Decision Directive 39 (PDD-39) on June 21, 1995 (as cited in Seiple, 1996). These terms describe the response to the use of weapons of mass destruction.

The FBI is the lead federal agency in the crisis management phase of response, regardless of the type of disaster. Crisis management refers to either identifying perpetrators before an attack occurs (such as preventing the attack) or taking steps to identify the perpetrators after an attack has occurred. The ultimate goal of crisis management is to capture the perpetrators and prevent additional attacks.

During consequence management, FEMA becomes the lead federal agency in charge. The ultimate goal of consequence management is to manage and minimize the impact of the event on the community and return to normal operations. Consequence management will entail patient management, resource management, and other recovery efforts.

Although it might seem that crisis and consequence management are two separate functions, they will probably occur simultaneously. The president and other top officials will decide when the crisis management phase is over. This will be important in establishing which federal agency has the lead in the investigation, but the response activities related to crisis and consequence management will parallel and overlap each other. It is also important to note that both the FBI and FEMA will follow the Federal Response Plan, during both crisis and consequence management.

In addition to the federal response, there will be local and regional teams available to assist in disaster response. Some of these teams include:

- American Red Cross
- Disaster medical assistance teams (DMAT)
- Disaster mortuary operations response teams (DMORTs)
- Urban search and rescue teams (US&R)
- National nurses response team (NNRT)
- Other local and regional agencies and teams

Infection control nurses must be familiar with the community, state, and federal responding agencies. This allows the ICNs to see the big picture of how response activities will unfold.

The central concern during the response phase will be patient management. What is the facility's surge capacity? How will the facility juggle a large number of acutely ill patients and deal with an influx of the worried well? Does the facility have the equipment to meet the needs of an increased patient population? Are decontamination strategies and supplies available and is staff trained to apply them? Where will the facility physically locate family members while patients are being triaged and treated?

Most morgues can house fewer than a dozen bodies. How will the facility or community morgue handle a greater number of victims? Does the facility's pharmacy have enough of the appropriate antibiotics on hand to dispense to employees, employees' families, and victims until the Strategic National Stockpile or other resources become available? Facility personnel should address all of these questions before a disaster occurs. Although not all of these issues are of concern to an infection control nurse, as a coordinator of the disaster plan, it will be essential that the ICN knows how to communicate the issues to the correct department so that effective plans are developed.

The duties of the infection control nurse during the response phase are essentially the same as those for the preparedness phase, but the implementation of these responsibilities differs. Following are duties of the ICN during disaster response.

- Assessment
- Education/training
- Surveillance
- Epidemiology
- Response plan implementation
- Communication
- Performance measurement

Assessment During Response Phase

Predisaster assessments are broad risk assessments of the community, whereas after disaster strikes, a more focused assessment must be performed to determine who in the community is at risk. For instance, prior to disaster, it may be determined that floods are a risk in certain subsets of the community; however, once a flood occurs, it is imperative to rapidly assess exactly which areas of the community are affected. The information gathered during the response is usually quick and dirty and is utilized to determine immediate interventions required to handle the response. Data collected often include logistical information and that which is specific to the disaster, such as a list of people or families that live or work in a flooded area so that tetanus vaccination needs can be determined.

Evaluation of available resources must also occur during response. Although resource assessment is performed during the planning phase, resource utilization can change at a moment's notice, especially during a disaster. It is imperative to constantly assess what resources are available and which are needed in order to mount an effective response. Infection control nurses may have to assess antibiotic prophylaxis or vaccination doses or PPE for isolation. They will also have to assess the amount of available drinking water and clean water for handwashing, bathing, linen management, sterilization of equipment, dietary maintenance, dialysis, and toilet facilities. Another critical aspect of resource assessment during a disaster response is the availability of sewage facilities to safely dispose of human waste.

Effective assessment during the response calls for coordination and communication skills. Infection control is often the liaison between hospitals and the public health department during disaster response. These relationships should be established prior to a disaster during the planning phase. If this is not possible, it will still be essential for the ICN to coordinate response efforts with both inside and outside agencies.

Education and Training During Response Phase

A second infection control responsibility during disaster response is education regarding the event at hand. If a contagious agent is involved, education will need to address control and isolation measures, treatment requirements, and prophylaxis or vaccination recommendations. Educational materials created by the ICN should address how staff, patients, and visitors can protect themselves and their community during the response. This education will be event-specific, and will concern the following:

- Water safety
- Sanitation control
- Proper food preparation (e.g., temperature control)
- Agent-specific information (e.g., route of transmission, treatment)
- Isolation precautions
- Prophylaxis
- Vaccination
- Control measures

Surveillance During Response Phase

Another responsibility of the ICN during disasters is surveillance. Depending on the type of disaster, sentinel surveillance (an active surveillance program initiated in response to a sentinel, or unusual, event) may be initiated. Thus, for example, following a known or suspected bioterrorism attack, a sentinel surveillance program would be initiated to look for additional cases of the causative agent. If the bioterrorism attack used *Yersinia pestis* (such as in cases of pneumonic plague), the active sentinel surveillance program would have to focus on identification of new cases of all forms of plague (bubonic, septicemic and pneumonic).

Surveillance is important for other types of disasters as well. For instance, diseases spread by contaminated water may be a concern after floods. A sentinel active surveillance program may be needed to detect new cases, since waterborne agents are not typical indicators collected. Surveillance programs implemented in response to a disaster are generally shortterm and end when the crisis ends or shortly thereafter. This in contrast to ongoing public health and nosocomial surveillance programs such as bloodstream infection surveillance or tuberculosis monitoring.

Epidemiology During Response Phase

Another role of the ICN during disaster response is epidemiologist. The epidemiological interventions necessary vary according to disaster type. An outbreak investigation may be warranted if a communicable disease is involved, or epidemiological information such as risk factor data may be collected and analyzed. Typically, the epidemiology performed during disaster response is limited. The response phase is generally relatively short and there is not sufficient time to establish and implement an epidemiological investigation (this occurs more frequently during the recovery phase).

This is not true for an unannounced bioterrorism attack, however, where the epidemiological investigation will be critical to mounting an effective response. If terrorists covertly release an aerosolized biological weapon, the event will not be detected until days to weeks after the incident, when patients become ill and begin infiltrating the medical system. When this occurs, rapid and focused epidemiological investigation will be needed to identify the possible date and location of the release. Victims' histories will be taken and examined for shared activities, such as attendance at a mutual event. It is essential that the release date and location be identified to determine other people or groups that are potentially at risk. This information can guide distribution of treatment, prophylaxis and vaccination.

If a contagious agent is used in a bioterrorism attack, the epidemiological investigation will be even more critical. Not only will the date and location of release need to be identified, but a list of contacts (i.e., people who came into contact with infected patients since the onset of infectiousness) must be identified as well. For instance, if smallpox is released as a biological weapon, the two groups at risk of exposure are those exposed to the initial release (which will be identified when the date and location of the release is determined) and those exposed to infected individuals (which will be identified in a thorough epidemiological investigation of potential contacts).

Either before or in conjunction with the epidemiological investigation to determine the date and location of the release, it will be imperative to establish the causative agent. Treatment, prophylaxis, and isolation depend on the causative agent. Time is of the essence because patients suffering from diseases caused by some of these agents can progress to death rapidly without appropriate treatment. For example, untreated pneumonic plague usually progresses to death within 36 to 72 hours (Inglesby, et al., 2000). Although diagnosis will not be a direct responsibility of the ICNs, it is likely that their infectious disease expertise will be consulted in the evaluation process and in deciding which, if any, isolation precautions should be implemented while awaiting confirmatory diagnosis.

Agent identification and patient diagnosis will depend a great deal on the effectiveness of the passive surveillance system implemented during the preparedness phase. If clinicians maintained a high index of suspicion and had a good knowledge foundation regarding the potential infectious diseases that could occur following a disaster, it is more likely that the event or outbreak will be rapidly identified.

Obtaining an accurate assessment and patient history will also be critical to the epidemiological investigation. The history should include symptoms, severity of illness, date of symptom onset, source, route, location, and date of exposure if known, and body site affected. For example, a new painless necrotic lesion on the arm might indicate cutaneous anthrax, whereas respiratory symptoms with an accompanying widened mediastinum on chest X ray would suggest inhalation anthrax. Both diseases result from exposure to the same agent, but the route of exposure is different.

Date of symptom onset will be important in determining approximate date of exposure, which may lead to information about the location and date of the release. This will require the application of epidemiological investigative skills and methods. Although this information will not help the patient currently being treated, it may prevent future deaths by identifying other high-risk groups that would benefit from prophylaxis.

Response Plan Implementation During Response Phase

The ICN is also responsible for implementing the response plan developed during the planning phase before the disaster. Response plans should be flexible, allowing the facility to expand or contract the extent of the response as needed. For example, in the case of small disasters, only per diem staff may be needed for work, whereas large disasters may require the facility to call on memorandums of agreements with outside agencies to help meet the staffing needs.

One of the most critical components of disaster plan implementation is the use of a disaster documentation log (McDonald, 2000). Every individual or department responding to the disaster should maintain a log to document events that occur during disaster response. This log should be started as early in the disaster response as possible, and used to document the date, time, and information that is currently known. It should be updated periodically as the disaster response progresses until the debriefing session after the crisis is over. The information documented in the disaster logs will be invaluable during the debriefing session, when writing the after action report, and during the disaster response evaluation process. In addition, the logs will help document the sequence of events and decision-making process throughout the response. Experience has indicated that the maintenance of disaster logs has been "the single most useful piece of information gained" (McDonald, 2000, p. 123-2).

In most disasters, patient decontamination is unnecessary. Patient decontamination recommendations vary, depending on the agent encountered and how soon the event is identified. In a chemical terrorist attack, patients begin experiencing symptoms minutes to hours after exposure. The event is easily identified and prompt decontamination is critical to saving lives. Other events, such as a bioterrorism attack, do not necessarily require patient decontamination, depending on how soon the attack is identified. For example, in the event of a covert release of a biological agent, patient decontamination may not be necessary. By the time patients become symptomatic and present to health care institutions days to weeks after the exposure, they will probably have bathed and changed their clothes, thus decontaminating themselves. However, if the bioterrorism attack is announced within 12 to 24 hours after the release, exposed individuals should be decontaminated by bathing with plain soap and water and changing their clothing.

The decontamination recommendations for biological terrorism are different than those for certain chemicals, such as blister agents, which may respond better to dry powder decontamination compounds (Hurst et al., n.d.). However, these powder agents are not widely available in the civilian population. For that reason, some hospitals or

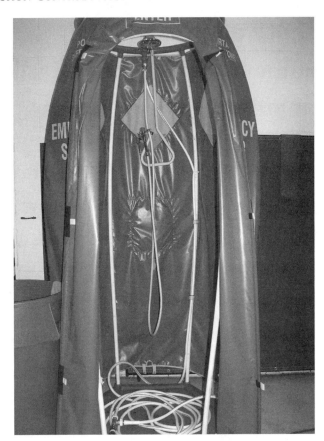

Figure 11-4. Decontamination shower for ambulatory victims. *(Photo courtesy of Terri Rebmann.)*

communities may choose to use traditional soap and water decontamination, regardless of the chemical agent to which the patient was exposed (Figures 11–4 and 11–5.)

Whatever decontamination strategies are chosen by a facility, or which group(s) of employees are designated to do the decontamination, the facility should practice decontamination strategies as part of the disaster response plan exercises. Staff who practice decontamination during an exercise are likely to be able to perform it rapidly and correctly during an actual event. In addition, practicing the procedure ensures that the facility has the equipment it needs to provide adequate decontamination services.

Environmental decontamination is another concern during some types of disaster response. Although the ICNs are unlikely to perform environmental decontamination, they will serve as the expert resource on which items require decontamination, and the proper procedure for disinfecting them. Recommendations for environmental decontamination depend on the location of the environmental source of concern, the causative agent, and the scope of the event.

Given existing knowledge, environmental decontamination is not considered necessary for streets, cars, or the outsides of buildings following a bioterrorism attack, because weather plays a key role in rapidly disseminating biological agents in outside air. In contrast, some outside

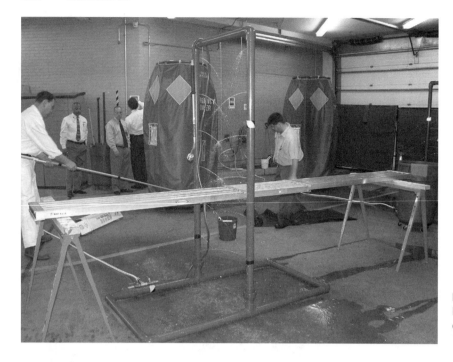

Figure 11–5. Decontamination shower for nonambulatory victims. Staff in background are preparing equipment for use during a drill. *Photo courtesy of Terri Rebmann.*

areas may require decontamination following a chemical spill or attack. Exact recommendations may be found in the educational materials on biological and chemical terrorism.

Indoor environmental sources will require decontamination strategies following a biological or chemical incident, but the interventions vary according to the agent utilized and the scope of the release. For example, more stringent decontamination methods are necessary for anthrax when it is released in spore form, due to the hardy nature of spores. Final recommendations regarding environmental decontamination following release of anthrax are pending investigation into the anthrax letters that contaminated United States postal offices in the fall of 2001.

Other agents, such as smallpox, require diligent environmental decontamination as well. Smallpox can be spread through hand-to-hand contact or contact with fomites, making decontamination of environmental surfaces imperative to prevent secondary transmission. EPA-registered, health care facility-approved disinfectants are required for environmental decontamination of smallpox, although a 0.5% hypochlorite solution may be used (this solution is made by mixing one part household bleach with nine parts water) (Henderson et al., 1999). In the event of a single smallpox case, decontamination of the inside of a health care facility would be critical to prevent secondary spread. Decontamination recommendations for other biological and chemical agents are available in training products that cover treatment and patient management of potential bioterrorism agents. Again, it should be noted that ICNs will most likely function as the expert resource consulted on decontam-

ination strategies, rather than the person or people performing the procedure.

Communication During Response Phase

Communication is perhaps one of the most critical responsibilities of the ICN during disaster response. Experience with disaster plan exercises has shown that the largest issue has been communication (Altman, & Kolata, 2002). Facilities must be able to communicate both internally between departments and externally with outside agencies. In addition, communication with the general public in the community will be critical. During a crisis, accurate consistent messages must be provided to the public, as well as information regarding who is at risk and how those groups can quickly obtain treatment. Infection control is unlikely to be the primary means of communication during disaster response, but will play a role in overall coordination of the response and in development of media messages for the general public.

Communication and reporting will also be vital within your facility and with outside agencies, including other health care facilities in your health care system or community. In order to maximize effectiveness of response, all health care and public health facilities and agencies should have a communications network in place before an incident occurs. Building this communications network will require the formation of key partnerships both within the organization and with outside agencies. The process of developing and exercising the response plan will aid in this endeavor.

The response to the anthrax-tainted letter incidents from fall 2001 (Seiple, 1996) highlights the need for good communications systems. During this period, communication between law enforcement and the medical profession was problematic. Prior to these incidents, the two groups rarely interacted. They had to learn to assist each other and work together rapidly in order to mount an effective response. The FBI had to learn to collect evidence without disturbing the medical process and physicians had to learn to treat patients without disturbing the chain of custody process. Miscommunications between agencies as well as between professions pointed out the need to develop communications systems prior to a disaster.

Communication needs include education that takes place within the organization, in outside agencies, and with the general public. In addition, communication will involve the sharing of patient-related information with the public health departments, both local and state. Due to new confidentiality regulations, such as HIPPA, patient information cannot be shared between hospitals or health care institutions, but certain information can and should be provided to the health department performing the epidemiology investigation (Health Insurance Portability and Accountability Act of 1996, 1996).

Another important component of communication during the response phase is assisting in the criminal investigation. Some disasters, such as biological or chemical terrorism, are crimes and will be extensively investigated by the FBI. As part of the investigation, the FBI gathers evidence, requiring participation from both health care and public health agencies. These procedures are new to most health care professionals; forming partnerships with federal agencies in advance will build a relationship and communications network that will make working together easier in the time of crisis. Infection control nurses do not need to know how to gather evidence correctly, but they do need to know how to communicate a potential event to the correct agencies so that the investigation can be initiated.

The rapid establishment of a reporting structure is crucial if you suspect a nonnatural (biological or chemical) disaster. The earlier the local and state health departments become involved and notify the FBI, the more likely that critical evidence is obtained and conserved. For example, if a facility has a patient that is suspected of having anthrax, that facility should not treat and release the patient before involving the health departments and FBI. There may be additional clinical samples or information to collect during the initial exam to facilitate the criminal investigation.

Risk communication is another issue that must be addressed during the response phase. According to Peter Sandman, Risk Communication Expert, "Risk communication tries to create a level of 'outrage' appropriate to the level of hazard" (Snow, n.d.). From a disaster standpoint, this means formulating communication that either alerts or calms people down, depending on the situation. One example would be media messages from a hospital explaining the following:

- Why community residents should obtain vaccination following a flood
- How community residents can obtain vaccination
- Where to obtain the vaccination
- The potential consequences of not obtaining vaccination
- Which groups need and do not need vaccination
- Which interventions are not helpful or harmful

Performance Measurement During Response Phase

The final role of the ICN in disaster response is performance measurement. As in the preparedness phase, measuring the effectiveness of response is difficult for most disasters. An overall perception of effectiveness may be easily determined, but actually using a measurable tool is problematic. What is the expected rate of morbidity and mortality in a foodborne outbreak following a hurricane? There are no easy answers or tools to calculate the expected incidence.

As with preparedness, the best approach may be to use a subjective tool. The response should be evaluated as a joint effort between infection control and other members of the planning committee in the facility. This is not a one-time action, but a continuous cycle of evaluating the response process. A thorough evaluation will require communication between the responding departments and agencies.

As with the preparedness phase, the interventions for disaster response vary, according to the type and scope of the disaster. Response activities following a large-scale chemical terrorism attack that affected thousands are much different than those for a flood that involved a few hundred families. Thus, while the principles of response are the same, the scope is different.

Recovery

The duties of the ICN during the recovery phase are essentially the same as those for the preparedness and response phases, but the implementation of these responsibilities differs. Following are the ICN's duties during disaster recovery.

- Assessment
- Education/training
- Surveillance
- Epidemiology
- Response plan evaluation/updating
- Communication
- Performance measurement

Assessments During Recovery Phase

Assessments in this case refer to evaluations of the facility and the community's needs in order to return to normal or baseline. This includes an assessment of facility or community mental health, resources, and the disaster response plan. From an ICN's perspective, assessment of facility resource needs following an emergency is critical. One of the central components of the recovery phase is the replacement of lost resources. The response phase is resource intensive and often leaves the facility or community depleted in physical and human resources as well as emotional and financial reserves.

A facility may have to restock personal protective equipment, medications, and other medical supplies. The facility may also need to deal with a loss of staff that fell victim to the disaster, as health care workers often make up a large portion of a community's population. In addition to replacing lost resources, the facility or community will have to address the mental health and spiritual consequences of a large disaster. See Chapter 4 for discussion of mental health promotion.

Education and Training During Recovery Phase
Education and training during the recovery period should focus on the following:

- Dissemination of information on the effectiveness of the disaster response
- Areas for improvement related to disaster response
- Changes or updates to the disaster plan
- Ongoing infection prevention strategies
- Results from data gathered during the epidemiological investigation

Surveillance During Recovery Phase
Surveillance during the recovery period will most likely consist of a return to routine surveillance activities. In some cases, facilities may choose to continue surveillance for indicators begun as part of sentinel surveillance. For instance, during recovery from a bioterrorism attack, facilities may choose to continue active surveillance for the causative agent (such as pneumonic plague or inhalation anthrax) until they are certain the outbreak is over. This is more likely when the agent used was contagious like smallpox, making it vital to continue to identify new cases, which is best accomplished through active surveillance. If a noncontagious agent such as anthrax is used, only patients exposed to the initial release are at risk (as opposed to contacts of infected patients), and therefore active surveillance may not be necessary after the outbreak is over.

In addition to possibly incorporating sentinel surveillance into routine surveillance, facilities also need to decide if new surveillance indicators are necessary. After recovering from a bioterrorism attack using anthrax, some facilities may choose to initiate a syndromic surveillance program to quickly identify a potential future bioterrorism attack. Obviously, this would be resource intensive and would require a joint decision between administration and infection control.

Epidemiology During Recovery Phase
Some facilities may use the findings of the epidemiological investigation to determine which surveillance should be maintained or initiated. Epidemiology during the recovery period will focus on the disaster situation. Once the crisis is over, a more in-depth investigation can be performed, focusing on risk factors, groups most affected, route of transmission, and interventions that worked or did not work. The results of the epidemiological investigation must be disseminated throughout the facility and public. Publication in a peer-reviewed scientific journal should be considered in order to share the results and lessons with a wider audience.

Response Plan Evaluation During Recovery Phase
Infection control nurses must assist in evaluating the disaster response plan. How effective was the plan? Was staff familiar enough with the plan to effectively implement it? Were there facets of the plan that did not work as effectively as possible? Are there areas that can be improved before the next disaster strikes? While the ICN probably won't be able to answer all of these questions alone, the evaluation process should be a joint effort of the facility planning committee, of which the ICN is a member.

It is critical for the facility to hold a debriefing session in which all of the responding departments and agencies discuss what was learned from the situation. Furthermore, this information should be used to generate an after action report. This will be greatly facilitated by the availability of any disaster logs that individuals or departments maintained during the disaster. Once the lessons learned from the event have been discussed and documented, the disaster response plan must be updated. If a facility discovers during response to a disaster that more decontamination gear is needed and more staff should be educated in its use, this information should be incorporated into the disaster plan. Thus, a facility might institute a mandatory quarterly drill for decontamination staff to practice donning protective gear and simulating the decontamination process. The debriefing, evaluation, after action report and updating the response plan may not all be responsibilities of the ICN, but as a responding department, infection control will be responsible for participating in these activities. In some facilities, the ICN may be in charge of these activities.

Communication During Recovery Phase
Communication during the recovery period will be less stressful and intense than what occurred during the disaster. Recovery communication will involve the following:

- Dissemination of the epidemiological investigation findings
- Sharing lessons learned between departments and with outside agencies
- Evaluation of communications that took place during the disaster response
- Gap analysis for future disasters

Performance Measurement During Recovery Phase

Performance measurement during the recovery period involves aspects of disaster recovery that have been previously discussed. Outcome measurement as it relates to disaster recovery involves the following:

- Participation in the debriefing session
- Evaluating lessons learned from the disaster
- Documenting gaps in the response plan and lessons learned during the disaster
- Assigning individuals or departments the responsibility of addressing the gaps identified during the evaluation process

Mitigation

Mitigation strategies seek to reduce the negative impact of a disaster or emergency. Mitigation is affected by national and international policies and the infrastructure of the health care and public health systems. A stronger health care and public health infrastructure will ensure a more rapid and effective response, which in turn will decrease the negative impact of the event.

From the perspective of an ICN, there are few interventions during the mitigation phase of emergency management. ICNs do not get overly involved in the mitigation phase of emergency preparedness. Part of the difficulty in describing the infection control nurse's role during this phase is that mitigation is similar to the preparedness phase in the emergency management model.

As in the other three phases (preparedness, response, and recovery), the role of the ICN during the mitigation phase can be summarized in the following seven duties:

- Assessment
- Education/training
- Surveillance
- Epidemiology
- Response plan
- Communication
- Performance measurement

Assessments During Mitigation Phase

Assessments during the mitigation phase include community and facility risk assessments of factors that affect the overall ability to respond to a disaster. For example, a risk assessment of a small rural hospital may determine that the facility does not have the resources necessary to respond to a large-scale disaster. This information should be weighed against the probability of a disaster occurring in that community (such as an earthquake). If the risk assessments determine that a large earthquake has a low to moderate likelihood of occurring, the facility may decide to explore or implement new policies and memorandums of agreement with larger facilities or companies to supplement the rural hospital's resources when disaster strikes.

Education and Training During Mitigation Phase

Education during the mitigation phase is very similar to that which occurs during preparedness. The ICN should create and disseminate educational materials about various types of disasters to the facility, community, and the general public. The general public must have a good basic understanding of the prevention and control of the spread of infectious diseases. This baseline of knowledge helps mitigate fear and panic when an infectious disease hits the community. We saw this occur more frequently in the past when public health took a larger role in educating the public about infectious diseases, especially prevention and control strategies. For example, in the massive educational campaign that public health undertook with smallpox, signs were posted in public areas describing control measures to protect one from the risk of disease.

Over the years, the impact of infectious diseases on the health of the citizens in the United States has lessened, thanks to diligent and more widespread vaccination programs, better infection control policies and procedures, and the availability of new medications and treatments. Subsequently, basic information on prevention and control of the spread of infectious diseases has almost disappeared. It is the role of the ICN to help educate the facility, community, and the general public about the basic principles of infectious disease control and prevention.

Surveillance During Mitigation Phase

Surveillance during the mitigation phase refers to building a surveillance infrastructure rather than to the specific recommendations regarding which indicators should be collected and analyzed. In practice, this means having the necessary infection control policies and procedures in place before a disaster occurs and providing the ICN the authority and autonomy to expand or contract surveillance indicators in preparation for or reaction to a disaster. In other words, day-to-day surveillance may have to be curtailed during a disaster in order for the ICN to conduct disaster surveillance (such as adding sentinel surveillance). Infection control policies and procedures must be broad and flexible to address these issues.

Epidemiology During Mitigation Phase

Epidemiology during the mitigation phase refers to the examination of general disease trends in a community and the policies, procedures, and epidemiological infrastructures that are in place. This is primarily the function of public health, but in some communities, the ICN may participate in or coordinate these assessments and procedures. For instance, quarantine laws and policies must be evaluated and instated before a disaster occurs in order to facilitate the implementation process. Although ICNs are unlikely to be involved in assessing or creating laws related to quarantine, they will be responsible for addressing the issue of quarantine and/or control of infectious diseases in the hospital or health care facility setting at which they work.

Disaster Response Plan Development During Mitigation Phase

The role of the ICN in disaster response plans during the mitigation phase involves building the necessary support system to develop an all-hazards, effective disaster response plan. This will require an adequate health care infrastructure and appropriate policies and procedures. The development of this infrastructure is a joint venture between Infection Control and facility administration. Administrative support is needed to encourage and allow departments to participate and funding must be allocated for these processes. In some regards, agencies such as JCAHO provide the impetus needed to prompt facilities to participate in this process (JCAHO, 2001).

Communication During Mitigation Phase

During the mitigation phase, communication networks and relationships must be established and maintained between infection control and other departments or agencies that would respond during a disaster. These relationships help build the infrastructure necessary for the other phases of emergency management. Thus it is helpful for the ICN to have a relationship with the local public health department in order to design, coordinate, and implement a syndromic or active surveillance program in case of disaster.

Performance Measurement During Mitigation Phase

Performance measurement during the mitigation phase includes development of the policies, procedures, and infrastructure that must be in place to ensure that evaluation of the disaster management process is successful. Both support and funding for evaluation of the disaster management processes must be available, and new policies or guidance are needed to develop and implement standardized methods for evaluation of disaster plan development and implementation. The subjective tools currently in place would be greatly improved by scientific research into the best approaches and methods to use when evaluating disaster management principles.

SUMMARY

It again should be emphasized that the four phases of the emergency management model are not processes that occur separately from each other, but that overlap and occur simultaneously. Infection control interventions for the mitigation, preparedness, response, and recovery phases are not broken out as cleanly as it would appear. For instance, the epidemiological investigation will begin as soon as the disaster is identified and will continue until all of the relevant data are collected and analyzed. It is unlikely that the facility or ICN will find a point at which either can say, "The disaster response is over; we're starting recovery now." Infection control nurses must be familiar with the principles of emergency management and their role in all aspects of this process in order to maximize the effectiveness of disaster response and minimize the consequences of a disaster.

CASE STUDY

Pneumonic Plague

The infection control nurse receives a phone call from a medical intensive care unit physician working at their hospital. The physician states that a patient just died in the ICU whom she believes might have had pneumonic plague. After checking the chart, the infection control nurse notes that the patient did not have any risk factors for plague (occupational or animal exposure, or recent travel to an endemic area). Bioterrorism is suspected. The infection control nurse also notes that the patient had not been in isolation while in the hospital.

1. To whom should the infection control nurse report this incident?
2. How should the infection control nurse determine the dates that the patient was contagious?
3. Who should determine the date and location of the suspected bioterrorism attack?
4. Who should develop the case definition for determining who else may have pneumonic plague?
5. How should the infection control nurse determine which hospital employees, patients, and visitors are at risk of secondary exposure?
6. To whom should the infection control nurse provide prophylactic antibiotics?

TEST YOUR KNOWLEDGE

1. Which of the following is not a phase of the emergency management model?
   A. Preparedness
   B. Planning
   C. Response
   D. Recovery

2. The infection control professional should always be in charge of writing the disaster response plan for a health care facility.
   A. True
   B. False

3. Which of the following is an example of active surveillance?
   A. A hospital that calls the local health department and states it has seen 20 patients with a similar disease presentation within the past 24 hours

    B. Tracking the number of patients seen in an emergency room each day

    C. Waiting for clinicians to report unusual changes in their medical community

    D. Communicable disease reporting

4. Which of the following assessments should take place during the preparedness phase?

    A. Self assessment

    B. Facility assessment

    C. Resource assessment

    D. All of the above

5. Which of the following describes the difference between epidemiological investigations during the preparedness and response phases?

    A. Epidemiological investigations during the preparedness phase are in-depth reviews of the incident, while those during the response phase are quick and dirty.

    B. Epidemiological investigations during the preparedness phase focus on rapid identification of an incident, while those during the response phase are quick and dirty.

    C. Epidemiological investigations during the preparedness phase are quick and dirty, while those during the response phase are an in-depth review of the incident.

    D. Epidemiological investigations during the preparedness phase are quick and dirty, while those during the response phase focus on rapid identification of an incident.

6. Which of the following describes the type of educational materials that should be provided during the response phase?

    A. Broad description of disaster response

    B. Description of potential types of disasters

    C. Description of event-specific agent

    D. Areas for improvement related to disaster response

7. Which of the following interventions would be performed during the preparedness phase?

    A. Developing a disaster response plan

    B. Creating educational materials related to disaster response

    C. Epidemiological investigation following a flood

    D. Development of policies and procedures related to quarantine

8. Which of the following is not assessed as part of resource assessment?

    A. Surveillance indicator selection

    B. Amount of on-hand pharmaceuticals at the health care facility

    C. Number of functioning ventilators at the health care facility

    D. Number and method for obtaining backup staff

9. The epidemiological investigation ends when the crisis is over.

    A. True

    B. False

10. Which of the following is not true about media communication?

    A. There should be one (or one per shift) designated spokesperson.

    B. Speculation on the event is appropriate when accurate information is not yet available.

    C. Information should be provided in short soundbytes.

    D. Qualifying statements should be avoided.

See Test Your Knowledge Answers in Appendix B.

EXPLORE MEDIALINK

Interactive resources and an audio glossary for this chapter can be found on the Companion Website at http://www.prenhall.com/langan. Click on Chapter 11 to select the activities for this chapter.

REFERENCES

Altman, L., & Kolata, G. (2002, January 6). Anthrax missteps offer guide to fight next bioterror battle. *NY Times*, 1.

American Red Cross. (1992). *Family disaster plan and personal survival guide*. Falls Church, VA: American Red Cross.

American Red Cross. (1998). *Providing health care in disaster*. Falls Church, VA: American Red Cross.

Association for Professionals in Infection Control (APIC) & Epidemiology and Institute for Bio-Security at Saint Louis University School of Public Health. (2001). *Mass Casualty Disaster Plan Checklist: A Template for Healthcare Facilities*. Available from APIC website at http://www.apic.org/bioterror/

Centers for Disease Control and Prevention (CDC). (2003a). *Biological Agents/Diseases*. Retrieved May 21, 2003, from http://www.bt.cdc.gov/agent/agentlist-category.asp

Centers for Disease Control and Prevention (CDC). (2003b). *National Pharmaceutical Stockpile*. Retrieved April 15, 2003, from http://www.bt.cdc.gov/stockpile/

Institute for Bio-Security at Saint Louis University School of Public Health (2001). *Bioterrorism toolkit: Key resources for infection control professionals and health care workers*. Available from their website at http://www.slu.edu/colleges/sph/csbei/bioterrorism/products.htm

Institute for Bio-Security at Saint Louis University School of Public Health (2002). *Bioterrorism toolkit II: Key resources for infection control professional and health care workers*. Available from their website at http://bioterrorism.slu.edu/bt/products.htm

Institute for Bio-Security at Saint Louis University School of Public Health (2003). http://bioterrorism.slu.edu/

Institute for Bio-Security at Saint Louis University School of Public Health (2003). *Smallpox: Clinical description & recommendations for a vaccination program*. Available from their website http://bioterrorism.slu.edu/bt/products/smallpoxcd.htm

Federal Bureau of Investigation (FBI). (2002, April). Symposium conducted at the meeting of the National Disaster Medical System Conference, Atlanta.

Federal Emergency Management Agency (FEMA). (1995). *An orientation to community disaster exercises* (IS SM 120). Washington, DC: U.S. Government Printing Office.

Federal Emergency Management Agency (FEMA). (1998). *Principles of emergency management student manual* (DHHS Publication No. 1998-622-686/93421). Washington, DC: U.S. Government Printing Office.

Federal Emergency Management Agency (FEMA). (2003). *Basic incident command system* (IS-195). Retrieved May 21, 2003, from http://training.fema.gov/EMIWeb/IS/is195.asp

Franck, J. (2002). *Anthrax: Protecting and preparing your family*. Available from APIC website at http://www.apicelearn.org/

Health Insurance Portability and Accountability Act of 1996. (1996). Retrieved March 4, 2003, from http://www.hep-c-alert.org/links/hippa.html

Henderson, D. A., Inglesby, T. V., Bartlett, J. G., Ascher, M. S., Eitzen, E., Jahrling, P. B., Hauer, J., Layton, M., McDade, J., Osterholm, M. T., O'Toole, T., Parker, G., Perl, T., Russell, P. K., & Tonat, K. (1999). Smallpox as a biological weapon: Medical and public health management. *Journal of the American Medical Association, 281*, 2127–2137.

Hurst, C. G., Newmark, J., Maliner, B. L., McMahon, M. A., McCarthy, R. L., Norton, P. L., Holland, R., Story, T. J., Alzamora, J. M., Henderson, E. M., Key, S. L., Logan, T. R., Norman, C. A., Ralls, D. L., Rimpel, L. Y., & Rotella, M. L. (n.d.). *The medical management of chemical casualties*. Aberdeen Proving Ground, MD: U.S. Army Medical Research Institute of Chemical Defense.

Inglesby, T. V., Dennis, D. T., Henderson, D. A., Bartlett, J. G., Ascher, M. S., Eitzen, E., Fine, A. D., Friedlander, A. M., Hauer, J., Koerner, J. F., Layton, M., McDade, J., Oster-holm, M. T., O'Toole, T., Parker, G., Perl, T. M., Russell, P. K., Schoch-Spana, M., & Tonat, K. (2000). Plague as a biological weapon: medical and public health management. *Journal of the American Medical Association, 283*, 2281–2290.

Joint Commission on Accreditation of Hospital Organizations (JCAHO). (2001, December). Emergency management in the new millennium. *Joint Commission Perspectives, 21*(12).

McDonald, M. R. (2000). Disaster response. In Association for Professionals in Infection Control and Epidemiology, *APIC Text of Infection Control and Epidemiology* (123, 1–7). Washington, DC: APIC.

Osterholm, M. (2002, November). *Putting syndromic surveillance into context (public health)*. Symposium conducted at the meeting of the National Syndromic Surveillance Conference, New York.

Rebmann, T. (2001). *Clinical description and epidemiology of bioterrorism agents: Anthrax, smallpox, and plague*. Available on the web at http://bioterrorism.slu.edu/bt/products/clinical.htm

Rebmann, T. (2002). *Assessing facility bioterrorism preparedness: A guide for infection control professional*. Available from APIC website at http://www.apicelearn.org/

Rebmann, T. (2003). *Role of the infection control professional in bioterrorism preparedness*. Available on the web at http://bioterrorism.slu.edu/bt/products/roleicp.htm

Rebmann, T., Shadel, B. N., Clements, B., & Evans, R. G. (2002). *Bioterrorism preparedness: Development of outcome/performance measurement tools* [Abstract]. Philadelphia: Association of Schools of Public Health.

Saint Louis University. (2003). *Disaster preparedness for nurses certificate program*. Available from Saint Louis University School of Nursing website at http://www.slu.edu/colleges/NR/cne_disaster_prep_home.html

San Mateo County Emergency Medical Services. (1998). *Hospital emergency incident command system update project*. Retrieved May 21, 2003, from http://www.emsa.cahwnet.gov/dms2/heics3.htm

Seiple, C. (1996). *Another perspective on the domestic role of the military in consequence management*. Retrieved May 19, 2003, from http://www.nici.org/Research/Pubs/98-2.htm

Snow, E. (n.d.). *Risk communication: Notes from a class by Dr. Peter Sandman* (Seminar at Hanford Nuclear Reservation). Retrieved January 6, 2003, from http://www.psandman.com/articles/risk.htm

Starling, C., & Stangby, A. (2003, March). *Hospital emergency incident command system*. Course conducted at the meeting of the National Disaster Medical System Conference, Reno, NV.

Thompson, W. (2002, November). *Aberration detection methods for influenza-like illness*. Symposium conducted at the meeting of the National Syndromic Surveillance Conference, New York.

U.S. Department of Justice, Federal Bureau of Investigation. (1999). Counterterrorism Threat Assessment and Warning Unit Counterterrorism Division. *Terrorism in the United States, 1999*. Available from FBI website at http://www.fbi.org

CHAPTER 12

Disaster as the Personal Experience

Joanne C. Langan and Vered Kater

LEARNING OBJECTIVES

1. Discuss the value of using stories as a strategy in learning the meaning of a disaster experience.
2. Describe similar themes among nurses' disaster stories.
3. Differentiate priorities discussed between the nurses' stories and those of bereaved parents.

4. Explore common responses offered to bereaved persons and discuss how each may be construed as helpful or hurtful to the bereaved.

MEDIALINK www.prenhall.com/langan

Resources for this chapter can be found on the Companion Website at http://www.prenhall.com/langan. Click on Chapter 12 to select the activities for this chapter.

CHAPTER OUTLINE

Know Your Terms
Audio Glossary
MediaLink Applications
    Dealing with Sadness
    Questions for Discussion

GLOSSARY

Burn tanks. Where the patients' burns are cleaned and the wound care is provided

Cell saver. A machine that stores the blood that the patient bleeds out to be given directly back into the veins

Comfort kit. Packages created for school-age children to have stored at the school in case of disasters, to include liquids, cans of food, change of clothes, and a blanket

Family room. A special area in the hospital designated to care for victims' families and friends by answering questions about the victims and providing updates about the victims' status

Kwashiorkor. A disease resulting from a deficiency of protein

Operation Moses. The transport and relocation of fragmented Jewish families suffering from a severe drought in Ethiopia, from the region of Gondar to Israel from 1983 to 1984

Safe room. An area in the home that is prepared for disaster situations by storing water, food, toys, games, gas masks and may even be taped to be airtight in preparation for a gas attack

Shiva. The traditional Jewish seven-day mourning period, a thoughtful and appropriate time for friends and family to visit in the home of the bereaved

Stories. Used as a strategy to learn about a phenomenon

Support group. People who meet together who have experienced the same kind of tragedy in their lives, formally or informally organized among friends or through a professional

INTRODUCTION

Previous chapters in this textbook have offered a myriad of definitions and information about planning for and responding to disasters and mass casualty incidents. Personal information and reactions were also shared regarding the theory and concepts presented. As we prepare nurses for practice in an increasingly complex world, it is essential to cultivate pedagogies that will help them apply critical thinking and caring to communities (Sorrell, 2002), and storytelling is one such method. Stories are used as a strategy to learn about a phenomenon. Those who have experienced disasters firsthand are able to tell the truth of what happened and what it meant to them to live through the disaster. Listening is a critical competency that nurses must continue to develop. We need to hear the truth, learn from it, and apply that learning to care more effectively for victims of all tragedies.

This chapter is a compilation of interviews with nurses, nursing faculty, and bereaved parents who have had intimate encounters with terrorist events and the victims of these events. When visiting Israel, we were struck by the courage and resolve people have to continue to live their lives to the fullest, as best as they can. They refuse to cut themselves off from living and give in to the terrorists. They use greater caution and their sense of normalcy is forever changed. However, they try to enjoy each day and each other. These are their stories and the stories of others from whom we can learn.

ISRAEL: INTERVIEW WITH L.

L. is a religious nurse educator. She is married and is the mother of four children and has two grandchildren. Her interview follows.

Given the economic and political milieu as well as the culture that deals with fear of terrorism in every day living, how do you get beyond what you are feeling to continue to live your lives, take care of your families, to work as nurses and teachers?

How do we function on a daily basis with the fear and the stress and anxiety associated with the country in which we live? I function better on some days and some days are worse. I must admit on some days I have awakened with physical symptoms, which I relate to this stressful situation. Sometimes I wake up extremely tired and headachy, and I attribute that to the situation. Sometimes I even feel panicky when I have to take a bus in the morning.

When I began to develop anxiety-like symptoms, I made the decision that I would not let it get the better of me. I consciously worked with myself to put it in the back of my mind. I do not listen to the news. I do not want to be bombarded with the news. I may listen to it once a day or less than once a day. And if anything has happened, I may ask my husband to tell me just very briefly about it and I bury my head in the sand and go forward. I try not to let the media affect me and I try not to relate to it on a personal level. I know it is happening around me. I know if anything is going to affect me personally, it will find me. And the way to function is by closing it off.

I don't think anyone really perceives that it is ever going to happen to them, otherwise you would never get into a car because you could get into a car accident. It is very worrisome though, in the morning when you say good-bye to five family members and they are all going in different directions. It is particularly difficult with adolescents. I have three adolescents at home. They don't cooperate. They really don't. Even during these times. I would think they would mature more quickly and say, "Mum, we understand. We'll phone you as soon as we get there." But they don't cooperate.

They will call very reluctantly. They'll forget to call and then I'll call them. That's the hardest thing for me, being the mother of adolescents. Adolescence is always a challenging time. They do not understand my level of anxiety.

It's like you would say, "What time will you be home?" They don't want to be asked that. Even under these circumstances they don't want to be asked that. They want to be able to act out their adolescence even in this environment. For me, it is very hard because I want them to understand the circumstance is different, and obviously, their adolescence is a barrier for them to understand that.

I think I can generalize that parents are reacting with more caution than their children. I worry for our youth. I really worry for them. I think when you're 40 or 50 you can make some sense out of all this, and I don't know if the adolescents are thinking about their future. I don't know what is going on in their heads.

I know from observing my own children and also their friends that they are just yahooing and getting on with it and acting out and going out to the movies, and to the malls in spite of it all. I don't quite understand it. You know, I would almost be happier if they were more fearful. I would regard that as more normal. But they are off being kids regardless. However, I really wonder what is happening on a deeper level because they must express and feel fear like we do, or maybe they don't?

When asked if the school children have any opportunity to speak with a counselor, or if the counselors go to the schools to give children the opportunity to discuss what is happening in their country and community, L. replied:

My daughter lost a classmate and a counselor came in for just one session to discuss it with the class. Anything that requires more than that, I suppose the parents would have to look into it and take more responsibility. But I remember myself growing up as a young person in my teens and early twenties. I remember feeling the whole world being ahead of me. And I don't know, I am just not sure how our kids look at that.

TEACHER, NURSE, AND CLERGY INTERVIEWS

Vered Kater, an Israeli faculty member at the Henrietta Szold Haddasah Hebrew University School of Nursing conducted several interviews in Israel, asking the following questions:

1. How have you prepared your families for disaster?
2. What is your personal disaster plan?

3. How do you continue to function in your work, families, and recreation or play activities in the midst of the fear of terrorist activities?
4. What is your role as a nurse in disaster response?
5. Are you ever responsible for students during a disaster response? What is your role and theirs in this situation?

* * *

The first educator has a one-year-old child and her husband is a police officer who will be called to respond in an emergency. She and her husband have not prepared anything. There is no special safe room and no extra food; however, extra water is stored. They have no personal disaster plan in place and continue to function normally. She states that in her role as a nurse in a disaster response, she goes where she is supposed to go. Her child will be in childcare at work. She is not responsible for students during a disaster response.

* * *

The second nurse educator is a mother of four. Her husband is a physician who will be on duty during a disaster. She has only prepared her family by storing up a lot of water. She states, "We do not believe the plastic [on windows] will do any good." Her personal disaster plan is to have the big kids take care of the little ones while she and her husband go to work. They continue to function "totally normally." She said, "We had a great Purim party." In a disaster response, she would go to the Ein Karem Hospital in her role as a nurse and her husband would report to Mount Scopus Hadassah Hospital. She is not responsible for students during a disaster response.

* * *

The third nurse educator interviewed had been in Israel for 8 months at the time of the interview. Her husband is a clergyman who travels to the United States occasionally.

NURSING VIGNETTE 12–1 "A"

I was born here in Israel. I usually work 12-hour days. During the last war, I had no children. You cannot have constant fear. My barrier to fear is to not think about the terrible things that happen. I read the paper sometimes to get information, but sometimes I cannot look at the pictures. It is overstimulating when they show the results of bomb after bomb explosion. It is too stressful. I try not to listen to the radio.

You are always frightened that it will be your family. There is always someone hurt. You are afraid to take the public bus. I drive the children. When I go to Tel Aviv, I drive instead of taking the bus. When I go to the market in Jerusalem, I go without the children.

Then I am not as frightened. When I was pregnant, I would not go to the market.

As a single parent, I go to California for a change of scenery, to visits my two sisters. I must consider what I would do with my son in case of my death. I want to keep him safe.

I am not afraid to go to work. At the kindergarten and preschool, there is a security wall, an electronic gate, and it is in an enclave. We have our masks at home. When we are on "high alert" we walk with the masks.

Sometimes I cry. I continue to live. I have no choice. I need to function and I must plan for the future.

They have three children, ages 2, 5, and 8. They have prepared their family by having a [safe] room ready with toys. Their personal disaster plan includes having the children play in the room, especially with video games. The children have decorated their own [gas] masks. One of the nurse educator's personal friends is pregnant and her husband is in the army. In the event of a terrorist attack or disaster, the pregnant friend would join them in their safe room. They all continue to function "normally." Her role in a disaster response is to take care of her family first. She is not responsible for students during a disaster response.

* * *

Another nurse educator and his wife have been in Israel for 2 years. Their grown children remain abroad. They have prepared a safe room with food and water and other necessary supplies. His personal disaster plan is to go to work. He continues to function normally in the midst of the fear of terrorist attacks. His role in disaster response is not entirely clear to him, but he knows he will be working in the hospital. He is not responsible for students during a disaster response.

* * *

Born in Israel, the next nurse educator has served in the army. She has a husband and one son in the army. They have prepared their family for disaster by having supplies in their home, yet they have not sealed a room. Her personal disaster plan is to go to work at the hospital, to serve in the family room. They too continue to function "normally." Her role in a disaster response is to work in the family room. She is not responsible for students during a disaster response.

* * *

The sixth nurse educator has been in Israel for 7 years. She states that she does not understand Hebrew very well and has no dependents. She has prepared for a disaster by sealing a room and has food and water and, "everything the government told me to do is ready." Her personal disaster plan is that she is ready to work at the hospital, or wherever needed, if she is called up. She states that she does not function as well during the constant threat of terrorist attacks when she must always go out with her [gas] mask. She states that she is a bit apprehensive when "going to town." Her role as a nurse in a disaster response is to work in the neurological intensive care unit. She has worked there for six years and teaches in that department. She is not responsible for students during a disaster response.

* * *

Another interviewee, a nurse educator for 20 years in Israel, has no dependents, but has one sister living with her. She has prepared for a disaster by having one room sealed and ready with everything in the room. Her personal disaster plan is to simply go to work. She continues to function "normally" in spite of the constant threat of terrorist attacks. Her role as a nurse in a disaster response is to "go

where I am supposed to be." She is not responsible for students during a disaster response.

* * *

As a single mother with a 3-year-old child, this nurse educator has prepared her family for disaster by having tape and "everything else including food and water." However, the safe room is not ready. Her personal disaster plan is to go to work and her child will go to the child care area in the hospital. She continues to function "normally" in spite of the threat of disaster. Her role as a nurse in a disaster response is to work in the emergency room. She is not responsible for students during a disaster response.

* * *

The ninth nurse interviewed by Ms. Kater is single, has no children, and has been in Israel since 1966. She admits that she has not prepared at all. "I continue to do everything as normally as possible." Her personal disaster plan is to go to work as soon as possible. She states, "Work is the best place to be, no time to think about personal dangers. Life is too precious to waste it. Fearing the fear is worse than the fear itself. I continue to go out and am not really afraid; I am a realist and at the same time an optimist. Last night, the evening of the latest war, I went out with a few friends and we enjoyed a very good meal (not our last!!)" Her role in disaster response is to work on one of the surgical floors. She is not directly responsible for nursing students. "They sign a waiver and know exactly where to go when called up. They are all adults and the majority has had army service."

* * *

Finally, a nurse supervisor, who is the third generation to live in Israeli, has prepared for a disaster by having the plastic from the previous Gulf War ready. She has no personal disaster plan. She continues to function as she normally does, regardless of the increased threats of disaster. Her role as a nurse in a disaster response is to "go to work." She is not responsible for students during a disaster response.

ADVICE FROM BEREAVED PARENTS

Malki was born in Melbourne, Australia and was brought to Israel at the age of 2, as the youngest of four children. As a 10th-grade student, Malki was one of 15 murdered (and hundreds injured) by a suicide bomber on August 9, 2001, in Jerusalem's Sbarro restaurant. Malki was the middle child with three older brothers who were born in Australia and three younger sisters who were born in Jerusalem. Her parents, Frimet and Arnold Roth spoke to us about their daughter, their other children, their grief, and what people say and do that is hurtful and what people can say and do that is helpful in easing their pain.

The murder of our daughter has changed our lives forever. Many families here in Israel have been

Vered Kater, RN, MSN
Clinical Nurse Specialist

To answer your questions in writing is not as easy as it was talking about it, but I will try. The answer is totally subjective and specific for me, as I am unmarried and without dependents. I am coping with feelings [about the political milieu] on a daily basis, often by denying my own feelings to surface. If I do not talk or think about them, they do not interfere with my life. In order to function normally, to teach and go on, it is necessary for me to deny the problems; not to think too much about what may happen, what could go wrong, and what is totally wrong with the system. I have some friends who believe the exact opposite. Extreme religious zealots scare me, Jews as well as Arabs. They have blinders on and can only see one way, their own, without conceiving that others can also think.

How can I continue to teach and meet employment requirements and obligations? Teaching pediatric nursing is a wonderful escape to normal life in this crazy place. To see the faces of my students when they concentrate on clubfeet or spina bifida is great. They are allowed to forget everything that is real and concentrate on concrete or abstract problems. This reinforces normal behavior. For most students it is hard to learn while things happen all around them. By more or less forcing them to listen and think about faraway problems of pediatric nursing, I feel that I can help them to hold on, to grow, and to face their family at the end of the day in a more peaceful manner. Perhaps it is an illusion, but it certainly helps me to cope. The feedback they give me is encouraging. I help them think, my classes are never dull, and the students take an active part in disseminating information. Even if only for a few hours they have to concentrate on something not terror related. They have a positive experience which is sorely needed.

I think that a visit to Israel, where man-made disasters are daily occurrences, shows bravery [of the authors]. For me, it was important to be able to share our experiences. I think that the fact that I was born in the middle of a war and have been through a lot of different wars influenced my involvement. In fact, when I was asked to coordinate your visit, I had to think if I really wanted to be confronted with the part of my life that I prefer to deny. I am glad I did agree, as it helped me talk about our lives here with such a warm group of colleagues.

By the way, yesterday all schools as well as preschools had a drill and the kids spent part of the day in shelters. The last few days were awful again. Fanatics killed children. Olive groves were destroyed and people are getting very angry again. There are also an increasing number of road accidents. I think that is partly due to the lack of concentration, as well as by young people needing an outlet for their energy. They may have lost the belief that planning for a peaceful future is possible.

On an everyday basis, I cope in my own consciously chosen manner. I do read the paper every day, but never the grisly details. I do look at least twice a day at the TV news. I try not to talk about political issues with friends, as the result will always be an awful argument. Lack of understanding different points of views is typical among the Jews living here. Everybody is convinced that his or her opinion is the correct one. I try to go out more than ever to see films, theatre, and concerts. Long-term planning seems rather unreal. I live now and try to live as intensely as possible. I miss the fact that I cannot spontaneously take a walk into the mountains behind my house; it is not safe. I miss the volunteer work I did with handicapped children in Idna (near Hebron), and I have not spoken for 2 years with friends I had in Beth Jala, Bethlehem, and Silwan. I am not afraid to travel on a bus or to go to the market. I believe that if I live every moment as well as possible and repair any damage I have caused as soon as possible, then I am also ready to leave this earth should my time come unexpectedly. I am not afraid to die; I hate the idea of becoming dependent upon other people due to a handicap. I do not think that I can cope graciously with that. My basic trust for other human beings is still rather wobbly. It is surprising, as my first 3 years were spent with wonderful war parents and the rest of my childhood with parents (two divorces) and brothers I did not even know I had. I worked hard to become what I am, and at present I am more or less accepting myself as I am. It took me almost all my life to get here. I would like to stay on this earth a while longer and enjoy the sunset and dawn of each day. But if this is not to be, then I will hope to leave with one big bang.

A disaster is, as mentioned in most dictionaries, a sudden or great misfortune. A misfortune is very personal, what one person views as disastrous, another may not. Living in Israel in these times may be seen as a disaster, as disastrous events happen daily. I have been living in Jerusalem, Israel, for over 30 years and must admit that my life is very normal in spite of regular abnormal incidents. Getting up in the morning while listening to the birds on my balcony and breathing in the scent of pine trees gives me the energy to live my life as best as possible. My philosophy is very personal—life is too short to be scared while living it. I live as if the whole world is good and kind; therefore, I try consciously to be kind and caring. This is my denial mechanism but at the same time, it enables me to enjoy living to the fullest.

Having experienced several wars, after being born during one, I hope one day to see peace around me. In my own small way I work towards this goal by accepting people as they are, without judging. As a nurse, I listen and talk to many different people, often this dissipates tension, because as long as one talks or listens, one cannot shoot nor kill.

I hope that there are many more that believe this universal truth, and hopefully peace may come one day to this corner of our world.

Keep well and shalom from Jerusalem.

affected by terrorism during the past 2 years. At the time of Malki's murder, about 300 Israeli civilians had been killed through these senseless acts of violence, and we wondered how society could keep functioning. One year later, that count is closer to 650. [In July 2003, it exceeded 800.]

The traditional Jewish 7-day mourning period, the *shiva,* is a thoughtful and appropriate time for friends and family to visit in the home of the bereaved. For some people it helps to have a house full of people. In accordance with Jewish tradition, visitors don't initiate conversation; it is up to the grieving family members to speak if they feel up to it. They may choose silence. Sitting in low chairs is customary. You feel crushed, devastated, and low. Clothing worn at the funeral is ripped, and mourners continue to wear the same garments for the entire 7 days, a period during which the magnitude of the loss has to sink in. If there is a Jewish holiday, the 7 days of mourning may be interrupted or abbreviated. It is so important to have those 7 days in which other people take care of your needs, the needs of your family, your home, and cooking. People come in to help. But once the 7 days have passed, that's when the next stage starts with a shock, a jolt, because you have to face the reality that for everyone else life has continued, life goes on.

Once the 7 day *shiva* is over, it is important and valuable to the mourners to have people continue to come and visit and, just by sitting there with you, show their concern and support. It was very disappointing to us as a grieving family to see that many people who were there initially found it impossible to come or call again. They may apologize and say, "I can't come—it is too painful." I thought, "*I* am in pain—how can *they* say that?" I feel it is an obligation to be there for the bereaved. A couple of our neighbors stayed in our house for hours while we waited to know Malki's fate. The bombing took place at 2 in the afternoon, but we didn't find out that she was one of the victims until 12 hours later. Those neighbors have never come back and spoken to us since then. I assume it's hard for them. But their silence and absence is harder, and sends a very painful message to us. Some friends continue to show their concern. I really appreciate that.

What People Should Not Say to the Bereaved

Many things are perfectly acceptable to say to the bereaved families. Some other things need to be avoided or at least carefully thought about before anyone says them. They can be hurtful, especially when they come from people who have not personally experienced this kind of loss—a loss that is deeper and harder than any other.

1. I do not like to hear neat explanations as to why this tragedy happened. People will say, "It happened according to a plan." Some say: "It's God's plan" or "The Lord only gives us a load that He knows we can carry." We do not know why this happened, no one does. I hope to some day understand it in a world or time to come, but it will not be here on earth.

2. Five months after the killing, a caring friend told me about one of my daughter's friends—about how she has managed to pull things together and get on with life. The subtle message was: "And so should you." This is something I do not need anyone to tell me.

3. We are told to concentrate on our other children. They say, "Don't dwell on her death." Since this is coming from someone who has never known the loss of a child, it is hard to accept. When advice of this kind comes from someone who has lost a child, it's expressed in a different way, and I can relate to it.

4. Some stop me and say, "Hi, how are you?" This can be especially troubling when it is accompanied by a big smile. I feel they do not really want to hear how I am feeling. I find it hard to put on a show and say, "Fine, and how are you?" Why do they ask me this question when we bump into each other in the street, but never bother to come to me at home and really talk to me about how I am feeling? I'm perfectly capable of saying how I feel, which is that I feel terrible. I don't think they want to hear. If I cry, they seem to feel they have caused me some harm—but crying is sometimes the only response.

5. You will also hear others, certainly here in Jerusalem, say: "We all had a hard year with a lot of fear because of bombings and terror. Isn't this hard on all of us?" Yes, it is hard for everyone, but not everyone has lost a child—and that's truly something different and far, far worse. One woman argued with me, said everybody suffers and my suffering is just one in the bag of suffering and my pain is the same as anyone else's. That is not helpful because,

frankly, it's not true. The death of a child, and certainly the *murder* of a child, is so unthinkable, it's just not the same as *anything* else that happens in life.

6. It is very hurtful when someone asks, "Is your whole family going to be home for the holidays?" All of our children will *never* be home again.

These types of comments throw us. They seem like harmless, innocent comments to the people making them, but they cut right through us, and cause us enormous pain.

What Is Helpful

Some professionals are very good and their advice is very helpful. Some professionals are not as helpful. *The Worst Loss: How Families Heal from the Death of a Child,* by Barbara D. Rosof, is a great book. The loss of a child is a terrible pain, unlike any other. It is helpful to be with other bereaved parents, especially those who have lost children around the same age under sudden, unexpected circumstances. At one moment, you have a beautiful, healthy child and the next moment, the child is gone.

The professionals may describe this grieving journey as a process. They say you are moving forward, your pain will be different, and it will be lessened. To me, the pain does not change. You learn to harbor it all. You learn to keep going. In an article I read recently, two girls were kidnapped and murdered in England. A professor said: "The families will integrate this experience eventually into their lives. This experience will change their lives profoundly but they will be able to eventually think about it without great pain and emotion." I do not believe that. A mother said, "You become a part of a group of people who are unimaginably hurt. They are left with a gaping wound that will never heal." This I believe.

It's most helpful to hear from those who have had similar losses. There is a saying that "The suffering of many is half a comfort." What I believe this means is that others who have suffered like me lighten the pain a little, their company gives me strength, makes me feel I'm not alone. You do not feel singled out. When you see others who have suffered the same loss and are still functioning and continuing with their lives, you suddenly realize it can happen. Earlier on you just do not think you can go on.

Support groups of people who have experienced the same kind of tragedy in their lives,

whether formal or informal, are very helpful. Whether the groups are formed among friends you have made or organized by a professional, they can be an oasis. However, people do not share the same feelings—they're different, we're all different and we need to accept that we will all react in our own individual ways. You may hear something and think to yourself, "I hope I never feel that way or say that." It helps to be aware of these feelings and pitfalls and try to avoid them. For example, there was a man in one group who talked about the youngest of his six children who was killed in an attack. It really makes no difference how many children you have; the pain of losing one child is intimate and extremely intense. He said the other children in the family ask, "What about me? Am I not important to you?" He told us that he said to his children, "You will never be as important to me as the child I lost." This struck me as devastating to the living children. I will always keep this in mind. I would not allow myself to hint that sentiment to the other children.

Siblings

What we found is that, in almost every family, at least one child is profoundly affected by the sibling's death. This seems to be especially true with the younger children. The child may not be able to concentrate, or does not function well socially or in school. The professionals may say that the child had these tendencies before the tragedy occurred, "That is just the way they were." Trauma of this kind can really throw them. My advice to parents is to look around for the right professional. It is hard to find excellent psychologists and social workers. You are so overwhelmed that it is hard, but you need to get organized. Children can be lost. They may go "off the track" easily. This loss is overwhelming for children.

Parents and Children

We have a sort of contract with our children. They might say, "I'll keep growing—you keep keeping me safe." As parents, we are not always on top of the situation. There are many things outside of our control.

The death of a child hurts tremendously. Please do not avoid the topic of the loss. We are always hurting for her, and yes, the topic hurts and we may cry, but that does not mean we don't want to speak about her. It hurts more when you avoid mentioning her. Do not deny that she lived. Share the memories of the deceased with those who love them— celebrate their lives.

NURSING VIGNETTE 12–3   Responding to the Call

Julie Benbenishty, RN

At 1:00 a.m. the phone rings. "There's a gun shot injury and he has received six units of blood—get here fast!" I quickly dress with the clothes that have been thrown over my desk chair, give a quick kiss to the kids, leave them a note on the table, and leave the house. Within 10 minutes I am dressed in green scrubs, taking blood for coagulation tests and quickly injecting the experimental drug—Factor 7, or placebo—intravenously into the patient with the open abdomen in OR number 17. I continuously take blood from the patient to be centrifuged and send it to the United Kingdom for testing as I continue to give him another two doses of Factor 7 or placebo. The bleeding is controlled, the abdomen is closed, and he is wheeled into the recovery room intubated and ventilated. His family is waiting anxiously outside in the waiting room for news from the surgeon.

By 5:30 a.m. I am back home. While driving the kids to school an hour later, a bomb explodes in an inner-city bus less than a mile from the hospital. A new battle begins. We barely have time to orient ourselves with the new patients from the night shift when we hear about the bomb and we quickly get ourselves ready. Extra emergency equipment is prepared, extra staff is notified, and patients who can be transferred are done so quickly. In a panic, the assistant head nurse looks for her kids. The bus exploded at the stop near her house.

As we quickly take our places, the wounded are rushed into the OR (Figure 12–1A and B). We see the trauma surgeon together with the open-heart team and we all silently calculate this information. Two more injured are rushed into the OR followed by vascular surgeons. We hear the OR intercom sounding off, paging all personnel to different rooms. There is a frantic call for Factor 7 to be given to a bleeding patient. As I walk into the room, I take a count—two vascular surgeons, two general surgeons, the director of open-heart surgery, three anesthesiologists, and two anesthesiologist assistants. An intern is rushing back and forth to the blood gas machine with a syringe in his hand, to keep close count of pH and pO_2.

In the corner near the door there is a pile of empty blood transfusion bags, plasma, and packed cells. Blood samples are taken for coagulation times and pharmacokinetics and Factor 7 or placebo is injected. The patient continues to bleed. She is connected to the cell saver, a machine that stores the blood that the patient bleeds out to be given directly back into the veins.

While everyone is concentrating in this operating room in saving this young girl's life, there are five other rooms frantically working to stop the bleeding in other blast victims. To stop the massive diffused hemorrhaging sometimes drastic measures need to be taken. Instead of using the trial medication of Factor 7, the real drug used in hemophilia is administered.

More blood samples are taken and all surgeons are frantically looking for the source of the bleeding. The blood pressure and heart rate continue to plummet. Two nurses enter the room and ask for identifying marks so that the patient can be identified by name.

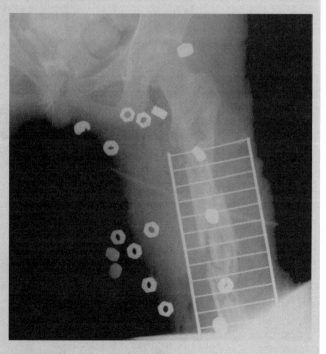

Figure 12–1A. Shrapnel wounds. *(Photo courtesy of Julie Benbenishty)*   **Figure 12–1B.** Shrapnel wounds X ray. *(Photo courtesy of Julie Benbenishty)*

Adrenaline is injected directly into the heart. "It's time to stop," states the anesthesiologist quietly. "The blood pressure is gone and the heart has stopped beating."

Without hesitation, the surgeon holds the heart in his hand and silently pumps it himself. The other surgeons still search for the source of the bleeding, trying desperately to tie off the open bleeding vessels. The anesthesiologist continues to take blood gas samples and inject adrenaline, calcium, and magnesium. Everyone steadfastly works at his or her tasks as if everything is going just as planned.

For another 15 minutes after time of death, the surgeon pumps the young girl's heart. He won't give up; he refuses to believe that there is nothing more to be done.

A young girl, after her morning coffee, kisses her mom good-bye and walks to the bus stop. The bus arrives; she gets in, takes a seat and thinks about the day ahead. Her day ends 3 hours later.

It's an unfathomable thought that this mother has lost her child. How does one break this devastating news to parents? This is how terror rips us apart.

The already full recovery room is pushed to the limit when five additional critically injured bomb victims are added. The walls are elastic. We accept all. No one is turned away.

But what is the price that the nursing staff has to pay? The physicians don't have the capacity to take care of all these extra patients. The morphine supply has long gone. We call the pharmacist. He will be there shortly. But what happens in the interim? We must find a pain solution. The nurses must revert to giving the patients any pain medication that they can find. Ampules of Ketamine are used for pain relief. Eight hours later the pharmacist arrives.

The entire nursing staff of the recovery room add extra hours and shifts to already overburdened schedules. When the phone rings, we are already more than just overexhausted. We get dressed, get the car keys, and go again. We all feel for these families. Maybe if we work extra hard, we can surely buy our children time, before the next attack.

We were all anticipating a relaxing weekend with our families. They too suffer from shock and anxiety when a bomb explodes in their home city. But instead of being with our young children and comforting their fears, we all go to work, where we use our skills to help the victims.

THE GLOBAL ROLE OF A DISASTER NURSE

This is the account of Elsie Roth, a public health nurse who has traveled far and wide serving communities facing disasters.

The career of nursing came to me very late in life. I graduated from Saint Louis University School of Nursing in 1983, at age 54. I knew in my senior year that the hospital setting was far too confining for me. I chose to be a public health nurse where I would have more autonomy. Little did I realize that my profession would lead me to one global disaster after another, in countries one only dreams of visiting. I will describe five events. Two were famines, two were front line wars, and one was a course preparing nurses for disasters.

1983, Operation Moses

In 1983, there was a severe drought in Ethiopia. The Jews of Ethiopia suffered from terrible discrimination and were dying. Israel wanted to receive them as citizens but had no diplomatic relations with the Ethiopian government. Word was sent to them, since they were all mostly in the region of Gondar, to start walking quietly at night to a designated place in neighboring Sudan. They would then be airlifted to Israel. Some 12,000 fragmented families

arrived in Israel from November 1983 to March 1984. It was called Operation Moses. I volunteered my services in March 1984 and stayed 8 months to help.

This was a whole new experience for Israel. Although they were used to receiving immigrants from all over the world, none had presented with such severe medical, psychiatric, and social problems, in such large numbers so quickly. Their absorption was very challenging. I created my own job, which was to care for 150 families (about 500 people). They lived in what was called an absorption center, which was a group of high-rise apartments. The culture change was shocking; one had to show them how to use a doorknob, turn on lights, use the bathroom, and eat new foods. I made rounds each day, 6 days a week. I would assess their wellness and show them how to be compliant with medications. I drew a little "sun up" for morning (A.M.) and "sun down" for evening (P.M.) medications. I was to identify real problems in all of the above areas, then take them to the appropriate person for help. Language was a real barrier, as they spoke the ancient language of Amharic. I overcame this by taking some of their young children who already had learned Hebrew to come with me on rounds. My dialogue was to the children in Hebrew who then translated the Hebrew into Amharic to their relatives, and then reversed the procedure. It worked very well and I found out all of the information that was necessary.

I never saw a complete family, or a person who was not ravaged by this experience. One recollection that I have was that many mothers started to feed their infants too much because they were afraid that a drought could happen in Israel. The babies looked like Sumo wrestlers. Ironically, we had to put them on diets 4 months after they arrived.

1986, The Gondar Region of Ethiopia

In 1986, I was invited to be the nurse on a trip to the Gondar Region of Ethiopia where 12 of us would assess the numbers and conditions of the Jews who, for whatever reason, could not be part of Operation Moses. We found terrible starvation. All of the children had kwashiorkor, a disease resulting from a deficiency of protein. We backpacked in corticosteroids for their very serious eye problems. We visited five villages. I then divided the population into groups, so that I could assess them separately, to treat eyes, wounds, and whatever else was needed. I had trained my friends to assist me. I will never, ever forget such poverty or such hopelessness of the human condition.

1991, The Gulf War

In 1991, the Gulf War began. I went to Israel to help as Saddam Hussein threatened to shoot scud missiles at Israel. A few minutes after our arrival in Tel Aviv, scuds hit. We had not even learned to put on the gas masks. We were quickly escorted to "safe rooms." These were rooms taped in preparation for a gas attack. We learned very quickly to put on our assigned gas masks.

I worked at the main trauma center on a geriatric ward in Tel Aviv. My job was to take care of the elderly, and in the event of an attack none of them wanted to put on their masks; they all had compromised breathing and were too weak to help themselves. It was very ironic that some of the patients were Holocaust survivors and here they were, caught in yet another disaster.

It is terrifying to hear scuds hit around you and not know if you would be next. No one complained; everyone just carried on. It was a real eye opener to see how a whole country came together with such spirit and bravery.

The Bosnian War

The Bosnian War came soon after. It was in 1993 to 1995 that I saw pictures of rape camps, mass graves, and starvation, to name a few horrors. I decided I had to do something about it. As a Jew, the Holocaust is always uppermost in my mind. This time, the Holocaust destroyed hundreds of thousands of *non-Jews.*

I was able to call an American Jewish women's organization called Hadassah. Their primary job is to support the Hadassah hospitals in Jerusalem. They are also involved in social reform in the United States. I am a lifetime member of Hadassah and a former President of the St. Louis chapter. At the time that I had asked for help from Hadassah, the United States had made no commitments to assist in Bosnia. The war raged on. Hadassah understood the immediate need to help on a national level. They gave me permission to go to Sarajevo with three other nurses to do a needs assessment. We wore flack jackets and helmets and left immediately as a lull in the war was only momentary. We came home and mounted a campaign from coast to coast for pharmaceuticals, medical supplies, and new warm clothing. It was a very ecumenical campaign; everything was donated and packed by all of us. I accompanied these supplies back to Sarajevo on two more occasions so that they would not be sold on the black market.

My congressman was able to get the supplies and me on a C-130 military transport plane. During the second trip back to Sarajevo, I stayed in a bombed out house with no heat, water, or food. It was winter. This condition was no different than anyone else had suffered. We delivered 150 tons of supplies, valued over $10 million.

2002, Disaster Preparedness Education in Israel

During a casual conversation with the dean of my nursing school, in August 2002, she mentioned that she wanted to institute a disaster preparedness program for nurses, but there was very little information on this subject. I told her that I knew exactly where to go for the best training in the world. Who would know better than the Israelis? They experience trauma every day. I again called Hadassah and their Nurses' Council went to work. Although the hospitals in Jerusalem had never done this before, they put together a 60-hour program, which we would take in 4 days, using their best and brightest people. Two nursing assistant professors, one public health professor, one infectious disease specialist, and I completed the course at the Henrietta Szold Hadassah School of Nursing. To my knowledge, we are the only group of Americans trained in Jerusalem in disaster preparedness.

In summary, the nursing process, to assess, plan, implement, and then evaluate, always guides my nursing career. This procedure is necessary and has worked effectively during all the disasters that I have had the opportunity to assist.

Finally, as a nurse, one sees people at their best and at their worst. A person's goodness, decency, and willingness to help in the worst of conditions seems to rise up over and over again. This never fails to renew my spirit.

DEPLOYMENT

Mark Foersterling, RN, was a member of MO-1 DMAT sent to the NYC burn unit as a Supervisory Nurse Specialist after 9-11. This is his story.

I was at the Noble Training Center for a medical weapons of mass destruction course scheduled September 10-14, 2001. I flew in on Monday morning. I was transported to the training base by bus and then housed in the fort's barracks. We had class that afternoon and evening.

Classes started early the next day at the training hospital. A short time after classes started, most of the beepers in the class all went off at once. A few moments later the director informed us that the World Trade Center had been attacked and that this was not a drill. The military base we were on was locked down by military on the inside and local police on the outside. One of the few planes that flew that day was one to a nearby airfield to return approximately a third of our class to work on the event. I was one of the 7,000 volunteers who kept running across the bottom of the TV screens. HHS Secretary Tommy Thompson had already sent four disaster medical assistance teams (DMATs) to New York and three DMATs to the Washington, D.C., area. In addition, HHS dispatched four disaster mortuary operational response teams (DMORTs) to New York and three DMORTs to Washington, D.C. This was the first time that the National Disaster Medical System had been fully activated and all 80 DMATs were ready to be deployed.

My team was activated along with the rest, but I stayed to complete the training that week. I was fortunate to find a TWA crew in Atlanta who wanted to fly back home to St. Louis. All the rental cars were already gone and the other modes of travel were all booked up. It was a very long week.

When I got home, my team was still on alert. We could possibly assist in receiving victims being landed at the local USAF base or go to one of the disaster sites. What happened was something else altogether, which is how I've found most of my deployments to be. You just never know what you'll get with a disaster or how you will be needed.

Approximately 1 week later, a request for nurses with burn experience was sent out to the DMATs.

Several members of our team worked in the largest trauma center in the region and volunteered to go. I went with two other nurses at the end of September to New York City. We had another nurse that later went to the D.C. burn unit.

I flew out of Lambert St. Louis International Airport on September 30 and landed at LaGuardia. I went by taxi to the NDMS Command Center set up in lower Manhattan. I presented travel orders and signed in at NDMS Operations. I received another special photo ID and completed all my paperwork. I was then taken to where we were going to stay for the next 2 weeks.

I was driven to the Helmsley Medical Tower next to the NYC burn unit (Figure 12–2). NDMS had arranged for rooms here. I was on the same floor as my two other team members. It was much better than our usual tent arrangement, like those found on the TV show *MASH*. One of the nurses was put into room 911.

I went over to the burn unit that evening. I wanted to know what was needed and the details. The William Randolph Hearst Burn Unit was on the eighth floor. I entered via a security officer at the door and the first person I met was a burn/trauma physician. He had worked back in St. Louis 10 years prior and it was great to see him. I then met the nurse manager who wanted us to start the next day. We had to also get hospital IDs and computer passwords before starting. They were very short on the night shift, so I started that next evening.

The entire west wing of the eighth floor was covered with get-well cards. The bathrooms were the only place where these cards were not found. Most were handmade from school-age children. They were from every state in the Union. Some were on a roll of paper and signed by every person in the school. It was a very impressive sight. The unit was a long corridor with patient rooms mostly on one side

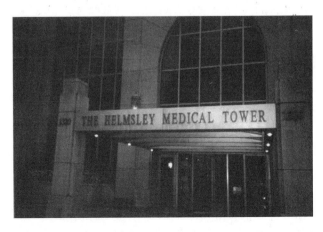

Figure 12–2. Helmsley Medical Tower. *(Photo Courtesy of Michael Foersterling)*

and the nurses' station and supply rooms on the other side. The first supply room had IV cases that were lined up against the whole wall and went almost to the ceiling. The rest of that room was filled with all kinds of equipment and linen. The other supply room had every type of burn care supplies you could think of in it.

I had one night of orientation to learn the hospital layout, practices, computers, and supplies. I was assigned to a very nice and knowledgeable NYC burn unit nurse. She was great. She also had a very heavy Brooklyn accent. She told me that her husband had recently been offered a job in Boston. She refused to go because she did not want her children speaking like them. I had a hard but successful time hiding my amusement with that statement, but I sure did not want to aggravate my lifeline 1 hour into my first shift!

The burn unit had wonderful equipment. The beds were gortex with every attachment. If you wanted to do chest PT on your patient, you just entered it on the control panel at the foot of the bed. Each room had top-of-the-line HP monitors in them. I think almost everything in that hospital was made by HP. The hospital had great community supporters and the FDNY took great pride in the 20-bed burn unit.

Most of the major burn injuries went to this one burn unit. It would provide burn care for the area. The unit only had three patients on the morning of 9-11. This was about the normal census for this time of year. It would generally increase during the late winter heating season. The unit filled that day. The smallest burn in that unit now was 50%. I think that unit may have had the sickest patients in the country that fall. The victims from the WTC generally made it out alive or did not survive. It was very similar to a large-scale flooding disaster where you find only a few injured and most either had made it out safely or had drowned. All the injured from the World Trade Center had been cared for and released by all the local hospitals, except for those in the burn unit.

The whole time we were there, we were referred to as the FEMA nurses. We were mostly DMAT nurses and some volunteer nurses from the Burn Association. They were federalized and assigned to NDMS, too. I think the reason for this name is due to the way we respond to disasters. FEMA evaluated the disaster and then requested the needed assets. If it includes medical needs, then DMATs are sent. Neither I nor anyone else was ever able to change us from the name of FEMA nurses. After awhile, we just gave up!

We had young healthy individuals who were fighters. This is not usually the case. Most burn patients tend to be at the age extremes of life. They also tend to be in less than good general health. We had a fight on our hands in this burn unit. I'm proud to say this country responded to the need. Most of the patients were injured by the burning jet fuel. Some had it fall on them while outside of the towers; others had it come down the elevator shafts into the lobbies. Most of the people that were burned higher up in the towers never had the time to make it out.

The patients' families were also not your typical families. They were there from the start of visiting hours until it was time to go home. Visiting time was very short and limited to only the spouse or parent. They had to keep all the others updated. Some families even called every night at a specific time for an update. These families were the best. I got to know some of the families very well. I got daily e-mails from one man all the way into March 2002 when his wife finally got to go home. I still get regular e-mails from him and a Christmas card with their photo together on it. I see her from time to time on one of the TV shows like *Oprah.* It's good to see her and remember that she won.

Different groups would come in for the visitors in the waiting room. They would bring dinner in for all of them. Most of the families never left that waiting room for extended periods of time. The hospital has multiple types of support people come to see them each day. You need to remember that you are taking care of more than just the patient.

The next 14 nights consisted of working 12+ hour shifts. The patients were so sick. They were mostly on ventilators with multiple IV drips and piggybacks. We gave IV fluids by the gallons. I had one patient that had 12 IV pumps plus all the piggybacks. You worked 1 hour at a time. You got everything that you needed done in that hour and then started on the next hour. Each hour was a very busy hour. The patients went to surgery as often as we could send them. Surgery was the only way they would get more skin. Skin is the name of the game for major burn patients. It is the barrier between the infections and exposures of the outside world and the life-sustaining body fluids that the patient needs to survive. We even made some special antibiotic impregnated fine mesh gauze for some of the patients' burns. The unit had several burn tanks where the patients' burns were cleaned and the wound care was provided.

I did not know it, but the tower where we were staying was being tuck-pointed. They would start chiseling at 0800, then stop for lunch, and then chisel until time to go home. We also had a pipe break down the hall several days after getting there. So, we also had plumbers working inside at the end of the hall. I did what every disaster responder must remember to do. You must adapt, improvise, and overcome. I was unable to change to any better locale in the tower. NDMS was checking but no current alternative was available to us. I reached a practical solution that would work for our short-term stay. I would leave in the morning as soon as possible. I would stop at the corner deli and get something for breakfast. I would then eat it going up in the elevator. I would then take a Benadryl for my sinuses that also made me sleepy. I would then put in my earplugs and go to bed. I would fall fast asleep and generally got several hours of sleep before the workmen woke me. I would then go back to sleep during their lunchtime. I would repeat the process once more after they went home. I would set the alarm for as late as possible and then run to the burn unit for my shift. I was very tired after 2 weeks of this, plus the work itself was exhausting.

I went to Ground Zero on Sunday morning, October 7, 2001, for a special FDNY service. It was a very solemn place. A horn would blow every time a body was found and all work would come to a stop. It was considered a good day when the horn sounded a lot. The FDNY Band and the U.S. Army Band were there. I think the saddest thing I've ever heard was when the fire department played "Amazing Grace" on bagpipes. It just echoed in that newly formed urban canyon. I attended the service with my St. Louis group and the members from the nearby DMAT tent. I visited the small park near us after the service. It looked out at the Statue of Liberty. It was lined with flowers where the families left notes about the victims. A small memorial was made next to the police memorial that was already there. It had pictures of the missing police officers with flowers and notes from their families. I was glad that I went, but did not really want to do that again anytime soon. I had to work again that night but at least there were no workmen on the weekend to interrupt my sleep!

I stayed an extra couple of days in the burn unit. I came home on October 14 to the most comfortable bed in America—mine. I was glad to have gone and helped. I would have gone back in a second if asked, but was glad that I was not needed. I saw what the worst in some people can cause and also the very, very best in others. I still think about it with mixed emotions. This is also part of going to a disaster.

Most of the 9-11 burn patients survived. This would not have happened in other places around the world. They have recovery times that will take months and even years to reach. All will have some limitations due to the severity of their injuries. I am sure they will overcome these as well. It was an honor to have met these people. The additional medical assistance stopped about the end of October due to patients being able to move to levels of lesser care.

NURSING VIGNETTE 12–4   Nurse Faculty Member in Northern Virginia

Marie Kodadek, PhD, RN

This faculty member was approximately 7 to 10 miles from the Pentagon when the Pentagon was struck September 11, 2001.

I was teaching a 3-hour lecture class in an annex building away from the nursing building. We were all oblivious to what was happening. When the class finished, I began to hear the students outside murmuring about a plane hitting something. It was about 12:30 or 1 p.m. before I found out what had really happened. The television was turned on in one of the nursing labs. All of us were glued to the TV watching what was happening. I had many messages on my cell phone when I finally checked it. Some parents were taking their children out of school but I figured the schools were safer than the roads at that point.

The parochial school, where we have one child, sent a note home that indicated that we were to prepare a "comfort" kit for our kids. They were to have seven plastic bottles of some kind of liquid, such as water, four cans of food such as Spaghetti-Os, a change of clothes, and a blanket. These were all to be brought to school in some type of backpack or large bag. Later, the school nurse asked parents to get separate containers of the children's medicines to be labeled and stored specifically for emergency situations. This was sort of a pain for the parents, but most parents complied. The school nurse also asked the teachers to have emergency supplies of their medicines at the school. She explained the importance of having diabetic medicines, supplies and antihypertension medicines available in case of a disaster where no one was able to leave the school building. The addition of the medicines added extra expense and created a bit of a problem with storage and security of medicines, but they worked it out.

Most of the parents had to spend some time talking with their young children about 9-11. They were all scared. As far as the family preparations are concerned, we always have loads of duct tape on hand in case that is needed. We probably have more bottled water on hand than before 9/11. We have taught the children where to find the lock

(continued)

box where all of the important papers are stored. They know who their legal guardian would be in case both of us are incapacitated. We also review this information each summer when we go on vacation. In case of a fire, everyone knows how to get out of the house and that they are to meet at the mailbox or at the house across the street. They know where extra keys to the house are stored.

My personal disaster plan is to stay at school, at work. My husband works in downtown D.C. and may not be able to get out in case something happens. The carpool would take care of getting the boys home; if it were my turn to drive, I would try to get them. However, we all keep each other's cell phone numbers handy in case we would not be able to pick up the carpool as scheduled. The boys are able to walk to friends' homes. They also have spare keys to get into the house. We all look out for each other as neighbors.

The kids really did not verbalize much fear about the events of 9-11. They were angry about events being canceled. When we had the sniper shooting at random people, school trips were canceled due to the heightened alert. One field trip destination was near Camp David. Some families were glad the trip was canceled. Not us. We did not feel real fear; but we were not going to do stupid things, either. We used common sense but did not

let it affect our lives too much; we were not about to give in to the terrorists.

I do not have a specific role as a nurse in disaster response. I still volunteer at the health department. I would be available as a field nurse. I volunteered to get the smallpox vaccine, but the vaccine was not available. The university was designated as a site to provide services such as administration of the smallpox vaccine or the anthrax antidote. Several faculty members volunteered to be on a response team. However, we have not received any training to date. There is also a concern about the nonavailability of sinks.

I am responsible for nursing students while we are in clinical agencies. If there were a disaster, and we were in one of the county schools during a clinical day, we would stay and help with the children. The university would probably close. We lecture about disaster planning but we do not have specific roles or a specific policy that I am aware of. The hospitals in this area really do not want to be responsible for the students because they already have so many levels of knowledge and skill available. They will not count the students in their work plan. If the students want to volunteer they will be welcomed, though. Faculty members are being asked to show up at the facility that we can reach and see if they need our help.

SUMMARY

The persons who shared their stories here are just a small representative sample of the millions of persons affected by disasters in recent years. Their stories are incredible in some cases, yet we can all relate to them on some level. Tragedy transcends all borders, cultures, socioeconomic levels and professions. We can look back at what has occurred in history, study the lessons learned and plan for the future. We cannot know what the future holds, but we have a responsibility to be prepared. By reading this textbook, you have taken a positive step forward. The authors hope that you will engage in lifelong learning. Being prepared for disasters involves a lifelong commitment to learning as we are continuously faced with new, different, and unknown challenges. We wish you great success in your learning endeavors and thank you for your willingness to join the collaborative effort in saving lives. But most of all, we wish you peace.

CASE STUDY

Losing a Child

Mr. and Mrs. L. live in the rural area of your town. You are the nurse who cared for their comatose son who was one of the victims of a mass school shooting. Their son died

17 days after the incident. Six months later you are alone at the shopping center when you catch Mr. and Mrs. L. staring at you. They approach you and ask, "Aren't you the nurse who helped take care of our Nicholas?"

1. What do you say to Mr. and Mrs. L.?
2. What do you avoid saying to Mr. and Mrs. L.?
3. Should you ask them how they are feeling?
4. Should you promise to visit them at their home?
5. How will you react if Mrs. L. begins to cry?

TEST YOUR KNOWLEDGE

1. Discuss how reading stories can be a valuable strategy in learning the meaning of a disaster experience.
2. What are some of the similar themes expressed in the nurses' disaster stories?
3. Review the nurses' stories and the story shared by the bereaved parents. What are the differences in priorities expressed in their stories?
4. Describe some of the effective expressions of condolence to bereaved families.
5. Discuss some of the expressions of condolence that may be perceived as hurtful by bereaved family members.

6. Many who have experienced terrorism compare the extreme changes in routines following a frightening event as giving in to the terrorists.

   A. True
   B. False

7. Following a terrorist event, the survivors may feel that their sense of "normalcy" is forever changed.

   A. True
   B. False

8. In general, nurses who survive disaster events feel that it is important to share their experiences with other nurses and nursing students.

   A. True
   B. False

9. Children living in a nation at war have a greater likelihood of experiencing accidents and abuse than children living in a peaceful society.

   A. True
   B. False

10. Those who have experienced a terrorist event often feel that repeated media reports and news coverage of the event cause over-stimulation and provoke anxiety.

    A. True
    B. False

EXPLORE MEDIALINK

Interactive resources and an audio glossary for this chapter can be found on the Companion Website at http://www.prenhall.com/langan. Click on Chapter 12 to select the activities for this chapter.

REFERENCES

Sorrell, J. M. (2002). Teaching through stories. An approach to student-centered learning. In G. Redmond & J. M. Sorrell (Eds.), *Community-based nursing curriculum: A faculty guide* (pp. 29–52). Philadelphia: F. A. Davis.

APPENDIX

Agencies and Acronyms

APIC	Association for Professionals in Infection Control & Epidemiology	HIPAA	Health Insurance Portability and Accountability Act
ARC	American Red Cross	JCAHO	Joint Commission on Accreditation of Healthcare Organizations
BSTs	Burn Specialty Teams	MOU	Memorandum of Understanding
CDC	Centers for Disease Control and Prevention	NACCHO	National Association of County & City Health Officials
DHS	Department of Homeland Security	NDMS	National Disaster Medical System
DMAT	Disaster Medical Assistance Team	NMRT	National Medical Response Teams
DMORT	Disaster Mortuary Operation Response Team	NNRT	National Nurses' Response Team
DoD	Department of Defense	OEP	Office of Emergency Preparedness
DOT	Department of Transportation	PAHO	Pan American Health Organization
EMS	Emergency Medical System	SEMA	State Emergency Management Agency
EOC	Emergency Operations Center	SNS	Strategic National Stockpile
ESF	Emergency Support Function	TARU	Technical Advisory Response Unit
FBI	Federal Bureau of Investigation	US & R	Urban Search and Rescue
FEMA	Federal Emergency Management Agency	VA	Department of Veterans Affairs
FRP	Federal Response Plan	VMATs	Veterinary Medical Assistance Teams
HHS	Department of Health and Human Services	WMD	Weapons of Mass Destruction

APPENDIX B

Test Your Knowledge Answers

CHAPTER 1: *Disasters: A Basic Overview*

1. b
2. d
3. d
4. a
5. b
6. a
7. b
8. a
9. c
10. c

CHAPTER 2: *Planning for Disasters*

1. a
2. d
3. b
4. a
5. d
6. d
7. a
8. d
9. b
10. b

CHAPTER 3: *Organization and Implementation of the Disaster Response*

1. Choices include: Administrators, ancillary support (laboratory, radiology, media, maintenance, engineering), infection control specialist, law enforcement, fire, EMS, American Red Cross, managers, nurses, physicians
2. b
3. Choices include: "Mass Casualty Disaster Plan Checklist: A Template for Health Care Facilities"; "Bioterrorism Readiness Plan: A Template for Health Care Facilities"; and "Bioterrorism Emergency Planning and Preparedness Questionnaire for Health Care Facilities."
4. Options include: Names and traditional identification methods; bar-coding triage tags with barcoded adhesive stickers; number coding with numbered adhesive tags
5. The ultimate goal of crisis management is to investigate the incident to determine who did it and deal with the immediate crisis. The FBI is always the lead agency, regardless of whether the agent is chemical, biological, or radiological.

   The ultimate goal of consequence management deals with the consequences from the incident, including handling the victims, resource management, and recovery efforts. FEMA will be in charge.
6. b. False
7. b. False
8. Triage
   Staging
   Extended medical care
9. a. True
10. b. False

CHAPTER 4: *Promoting Mental Health Predisaster and Postdisaster*

1. d
2. c
3. b
4. c
5. c
6. d
7. c
8. b
9. d
10. c

CHAPTER 5: *Preparing Nursing Administrators, Faculty, and Students for Disasters*

1. a
2. a
3. c
4. e
5. b
6. e
7. e
8. d
9. True
10. False

CHAPTER 6: *Preparing Staff and Inactive Registered Nurses to Manage Casualties*

1.
   - Providing a coordinated, comprehensive federal response to any large-scale crisis
   - Mounting a swift and effective recovery effort
   - Prioritizing citizen preparedness
   - Educating families on the best ways to prepare their homes for disaster
   - Providing suggestions for citizen's response to a crisis

2. During times of mass casualties, less severely injured victims are treated first, leaving those with severe injuries requiring large amounts of resources to be treated afterwards.

3. Following a mass casualty event, you can expect that *one third* of the victims will be critical, and *two-thirds* of the victims will be treated and released from the hospital.

4. Determine how many operating rooms are available with personnel to staff them. Determine how many X ray machines are available, calculating that all victims of blast injuries will require a chest X ray at 10 min/X ray.

5. False

6. False

7. Knowing about the ways in which bombs cause injuries helps the nurse anticipate the types of injuries. High order explosives cause a *defining, supersonic over-pressurization shock wave* that results in injuries to *gas filled organs, such as lungs, GI tracts, and tympanic membrane*.

8. Develop a database of licensed health care providers and recruit these workers as a reserve pool. It requires that the institution conduct regular educational offerings and exercises. Consider using health care students to provide basic level care during an emergency.

9. Designate a separate area for those with minor injuries, such as schools, clinics, hotels. Incorporate security personnel into the response plan so that all family and friends are taken to a designated area to obtain status reports and assist in the identification of victims. Keep the triage and treatment areas for personnel and victims only.

10. Assign nurses with emergency department, intensive care, and OR experience to the more critical patients. Since many people will be present, and PPE may be required, consider using vests, bright labels, or hats to group teams and identify the type of worker, i.e., physician, nurse, recorder, transport, etc.

CHAPTER 7: *Management and Preparation for Battlefield Casualties*

1. MEDIC M = Minimal—T3: Minimal. Minor injuries. Managed by minimally trained staff.
   E = Expectant—T4: Expectant. Serious, multiple injuries. Treatment is complex and time consuming. Treatment consumes considerable personnel or resources.
   D = Delayed—T2: Delayed. Time consuming surgery. Life not jeopardized by delay. Stabilization minimizes effects of delay.
   I = Immediate—T1: Immediate Surgery to safe life or limb. Minimal operating time. Expected good quality survival.
   C = Contamination

2. d.
3. EMEDS (Expeditionary Medical System)
4. a
5. Clara Barton
6. False
7. Geneva (known today as the Geneva Convention)
8. c
9. d
10. d

CHAPTER 8: *Preparing Community Health Nurses and Nurses in Ambulatory Health*

1. Planning assumptions are based on where your students come from specifically looking at the distance, bridges, and viaducts. How long do you feel your students could be stranded? If you believe that students will be picked up within one day, half the remainder within a day, and the remainder within another day; you should stock supplies for 100% for day one, 50% for day two, plus 25% for day three. Factor in the number of staff and other adults who may be on campus.

2. Set the item on the ground and clear all students, faculty, and staff from the area. Call 911. The authorities will assume command of the area when they arrive.

3.
- Establish a relationship with the Supervisory Agent in Charge of the nearest FBI field office, or the regional Joint Terrorism Task Force (JTTF), so that the institution receives information about threats.
- Appoint Liaison officers between international student groups may elicit information and build trust and reduce fears among international students.
- Take all necessary actions to create a safe environment.
- Review and direct the implementation of the emergency operations plan, as well as the terrorism incident annex, and mutual aid agreements with local partners.

4.
- Increased visibility of security officers may provide additional security.
- Increasing physical checks of critical areas
- Establishing single point of access for critical facilities
- Strict identification checks
- Limitations on public access
- Increase inspections of persons and vehicles through video monitoring

5. The four steps included in the FEMA plan include:
- Establishing a planning team
- Analyzing the capabilities and hazards of the organization
- Develop the plan
- Implementation of the plan

6.
- Determine the current state of planning
- Examine all current plans, such as fire, safety, as well as meeting with outside groups, review existing codes and regulations, identify critical products, services, and operations
- Review the internal resources and capabilities
- Review the external resources and insurance coverage.
- Conduct a vulnerability analysis, listing potential emergencies of all types, such as geographic, technological, physical, and human error
- Assess the vulnerabilities

7. The process is the same as sheltering in place at home. The windows and doors are closed and locked, air conditioning turned off, all occupants move to a pre-specified room, the windows and doors sealed with plastic and duct tape, and listen to TV or radio for updates.

8. Structural vulnerabilities include sprinklers, air ducts, and the blast resistance of the building. Structural vulnerabilities include what is intrinsic to the building that could be exploited, whether the structure can withstand the blast of bombs of different sizes, placed in varying locations.

   Operational vulnerabilities refer to the dynamic building-specific characteristics that motivate a terrorist, as opposed to the static structural vulnerabilities. Operational vulnerabilities may be the occupants that make it attractive to terrorists, for example, embassies, government offices, the ease of entry, and the occurrence of regular evacuation exercises.

   Contextual vulnerabilities include the building's proximity to other targets and the overall risk level for an attack as determined by the Office of Homeland Security. If nearby buildings are attractive targets, the building owners in close proximity should plan for the aftermath of an attack on the attractive target

9. Closest emergency exit, and an alternate route in case the original choice is destroyed. Protect yourself from falling debris by taking shelter under a desk or table.

   Avoid areas near file cabinets, bookshelves or other structures that may topple and injure them.

   Avoid facing areas with large amounts of windows or glass to prevent being cut by flying shards. Distance yourself from exterior walls that may crumble or be destroyed.

   Locate a battery powered radio or television so that you can listen to news and emergency directions.

   If a decision has been made to leave the building, do not use the elevators. As you descend the stairs, stay to the right side so that you do not hinder emergency workers ascending. If it has not been contaminated, carry your emergency supply kit with you.

10. Identification of those who would require additional assistance.

   Alarms signage for the emergency exit routes, a buddy system or team approach, or designated areas of rescue assistance, such as an operating telephone, cell-phone, closing door, smoke-blocking supplies, or a window with help sign

   May require evacuation devices to move people down stairs or over rough surfaces remove all physical barriers on the exit route, and perhaps heavy gloves for the manual wheelchairs and removal of debris

May need visual or vibratory alarm devices and tactile signage and maps. If a guide or service dog is used, plan for the evacuation of the animal also

Persons with cognitive or psychiatric impairments may find picture signage or color coding of escapes helpful

Break down information into simple steps. Do not talk down to people or treat them like children

CHAPTER 9: Considerations for Vulnerable Populations

1. False
2. False
3. True
4. False
5. True
6. True
7. True
8. False
9. False
10. True

CHAPTER 10: Preparing Nurses to Plan and Care for Children During Disaster Situations

1. b
2. c
3. d
4. a
5. d
6. b
7. e
8. d
9. c
10. e

CHAPTER 11: Role of the Infection Control Nurse in Disaster Preparedness

1. b
2. b
3. b
4. d
5. b
6. c
7. a
8. a
9. b
10. b

CHAPTER 12: Disaster as the Personal Experience

1. As we prepare nurses for planning and responding to disasters and increasingly complex roles in community-based nursing practice, methods are needed that foster critical thinking and caring behaviors. Reading the stories of nurses who have lived through these disaster experiences can offer insights into what disasters meant to them and how they responded.

2. Disbelief, fear, courage, life-changing experience, not allowing the terrorists to ruin their lives, sensible planning in anticipation of disasters, caring for others, a need to share "words of wisdom" to teach others, hope for peace.

3. Nurses' priorities—caution and planning, preparation for disasters, professionalism, caring and compassion, listening and understanding the needs of others, active participation in disaster relief efforts. Bereaved parents' priorities—sharing the pain of their loss and teaching others, especially nurses, about therapeutic responses and non-therapeutic responses to bereaved family members, religious customs, the grieving process for different family members

4. I am sorry this has happened to you. I suspect this may be an upsetting time of year for you. It may take some time for you to feel better. I am here for you. Would you like to talk about your (deceased) loved one? I realize that today is your (deceased) loved one's birthday. I suspect it must be hard for you to do your regular activities today without thinking about him/her.

5. It happened according to a plan. It is God's plan. The Lord only gives us a load that He knows we can carry. My family member has recovered since the tragedy, you should be able to pull things together and get on with life by now. Don't dwell on your child's (loved one's) death, you have other children (family members) to think about. Is your whole family going to be home for the holidays?

6. True
7. True
8. True
9. True
10. True

APPENDIX   C

Decontamination Forms & Volunteer Log

Saint Louis University Hospital

TeneT

DECONTAMINATION PRE-SCREENING FORM

Screening form must be completed on all staff members PRIOR to dressing into a Level A, B or C suit.

DATE/TIME:	NAME:	TITLE:	B/P	TEMP.	PULSE	R.R.

Saint Louis University Hospital

Tenet

DECONTAMINATION POST-SCREENING FORM

Screening form must be completed on all staff members UPON REMOVAL of a Level A, B or C suit.

DATE/ TIME:	NAME:	TITLE:	B/P	TEMP.	PULSE	R.R.

SLMMRS DISASTER TEAM LOG VOLUNTEER WORKERS				
Name	**Address**	**Primary Hospital**	**SLMMRS Badge #**	**Profession**

Source: St. Louis Metropolitan Medical Response System

INDEX